# EVER
## WOMAN
## HEALTH
# GUIDE

# About the Authors

## Maryon Stewart

Maryon Stewart studied preventive dentistry and nutrition at the Royal Dental Hospital in London and worked as a counsellor with nutritional doctors in England for four years. At the beginning of 1984 she set up the PMT Advisory Service which has subsequently helped thousands of women worldwide. In 1987 she launched the Women's Nutritional Advisory Service which now provides broader help to women of all ages. Maryon Stewart is the author of the best-selling books *Beat PMS Through Diet*, now in its third edition, *Beat Sugar Craving*, *Beat the Menopause Without HRT* and *Healthy Parents, Healthy Baby*. She is the co-author of The *Vitality Diet*, *Beat IBS Through Diet* and *The PMS Cookbook*. She has had her own weekly radio programme on health and nutrition, she has co-written several medical papers, and has written articles for many glossy magazines. She has contributed regularly to many TV programmes including 'Capital Woman', has done a series of programmes for Yorkshire TV's 'Help Yourself' programmes and has helped Anglia TV with their 'Bodyworks' series. Maryon has written her own regular page in the magazine *House and Garden* and has written regularly for *Healthy Eating Magazine*. She is on the panel of advisors for *First Steps* magazine and frequently lectures to both the lay public and medical profession. She is married to Dr Alan Stewart and they live in Lewes, Sussex, with their four children.

## Dr Alan Stewart

Alan Stewart qualified as a doctor at Guy's Hospital, London, in 1976 and spent five years specialising in hospital medicine. He became a member of the Royal College of Physicians. He worked at the British Homoeopathic Hospital in London and qualified as a Member of the Faculty of Homoeopathy. For the last twelve years he has specialised in nutritional medicine and was a founding member of the British Society for Nutritional Medicine. He is also a medical advisor to the Women's Nutritional Advisory Service and is actively involved in educating other doctors on the subject of nutrition. Dr Stewart co-wrote several best-selling books, including *Nutritional Medicine* and *Tired All the Time*, has written several medical papers, and regularly gives lectures to doctors and health visitors. He has also written articles in both the medical and popular press on various aspects of health and now writes the Doctor Page for *Healthy Eating* magazine.

# EVERY WOMAN'S HEALTH GUIDE

**Optimum natural health and well-being**

## MARYON STEWART & DR ALAN STEWART

Hodder & Stoughton

A Hodder & Stoughton book

First published in Australia and New Zealand in 1997
by Hodder Headline Australia Pty Limited.
(A member of the Hodder Headline Group)
10–16 South Street, Rydalmere NSW 2116

Reprinted 1997

**National Library of Australia Cataloguing-in-Publication data**

Stewart, Maryon.
Every woman's health guide: optimum natural health and well-being.

Includes index.
ISBN 0 7336 0267 3.

1. Women—Nutrition. 2. Women—Health and hygiene.
3. Diet therapy. I. Stewart, Alan, 1940–   . II. Title.

Typeset by Midland Typesetters, Victoria
Printed in Australia by McPherson's Printing Group

# Acknowledgements

Setting out to write a comprehensive self-help guide for women was indeed a daunting task. The first challenge was finding the time to put pen to paper with our busy practices, and four demanding children. The second hurdle was gathering all the relevant published medical literature to ensure that the book was scientifically based. Our task was made significantly easier because of the medical researchers and pioneers who have gone before us. Studying the wealth of published medical literature, on almost every subject we have written about, was enlightening. So our first thanks must go to the authors of the medical papers and textbooks we have quoted in our reference section, we are deeply grateful for their contribution to the overall picture.

Special thanks must also go to our wonderful patients who have been happy to share their 'stories' in this book with the aim of helping others who are suffering similarly. We decided to change their names, despite the fact that many were happy to be identified.

We are also grateful to the team at the Women's Nutritional Advisory Service for their support, particularly Cheryl Griffiths for her cool organisational skills and nifty fingers, and Margaret Knight, an experienced researcher, who spent many hours clawing through the journals in the postgraduate library gathering medical papers.

We would also like to acknowledge the skills of Lavinia Trevor, our agent, Sue Fleming, our treasured editor at Headline, for her expertise and wisdom, and to Mary Howell at Hodder Headline Australia and Philippa Sandall for their vision and their support.

Physical support came from Peter Loe who supplied us with wonderful ergonomic chairs to try out whilst we burnt the midnight oil, and to Wendy Cockerill for her expert back massage.

We would not have been able to complete our task without the help and support of our wonderful nanny Clare FitzGerald, who rose to the challenge without losing her cool, despite being tested, and for the additional support we received from Margaret Moon and Rosa Kingston, Grandma.

Last but not least, we must thank the children themselves—Phoebe, Chesney, Hester and Simeon—for being patient and supplying us with encouraging words and hugs when the end seemed like a long way off.

'I make no apology for saying that the health of the majority of human beings depends more on their nutrition than it does any other single factor. However important and dramatic have been the advances of hygiene, medicine and surgery, it is still true that even more important would be the effects that proper nutrition would have on morbidity and mortality. For this reason, I believe that the ultimate objective of nutritionists must be the nutrition education of the public.'

Professor John Yudkin, 1981

# CONTENTS

..............................................................

# Part Three — The Nutritional Answers 441

## Appendices

## Index – 558

# INTRODUCTION

Professor Henry Higgins, in *My Fair Lady*, once said, 'Why can't a woman be more like a man?' Perhaps it would be a great deal simpler if that were the case, but women are very different from men. Physically that may be stating the obvious, but what is not so widely appreciated is that women are *biochemically* different: they are governed by a hormonal cycle which is programmed from birth and continues through until they reach menopause and old age.

The demands placed on a woman's body throughout the many stages of her life are great and varied. All too often these demands are not met, resulting in poor health of one form or another. Women's bodies are very sensitive 'machines' with very specific requirements in order to perform optimally. When health trouble is brewing, the body is very good at sending warning messages, but the problem is that many women are not educated, and fail to interpret the message in time.

Lack of education relating to health is a subject which deserves its own book; there is so much to be told. General practitioners in the UK, by their own admission, have little or no knowledge about nutritional approaches to health, with the average time assigned to this subject being somewhere between two and four hours out of a whole medical training course. And yet the nutritional state of the human body, male or female, is as fundamentally important to health as good foundations are to a builder. We could be forgiven for being ignorant about health matters, but when doctors fail to provide the vital information needed to overcome the problems in question, we may be forced to use long-term medication, or may be left to our own devices, feeling thoroughly frustrated and miserable.

(It is interesting to note that in the 1992 *Journal of the Royal Society of Medicine* we learnt that 98 per cent of the final year medical students failed all the questions on nutrition, whereas in Australia 94 per cent of medical students answered one of the two parts correctly and 53 per cent answered both parts correctly. In Australia nutrition is regarded as an integral aspect of nutritional medicine whereas in the UK this does not apply.)

In the thirteen years of working with patients at the WNAS we have been able to help literally thousands of patients over their long-term ills, and removed unwanted and unjustified 'labels' that they thought they would have for life. To cite a few examples, we have dealt with busloads of patients who have been labelled psychologically or even psychiatrically ill, and have left them symptom-free after three or four months. Patients who have had severe migraine for years no longer even have headaches, we have former acne sufferers without spots, and irritable bowel victims who no longer have to pay attention to their digestion. The violent and often suicidal PMS sufferer who described herself as Jekyll and Hyde, feels like her old self again all month, ongoing problems with thrush and cystitis have abated, and the turbulent symptoms of menopause have been replaced in many patients by a new vitality for life.

These are some of the weekly achievements of our work at the WNAS. They are not miracles, just the result of the application of existing medical science. The published medical papers on which we base our recommendations are all to be found in postgraduate medical libraries. They are there for the taking, but very few doctors are familiar with them. As their application would very often result in the resolution of most of our chronic symptoms, you may well consider it a scandal that these papers remain behind closed doors.

We now know that we can positively influence both brain chemical metabolism and hormone function by replacing the essential nutrients which time, nature and lack of education have denied us. It is actually not a very difficult task, and a real case of the old adage 'a little knowledge goes a long way'. Science now also quite clearly demonstrates that we can influence the health of our children, both as babies and as adults, before they are even conceived.

There are many myths about the ageing process. In fact with adequate care and attention along the way, most women should be able to look forward to a very active and healthy old age with most of their 'bits' intact. However, in current practice this is not always the case. We often hear of women having a hysterectomy prematurely, or having their healthy ovaries removed. It is also not unusual to encounter patients who have been on sleeping tablets, or antidepressants, for as long as they can remember. In many cases these measures were not necessary, as can be shown when they are helped back to health by natural means.

It would be narrow-minded of us to claim that good nutrition is the only answer to good health. Whilst it is a fundamental issue, there are many other factors to consider. A woman's lot at the end of the twentieth century is for many a far greater burden than it might have been in times gone by. Women continue to be home-makers and mothers, without necessarily having the extended family to support them. Many also work for a living and share the financial strains with their partners. The result of this increased case load is that they tend to spend less time in the kitchen pre-paring wholesome meals, and instead they cut corners and use pre-prepared food. You may be surprised to learn that as recently as the mid 1930s our families were eating on average four proper meals per day, with only one in-between-meal snack. Now in the late 1990s we consume on average one or two proper meals per day with as many as five in-between-meal snacks. Our bodies were not designed for this.

It is quite common for over-committed working mothers to neglect their own needs, failing to find time to exercise or relax, and eating the wrong foods for comfort, or skipping meals alto-gether. There are others who are perhaps not leading such a pun-ishing schedule, but who would prefer to have a magic pill rather than put in effort in either the kitchen or the gymnasium.

At the WNAS we encourage women to re-evaluate their whole lifestyle. Their current complaint is seen as a warning light which starts off the process. Our programmes always incorporate dietary and lifestyle changes, the use of relevant nutritional supplements, an exercise regime and regular relaxation. We often incorporate other complementary therapies like homoeopathy, osteopathy, herbal medicine, massage, and acupuncture.

Many women's ills are the result of past traumatic emotional experiences which get buried away, either because they can't con-front them at the time they occur, or because they are too busy to deal with them. Difficulties with relationships, both in childhood and in adulthood, get locked deep inside, and unless these can somehow be come to terms with rationally, they may damage health later in life.

However, inadequate nutrient levels often affect brain chemistry, which in turn can affect mental processes. So perhaps trying to solve life's troubles *prior* to getting the body into optimum condition is not a good idea. The majority of our patients have been delighted to discover that problems which had seemed almost insurmountable prior to undertaking our programme, looked more like molehills that were relatively easy to confront and deal with afterwards.

The purpose of this book is to provide you with the education that you have missed out on, and to empower you with the information necessary to make a fully informed decision about your life, your health and your treatment plan. It is important to understand the strengths and weaknesses of what your doctor has on offer, as well as to have an overview of what self-help measures are available to you, plus the role of other complementary therapies for specific conditions.

The first part of the book will give you the missing background information and some food for thought. You then have the A–Z of key conditions, followed by suggested dietary and nutritional plans. The scientifically minded will find the medical references for each condition in the reference section in Appendix II. There is also a recommended reading list (Appendix III) and a useful address directory (Appendix V).

For those who feel they could use some expert help, we provide a tailor-made service which you can read about in Appendix IV.

We all have the power in our hands to influence not only our own health, but that of our family and future generations. Armed with new knowledge we are confident that you will find that the quality of health you enjoy is for the most part actually in your own hands. In our view we will be well into the twenty-first century before we can expect the medical profession to provide us with all the answers, and even that assessment may be optimistic.

Maryon and Alan Stewart
July 1996

# PART ONE

*Your Diet and Lifestyle*

# What's Wrong with Present-day Diet and Lifestyle?

In the last fifty years diet and lifestyle have altered dramatically. The whole of society has changed, and not necessarily for the better. At one time culinary skills were passed from one generation to another, and the woman's role was very definitely the 'home-maker'. She was not expected to go out to work whilst her family were growing, and more often than not she had her mother and other female relatives living close by as back-up. The motor car was a luxury, so her daily shopping was usually done locally on foot. She would expect to purchase fresh food regularly, which would have contained far more nutrients than produce purchased from the supermarket weekly. As fast food didn't exist, part of her role would be to cook wholesome meals for the family on a daily basis.

Fifty years on, the picture is quite different. Women have learned the art of the shortcut, very often through necessity. They drive to the supermarket once or twice per week to purchase food. They are presented with fast-option choices, which when short of time and adequate information, seem both convenient and appealing. Most of the food they buy has been preserved, sprayed with chemicals, injected, or indeed grown in chemically rich soil. They now expect food to be treated with pesticides and insecticides, and animals to be pumped full of antibiotics and growth hormones, with environmental pollution being the cherry on the top.

Human bodies were not designed to be treated in such a fashion, or to cope with modern-day stresses, so it is no wonder that our bodies develop problems. We probably treat our domestic appliances or our motor car with more respect. Few of us would dream of denying our car the appropriate fuel or oil, so how is it that women neglect their bodies so? In our experience at the WNAS it is the 'education gap' that is responsible for the wearing of blinkers, but when women are confronted with the real facts about diet and lifestyle, they usually take stock. Few of them, once enlightened, revert to their old habits as they are so pleased with their renewed health, and surprised at how enjoyable their new diet and lifestyle are. As an added bonus they are then able to pass their new-found knowledge on to other members of their family.

Let us examine more closely how eating habits have changed. A century ago, meat, animal fat and sugar formed a much smaller proportion of our diets than today. The consumption of cereal fibres has also dropped considerably.

♦ We have increased our consumption of sugar. On average, people in developed countries like Australia and New Zealand now eat around 50 kg of cane sugar each year. Sugar consumed in packaged and processed foods and drinks has increased from 30 to 70 per cent over the past fifty years. The last 100 years have seen a twenty-fivefold increase in world sugar production. In reality refined sugar is not something that we actually *need*, and the human race managed quite happily without it for centuries. Mother Nature, with her usual wisdom, has designed it so that the body can convert complex carbohydrates and proteins into the sugar required. Table sugar, sucrose, contains no vitamins, mineral, protein, fibre or starches; it may contain tiny traces of calcium and magnesium if we are really lucky, but apart from that it just provides us with 'empty kilojoules'. We have to really go out of our way these days to reduce our sugar consumption as food manufacturers often add it to some of the most unlikely foods: *cheese, fruit yoghurt, tomato sauce, baked beans, pickled cucumbers, muesli, Worcestershire sauce, sausages, peas, cornflakes, and canned drinks.*

♦ Excessive consumption of saturated animal fats results in a gradual blocking of the arteries that supply the heart, brain and other major organs. This leads to poor circulation, and then to heart attacks and strokes. It is worth noting that smoking accelerates this process. The increased incidence of breast cancer has much to do with animal fat consumption as well.

♦ We eat far too much salt—ten to twenty times more than our bodies really require each day—which can contribute to high blood pressure.

♦ We often drink far too much coffee and tea which can impede the absorption of essential nutrients, and aggravate symptoms of nervous tension, irritability, insomnia and headaches. On average we consume four mugs of tea and two mugs of coffee each day, which delivers approximately 800 mg of caffeine into our system. That doesn't include other sources of caffeine like chocolate, cocoa, cola and other caffeinated drinks. It certainly means that there are many women walking about with symptoms of caffeine excess. Count how many cups or mugs you have had today—you may be surprised.

◆ We consume volumes of foods with a high level of phosphorus, which again impedes the absorption of good nutrients and interferes with calcium absorption by bone tissue. Examples of these foods are soft drinks (low or normal kilojoule varieties), processed foods, canned, packaged, prepacked convenience foods and ready-made sauces.

◆ Alcohol consumption has increased since the end of the Second World War. Alcohol also impedes the absorption of good nutrients and in excess can cause all sorts of other health problems (see Alcoholism).

◆ Unbelievable as it may seem, we actually eat *less* food than we did thirty years ago and more. It seems that today's women actually expend less energy than those of a generation or two ago, and this has resulted in a 10–15 per cent reduction in food intake. This also means that intake of essential nutrients has fallen, particularly if eating refined or convenience foods.

◆ Many of the foods available contain chemical additives in the form of flavour enhancers, colouring and preservatives. While some of these are not harmful, some of them are, and our bodies are certainly not designed to cope with them.

◆ These days our meat animals are bombarded with antibiotics, to the point where they often become resistant to them. They are used as a preventative measure and often used for growth promotion.

◆ Nitrate fertilisers have been used to obtain fast-growing and abundant crops. It is now recognised that nitrates are harmful and can produce cancer, at least in animals.

◆ Almost all our fresh fruit, cereals and vegetables are sprayed with pesticides at least once. In addition, milk and meat may retain pesticides from feed given to livestock.

All these processes in the rearing and growing of food mean a reduction in basic nutrition, and the answer must lie in organic foods.

Although organic food is harder to obtain (unless you grow your own) and more expensive weight for weight, by consuming it you will be decreasing the number of chemicals you consume, and thus increasing your nutrient intake. According to The National Association for Sustainable Agriculture Australia (NASAA), organic vegetable foods are more nutrient dense for the equivalent weight. As they have not been tampered with chemically they deliver much more of what nature promised.

The same is true for meat. Additive-free or organic meat has not been subjected to drugs, growth promoters or contaminated foods. If you find 'clean' meat, it can be included in your diet approximately three times per week, unless of course, you are vegetarian. An alternative is to limit your intake to lean meat, eat more fish, or become a vegetarian.

There are numerous dietary guidelines for you to follow, depending on your needs, in Part Three. If you haven't already started reading labels in the supermarket, have a go next time you shop; there are a few surprises in store. Make sure you have plenty of time to spare as, sadly, many of the labels are pretty long.

## The Truth about Social Substances

Why is it that the things we enjoy the most seem to be bad for us? When we are in good health the general rule is that 'a little of what you fancy does you good'. However, when a personal health crisis appears, it may be necessary to make some sacrifices. Often the thought of making the changes is worse than actually taking the plunge. Surprisingly, people find the alternatives relatively acceptable, and prefer the health benefits they quickly feel delighted to be free from the 'addiction' or dependency. These may sound strong words, but it is not uncommon to find that the withdrawal of regular, but relatively small, amounts of caffeine—one or two mugs per day, say—can result in withdrawal headaches and other symptoms for a few days. The increased sense of well-being which follows the withdrawal symptoms, is certainly worth waiting for. Let us look at these social 'poisons' and see just where they fall down.

## Caffeine

Many of us have become slowly dependent on caffeine over the years, and our children follow in our footsteps. You will find caffeine in coffee and tea, but also in chocolate, chocolate drinks, cocoa, cola-based drinks, Lucozade, and some painkillers.

Caffeine is one of the substances known as methylxanthines, which act as both physical and mental stimulants. Although small amounts of caffeine can be of benefit in waking us up and stimulating our thought processes, it can have many adverse effects when used to excess. Over the years caffeine has been linked to heart disease, high blood pressure and even infertility. We know that caffeine worsens nervous tension, anxiety, insomnia and aggravates breast tenderness. It can also make you feel restless, nervous, with a rapid pulse and palpitations. High consumers will probably experience withdrawal symptoms when trying to kick the habit, rather like the symptoms produced by alcohol or nicotine withdrawal. If you depend on the caffeine 'buzz', then the road to good health will undoubtedly involve reducing your intake.

## Coffee

Coffee is the most widely used drug of our time. We are consuming more coffee than ever before. A 1992–93 survey by the Australian Bureau of Statistics found that average coffee consumption was 2.2 kg per person—the highest on record. There are many unacknowledged 'addicts' who would find it a challenge to give up, and even foregoing that last cup can produce symptoms of restlessness, nervous tension and headaches.

Ground coffee contains approximately 150 mg of caffeine per mug, and a mug of instant coffee roughly 100 mg. When we are well, moderate doses of up to 300 mg may be acceptable, but large doses can produce symptoms that could be mistaken for anxiety neurosis, including headaches, tremors, nausea and diarrhoea.

Weaning yourself off coffee can sometimes be a traumatic experience, but sadly there is no real shortcut. Cutting down gradually over a few weeks is the best option, and even when parting with those last few cups, set aside a few days so that you can hide away if you feel really uptight or out of sorts.

## How to Kick the Coffee Habit

◆ Reduce your intake gradually over the space of a week or two.
◆ Limit yourself to no more than two cups of decaffeinated coffee per day.
◆ Try some of the alternative drinks like dandelion coffee, Ecco, Caro or Nature's Cuppa which you can obtain from health-food shops.
◆ If you enjoy filter coffee, you can still use your filter, but with decaffeinated versions or with roasted dandelion root instead, which you can buy from the health-food shop. Simply grind it and put it through a filter, treating it just like ground coffee. It makes a 'coffee-like' strong malted drink.

## Tea

The bad news is that tea, the great Australian and New Zealand beverage, is not much better than coffee. It contains about 70 mg of caffeine per cup and approximately 100 mg per mug. However, it also contains tannin, another nasty, which inhibits the absorption of nutrients, zinc and iron in particular. Excesses of tea can produce the same withdrawal symptoms as coffee, but tea also can cause constipation.

Drinking tea with a meal will reduce the absorption of iron from vegetarian sources by one-third, whereas a glass of fresh orange juice, rich in vitamin C, would *increase* the iron absorption two-fold. Vegetarians and vegans need their iron, so drinking anything other than small amounts of weak tea, in between meals, may mean they risk becoming iron deficient.

## Acceptable Alternatives to Tea

Herbal teas are a good substitute. Unlike conventional Indian or Chinese leaf tea, most of the herbal varieties are free of caffeine and tannin, and can be both cleansing and relaxing. A good herbal tea 'lookalike' is Rooitea, which looks just like ordinary tea when made with milk. As an added bonus it contains a muscle relaxant and has been used in trials on babies with colic. Many of our patients prefer it to ordinary tea after a few weeks, but it does take a while to get used to. Apart from that there are many delicious varieties of herbal tea, and these days you can buy small packets to try, which means you don't get left with a box full of teabags you dislike. If you can't find these, look for brands like Celestial

Seasonings or Norganic. Our current favourites are Milfords Raspberry and Ginseng tea, Fennel, Lemon Verbena, and the Crabtree and Evelyn Mixed Berry Cup.

## Caffeinated Fizzy Drinks

We used to have only cola-based drinks to contend with, but these days there are a new generation of caffeinated drinks to tempt us. Apart from caffeine there is also sugar to consider, approximately 8 teaspoons per can of cola, or the chemical substitutes, and other additives. Sadly many young people get hooked on these drinks early on in life as the admen would have them believe the drinks are 'cool' and will enhance their image.

We are all much better off with the healthy varieties of fizzy drink, which are now given some space on our supermarket shelves. Or you can simply dilute some fruit juice with some fizzy bottled water yourself.

If you have been a large consumer of the caffeine varieties, you will have to follow the weaning instructions for coffee. We have had patients who consume 2 or more litres of cola per day, and know that the withdrawal symptoms are likely to be quite similar.

## Decaffeinated Drinks

Decaffeinated drinks usually still contain small amounts of caffeine as well as other members of the methylxanthine family, and decaffeinated tea also contains tannin. The regulations for decaffeinated cola are no more than 125 mg per litre.

The decaffeination process uses one of two methods, either water and carbon dioxide, or the Swiss water process which uses hot water, charcoal and the use of chemical solvents. In the latter process small residues of chemicals remain, but they are minimal. So decaffeinated drinks are better but not marvellous. At the WNAS we recommend restricting decaffeinated drinks to no more than two mugs per day.

## Alcohol

Whilst small amounts of alcohol on a regular basis do not cause us harm, unless you are planning a pregnancy, or are already pregnant, we know that alcohol knocks most nutrients sideways. (We shall cover how alcohol affects each condition in the relevant sections.)

Alcohol in excess destroys body tissue over the years, and can cause or contribute to many diseases, among them:

◆ cardiovascular diseases
◆ digestive disorders
◆ inflammation and ulceration of the lining of the digestive tract
◆ liver disease
◆ cancer, including breast cancer
◆ brain degeneration
◆ miscarriages
◆ damage to unborn children
◆ heavy drinking can be a risk factor for osteoporosis

One-third of divorce petitions cite alcohol as a contributory factor. Women under stress do sometimes hit the bottle in order to escape from reality, and as most of the above conditions come on gradually, we often don't perceive the real dangers of alcohol until it is too late. If your drinking has been escalating slowly it is advisable to seek help. It is important to cut your consumption to the recommended limits.

## Tobacco

Earlier this century, cigarettes were actually recommended by doctors, but more recent research has shown that in all but a few circumstances, they are bad for our general health. In addition, smoking during pregnancy affects the unborn child, and women who smoke more than fifteen cigarettes per day can expect to experience menopause two years earlier than non-smokers. Smoking also affects bone density, and even stopping smoking at the time of the menopause can reduce a hip fracture risk by 40 per cent—so it's never too late.

Despite Government health warnings and health-promotion campaigns, women still go on smoking. Research shows that the better educated women have cut back, but younger women, who are perhaps not so well educated, are still puffing away. Being parents of teenagers we know that it is still considered 'cool' to smoke behind the bicycle sheds! Thankfully, however, there has been a marked decline in the number of smokers overall since the late 1970s. It's now estimated that about 25 per cent of women over the age of eighteen smoke cigarettes. In 1977 it was 29 per cent.

## Giving Up Smoking

Giving up smoking has never been easy. The first step is to make the decision to quit, knowing that you may well experience true withdrawal symptoms, just as drug addicts and alcoholics do when they try to stop. Here is a plan to help you.

◆ Choose a day on which to give up, and write down the date.
◆ On the day before, smoke as many cigarettes as you can until you feel sick. Make sure you stub them out in the same dirty ashtray.
◆ Go to the library and get a book that contains pictures of the consequences of smoking.
◆ On the morning of your chosen day, pour yourself a glass of freshly squeezed orange juice, and sit and write down all the reasons for your decision to give up smoking.
◆ Pin your list of reasons up on the wall so that you can read it at weak moments.
◆ Put your cigarettes away in a drawer, and tell yourself you can have one whenever you want one.
◆ When you crave a cigarette, tell yourself you can have one but first consider the reasons why you decided to quit. Make a new decision not to light up.
◆ Go shopping and stock up with some of your favourite wholesome food, including some fruit and some raw vegetables and dips.
◆ Tell your close friends and family that you are giving up smoking.
◆ Take a good multi-vitamin and mineral pill each day, in addition to improving your diet.
◆ Try to avoid situations that are likely to make you feel like lighting up. For example, drink fruit juice instead of alcohol.
◆ If possible, go away for a few days to help you break your daily routine.
◆ Chew some sugar-free gum rather than sweets or chocolate.
◆ Put the handle of your toothbrush in your mouth whenever you miss your hand-to-mouth habit.
◆ Each time you feel you need a cigarette, stop, relax and breathe deeply, so that you get a good supply of oxygen into your lungs.
◆ Join a gym, and make sure you exercise regularly.

- Don't spend evenings alone, instead arrange to go to cinema, bowling or out for a walk.
- If you feel edgy in the evenings, have a few early nights.
- Keep a progress chart, ticking each day that you have remained a non-smoker.
- Save your cigarette money in a jar, and spend it on treats for yourself.
- Practise some formal relaxation like yoga or meditation.
- If you have a partner, ask for a massage when you feel tense or a bit ratty.
- Picture your lungs recovering now that they are smoke free.

It is never too late to give up smoking. Whenever you do decide to take the plunge you will be helping yourself to better health and preserving yourself for your loved ones. If you find it difficult to quit, contact one of the organisations listed in Appendix V and read some of the suggested books in the Recommended Reading List (Appendix III).

## Other Drugs

Natural remedies were passed down from one generation to the next, until the advent of the pharmaceutical industry post-Second World War. Drugs in general have revolutionised medicine and medical practice, to the point where they are hardly recognisable, which has both advantages and disadvantages. Whereas in years gone by we could easily have died of pneumonia, for example, modern antibiotics make that unlikely now. On the down side, however, many of us have come to rely on pills to help us cope with life, induce sleep, and indeed counteract the side-effects of another drug. So whilst some drugs can be life-saving, others can equally wreck the quality of existence, and it is therefore imperative to be discerning.

## Street Drugs

These have become increasingly popular in the last fifteen or twenty years. They are readily available and can sometimes be a tempting option for those whose lives are not going as planned. Women of child-bearing age should avoid all street drugs as they undoubtedly harm the unborn child, and in some case babies are born addicted. Drug users, even more so than smokers, tend to

us diet than non-users, and are not so concerned
eir health, as they are in the process of spoiling

and cannabis are both widely used substances and
...s of the hemp plant. The pro-marijuana lobby claim that
... is as safe as smoking cigarettes or drinking alcohol. Whilst marijuana does seem to have some medicinal uses, we are not advocating regular use, any more than we are recommending alcohol
or tobacco.

## Prescribed Drugs

Some fifty years ago Sir Robert Hucheson, President of the Royal
College of Physicians, London, was writing books about how diet
and nutrition were used as a mode of treatment at the beginning
of the century, it seems hard to believe that nutrition is no longer
considered a major part of conservative medicine. One wonders
how we became such a drug-oriented society. With the post-war
boom in the pharmaceutical industry, and the power and influence
the industry has been allowed to assume over doctors' education,
it is hardly surprising.

In the USA in 1993 nearly 75 000 million dollars was spent on
medicines by a population of 250 million (some 280 dollars per
capita), and in the UK in 1994 it was 3844 million pounds, roughly
69 pounds per man, woman and child. Australians spend twice as
much on alternative medicine out of their own pockets as they do
on conventional drugs, according to the world's largest survey on
the use of alternative medicine.

The survey published in the *Lancet* (2nd March 1996) found
that Australians spend approximately 1 billion dollars on alternative medicine, compared with 360 million dollars spent on patient
contributions for pharmaceutical drugs.

The survey also found that nearly 50 per cent of those surveyed
use at least one alternative medicine. This excluded the use of
calcium, iron and prescribed vitamins, making the results more
impressive.

Approximately 20 per cent of the population had visited one or
more alternative health care practitioner in the past year, however,
the majority self-prescribed alternative medicines, purchased most
commonly through retail health food stores and pharmacy.

Even doctors themselves, worldwide, now express concern

about the excessive use of benzodiazepine tranquillisers and sleeping tablets. The current recommendation is that these drugs, which include diazepam (Valium), nitrazepam (Mogadon) and lorezepam (Ativan), should be used as a temporary measure for only a few weeks, rather than in the long term. Those who have been taking them for any length of time should, if at all possible, have their dosage and frequency gradually reduced under medical supervision.

When we run into health difficulties, our body depends on us to clean up our act so that the immune system can function properly and do its job. The body has exceptional natural healing powers, but you wouldn't expect a wound to heal with a nail in it, any more than you can expect to be well without treating your body with respect.

# NUTRITION IS THE KEY TO HEALTH

The major causes of death in developed countries are heart disease and cancer, and both are influenced to a large degree by the type of diet we eat. Up to 50 per cent of people with heart disease or cancer could probably have prevented or delayed the onset of their illness if they had eaten a better diet (or stopped smoking). This is particularly important for those who become ill at a relatively young age, i.e. before sixty-five years. Furthermore, many minor ills are also influenced by diet and these include problems such as migraine headaches, high blood pressure, arthritis, kidney stones, premenstrual syndrome, eczema, fatigue, irritable bowel syndrome, insomnia and anxiety. These are only the tip of the iceberg as you will see, and in this book alone we have covered some 120 conditions.

When we are children our parents teach us how to eat, dress, wash and generally look after ourselves, and we are taught at school how to read, write and add up. But where and how do we learn about our bodies' requirements? Well, it is not at school, neither is it at evening classes, as they seem to concentrate there on car maintenance and the secrets of computer mechanics. The woman, who is often regarded as the 'nutritional head of the household', and is expected to meet the demands of her family's nutrient needs as well as her own, has little or no training for this job. When we consider this rationally, it seems so outrageous, especially as we trade both our cars and our computers in from time to time, but only have one body to last a lifetime.

Because we are so often told by our doctors that a balanced diet is all that we need to maintain our health, the WNAS conducted a random survey a few years ago to find out what people understood by the term 'a balanced diet'. We also asked which foods contained key vitamins like A, B, C, D and E, and some key minerals like calcium, magnesium, zinc and iron. The negative results of this survey would have been entertaining were it not for the fact that the consequences of an unbalanced diet may severely affect the quality of health. The only information that people seemed to have about their diet was the basic lesson from school, if they could remember it. Apart from knowing facts such as 'oranges contain vitamin C' and that 'liver contains iron', hardly anyone had a clue as to what actually constituted a sound balanced diet, or how much of each nutrient was required each day for their body size (or anyone else's body size for that matter).

Although magazine articles are one of the key sources of information about diet, confusion abounds as we lurch from one diet scandal to another. First we hear that alcohol is bad for us and that animal fats will cause our cholesterol levels to rise. Then we hear that we should be drinking two or three glasses of wine each day to prevent heart disease, and that fats have little influence on our cholesterol levels. Should we be eating liver regularly, or does it contain too much vitamin A? Will soft cheeses and uncooked eggs give us listeria and salmonella? Is decaffeinated tea and coffee *really* better for us or will the other methylxanthines get us anyway? We could well be forgiven for putting our heads in the sand and hoping for the best. Trying to sort out the dietary myths from the facts is an arduous task for anyone.

## Essential Nutrients

In order to fully understand the role of vitamins and minerals in health, it is necessary to have some idea about the part that each nutrient has to play. A truly balanced diet must provide an adequate supply of energy and protein, plus essential vitamins, minerals and specialised fats called essential fatty acids. The majority of energy comes from fats and carbohydrates in the diet, and a small amount from protein-rich foods.

Proteins, fats, carbohydrates and fibre are all essential for normal body function. Let's look briefly at the function they serve.

## Protein

This term is used to describe a series of complex chemicals that are widely found in many nutritious foods. Proteins are made up of amino acids, the essential building blocks, as well as many hormones, enzymes and other agents involved in the intricate metabolism of living organisms. If protein intake is not adequate in the diet, then tissue growth and repair cannot take place, and protein-rich tissue breaks down, especially muscle.

### Sources of protein

Protein can be found in both animal and vegetarian sources—meat, eggs, dairy products including milk and cheese, peas, beans, lentils, nuts, seeds and, to a very small extent, rice and potatoes. It is wise to have a wide variety of protein sources in your diet, especially if you are a vegetarian.

## Fats

Fats provide us with energy. There is a wide variety of different fats, which are all chemically similar, and per gram weight they provide us with over twice the energy content as carbohydrate or sugar.

### Animal fats

The majority of animal fats are saturated and serve only as a source of kilojoules. Animal fats are not essential and have a chemical structure that is saturated with hydrogen. This chemical nature means that they are usually solid at room temperature. A diet rich in these saturated animal fats, and lacking in fibre, vitamins and minerals, will often predispose to heart disease.

### Vegetable fats

Many, but not all vegetable fats are polyunsaturates and these include the specialised essential fatty acids, or EFAs, which are used in the building structure of our cells, especially those of our skin and nervous system, as well as being a source of kilojoules. Chemically these fats or oils are unsaturated and are able to accept more hydrogen molecules. This means that they are usually liquid at room temperature. Olive oil and canola oil are rich in mono-saturates which are not essential but they do not add to the risk of heart disease in the way that saturated fats do. Good sources of the essential fatty acids are corn, sunflower and safflower oils which provide the Omega-6 series of EFAs; oily fish such as mackerel, herring and salmon together with soy bean and walnut oil, and to a small extent, canola oil, provide the Omega-3 series.

## Carbohydrates

The term carbohydrates is a collective term for the different sugars and starches in our diet. Starches are composed of many individual sugar molecules, predominantly glucose, and are broken down by our digestive system into these simple sugars, some of which are better for us than others. The simple sugars are glucose, fructose and galactose which is part of the sugar found in milk. Table sugar, which is also called sucrose, is made up of one glucose and one fructose unit joined together. Its commercial production from sugarcane and sugar beet leads to the complete loss of vitamins and minerals found in these parent sources. A similar refining process to prepare white flour from wholemeal leads to a substantial reduction in essential vitamins and minerals. Sugars and starch-rich foods all require vitamin B and magnesium in order to be metabolised. Sucrose and to a lesser extent fructose also predispose to tooth decay.

### Sources of refined carbohydrates

Cakes, biscuits, sweets, chocolate, table sugar, white bread, white pasta and many breakfast cereals are all refined products that have been depleted of many essential nutrients. Fortunately white flour and some breakfast cereals are fortified with vitamins, and flour has added calcium. This helps to make up for these nutritional losses.

### Nutritious carbohydrate sources

All cereals, potatoes, rice and root vegetables. Fresh fruits and vegetables also provide a mixture of sugars—mainly fructose—and a small amount of starch.

## Fibre

Fibre is a type of carbohydrate that comes from the cell wall of plants, cellulose, and remains undigested in our gut. Because of its water-retaining properties, it forms the bulk of our stool. There are many types of fibre with differing properties. Most of us associate fibre-rich foods with those containing bran, for example, but bran may inhibit the absorption of certain essential nutrients including calcium and other minerals. It has little effect on blood cholesterol whereas the fibre in fruit, vegetables and oats helps reduce a high level.

### Good sources of fibre

A diet rich in fruit, vegetables, salad and cereals lowers blood cholesterol and the risk of heart disease, as well as providing many essential vitamins and minerals.

## Vitamins and Minerals

There are some fifteen vitamins, fifteen minerals, and eight to ten amino acids that have been isolated as being essential for normal body function. These nutrients are synergistic, which means they rely on each other in order to keep the body functioning at an optimum level. If you liken the body to a computer for a moment, the computer can only function when it has the correct data and commands fed to it; otherwise it refuses to work or breaks down altogether. Similarly, our bodies require the correct input of nutrients. When one or more nutrient is in short supply the body cannot function properly, and symptoms, be they physical or mental, occur.

Whilst it is true that severe nutritional deficiencies are rare in countries like the UK, Australia, New Zealand and the USA, poor intakes of a number of nutrients are acknowledged in some 20 per cent of women of child-bearing age. Combined nutritional inadequacies are likely to have an adverse affect on hormone function and on health in general during the ageing process.

# Nutritional Needs through the Ages

Our bodies are indeed very complex machines that have very specific requirements in order that they may function efficiently. Women particularly have varying needs, not just through their years of physical growth and development, but through each phase as it presents itself. The nutritional requirements for pregnancy are quite different, for example, from those needed by a woman at the time of the menopause.

The following table will give you some idea about the changing needs throughout life.

| | |
|---|---|
| Growth and development | All known nutrients |
| Puberty | All nutrients, and particularly iron, zinc, calcium and magnesium |
| Premenstrual syndrome | Particularly magnesium, B vitamins, iron and essential fatty acids (EFAs) |
| Preconception | Folate, other B vitamins and EFAs |
| Pregnancy | All nutrients, particularly EFAs |
| Breast-feeding | EFAs, calcium, magnesium and iron |
| Menopause | Calcium, magnesium, vitamin E, and EFAs |
| Post-menopause | Calcium, magnesium, EFAs, and vitamin D if deficient |
| The elderly | Vitamins B, C, D, calcium and iron |

# Essential Nutrients—Are We Deficient?

To continue the 'machinery' metaphor, learning what your body needs in order to function properly is a bit like trying to work a complicated computer without a manual. In fact, if the computer arrived without a manual, you would probably either leave it in the box until the manual arrived or, failing that, send it back to the shop. Becoming familiar with your body's needs demands a little patience and determination, because it is not that simple. It's almost like learning a new language.

Although we all have a body, that is where the similarity ends. Each individual body has slightly different requirements. The type of metabolism we have is inherited. There are the lucky robust minority who appear to be able to eat what they like, to maintain their weight and good health, and who seem to be oblivious to environmental and social stresses and strains. They must come from unusually strong stock. As for the rest of us, we have to come to terms with the fact that subtle differences determine the strengths and weaknesses of our make-up, and that one balanced diet for all is a myth. To understand your own nutrient needs you need to know a little about each individual nutrient. This is presented in the table on pages 19 to 25. Look through it and follow

UNDERSTANDING YOUR NUTRIENT NEEDS

| NUTRIENT | FOOD SOURCES | WHAT THEY DO | WHO IS AT RISK | SYMPTOMS | VISIBLE SIGNS |
|---|---|---|---|---|---|
| Vitamin A | *Retinol (animal vitamin A)* Liver, all dairy products and margarine *Beta-carotene (vegetable vitamin A)* All yellow, green, and orange fruits and vegetables | Essential for vision, especially in the dark, for growth and resistance to infection. | The ill, elderly and poorly fed pre-school children | Poor night vision, recurrent chest infections | None |
| Vitamin B1 (Thiamin) | Meat, fish, nuts, wholegrains and fortified breakfast cereals | Essential in the metabolism of sugar, especially in nerves and muscles | Alcohol consumers, women on the pill, breast-feeding mothers, high consumers of sugar | Depression, anxiety, poor appetite, nausea, personality change | None usually! Heart, nerve and muscle problems if severe |
| Vitamin B2 (Riboflavin) | Milk, meats, fish and vegetables | Involved in energy release from fats and carbohydrates | Those on a poor diet. | Deficiency rarely severe | Mild fatigue and possibly burning feet Peeling of the skin on the lips. Red ring around the iris of the eye |

UNDERSTANDING YOUR NUTRIENT NEEDS *continued*

| NUTRIENT | FOOD SOURCES | WHAT THEY DO | WHO IS AT RISK | SYMPTOMS | VISIBLE SIGNS |
|---|---|---|---|---|---|
| Vitamin B3 (Nicotinamide) | All forms of meat and fish, liver, fortified breakfast cereals and bread | Energy release from fats and carbohydrates, health of the skin and nervous system | Alcoholics, those on a poor diet, and with poor digestion | Diarrhoea, depression and dermatitis | A sore tongue and red scaly rash in light-exposed areas |
| Vitamin B6 | Meat, fish, nuts, bananas, avocados, wholegrains | Essential in the metabolism of protein and the amino acids that control mood and behaviour. Affects hormone metabolism | Women, especially smokers, 'junk-eaters' | Depression, anxiety, insomnia, loss of responsibility | Dry/greasy facial skin, cracking at corners of mouth |
| Vitamin B12 | All forms of meat, liver, eggs and milk, yeast extract | Involved in the chemical functioning of the nervous system, and the blood cells | Long-term vegans, those who have lost part of their stomach, and the elderly with digestive problems | Anaemia, loss of balance and a sore tongue | Smooth sore tongue, pale appearance, and unsteadiness |

| NUTRIENT | FOOD SOURCES | WHAT THEY DO | WHO IS AT RISK | SYMPTOMS | VISIBLE SIGNS |
|---|---|---|---|---|---|
| Vitamin C (Ascorbic acid) | Any fresh fruits and vegetables | Involved in healing, repair of tissues and production of some hormones | Smokers particularly | Lethargy, depression, hypochondriasis (imagined illnesses) | Easy bruising, look for small pinpoint bruises under the tongue |
| Vitamin D | Milk, margarine, sardines, cod liver oil, eggs (and sunlight) | For the balance of calcium in bones and teeth, and for muscle strength | Urban-dwelling, dark-skinned immigrants, especially young children and pregnant women, those with little sunlight exposure | Softening of the bones, poor teeth and weakness of the hip muscles | Enlarged skull, bowing of the legs and a waddling gait |
| Vitamin E | Most nuts, seeds and vegetable oils and dark green leafy vegetables | Protect tissues from wear and tear, keep cholesterol and other fats from deteriorating inside the body | Those on a very poor diet, or with serious absorption problems | None. Damage to the nervous system if severe | None |
| Vitamin K | Green leafy vegetables, and the bacteria in our intestines | Help with blood clotting | Those with a poor diet or on long-term antibiotics | Prolonged bleeding | None |

UNDERSTANDING YOUR NUTRIENT NEEDS *continued*

| NUTRIENT | FOOD SOURCES | WHAT THEY DO | WHO IS AT RISK | SYMPTOMS | VISIBLE SIGNS |
|---|---|---|---|---|---|
| Folic acid | All green leafy vegetables, liver and fortified cereals | Help maintain the health of the nervous system and the blood | Those on a poor diet, those taking anti-epileptic medication, coeliacs, and a percentage of the normal population of child-bearing women who are at increased risk of having a child with a neural tube defect | Often none. Possibly depression, fatigue and poor memory | None unless anaemic |
| Iron | Meat, wholegrains, nuts, eggs and fortified breakfast cereals | Essential to make blood-haemoglobin. Many other tissues need iron for energy reactions | Women who have heavy periods (e.g. coil users), vegetarians, especially if tea or coffee drinkers, women with recurrent thrush | Fatigue, poor energy, depression, poor digestion, sore tongue, cracking at corners of mouth | Pale complexion, brittle nails, cracking at corners of mouth |

| NUTRIENT | FOOD SOURCES | WHAT THEY DO | WHO IS AT RISK | SYMPTOMS | VISIBLE SIGNS |
|---|---|---|---|---|---|
| Zinc | Meat, wholegrains, nuts, peas, beans, lentils | Essential for normal growth, mental function, hormone production and resistance to infection | Vegetarians, especially tea and coffee drinkers, alcohol consumers, long-term users of diuretics (water pills) | Poor mental function, skin problems in general, repeated infections | Eczema, acne, greasy or dry facial skin |
| Magnesium | Green vegetables, wholegrains, Brazil and almond nuts, many other non-junk foods | Essential for sugar and energy metabolism, needed for healthy nerves and muscles | Women with PMS! (some 50 per cent may be lacking), long-term diuretic users, alcohol consumers | Nausea, apathy, loss of appetite, depression | |
| Calcium | Milk, cheese, bread, especially white, sardines, other fish with bones, green vegetables and beans | Needed for strong teeth and bones, also for normal nerve and muscle function. Lack leads to osteoporosis—bone thinning | Low dairy consumers, heavy drinkers, smokers, women with early menopause, lack of exercise increases the rate of bone loss-calcium in later years | Usually none until osteoporotic fracture of hip or spine. | Back pain, loss of height |

UNDERSTANDING YOUR NUTRIENT NEEDS *continued*

| NUTRIENT | FOOD SOURCES | WHAT THEY DO | WHO IS AT RISK | SYMPTOMS | VISIBLE SIGNS |
|---|---|---|---|---|---|
| Potassium | All vegetables and fruit | Needed for the health of all cells, especially muscles and the nervous system | The elderly, after prolonged vomiting, with use of some diuretics and poor diet | Weakness, low blood pressure and muscle cramps | None |
| Selenium | Most wholesome foods, especially seafoods | Involved in two enzymes that protect inflamed and damaged tissues and help thyroid function | The ill elderly, those on a very poor diet, possibly those with heart failure, alcoholics and long-standing malabsorption | None that are specific, just not well | None |
| Chromium | All wholesome foods, not sugar and other refined carbohydrates | Helps in the action of insulin. Deficiency causes a diabetic-like state | The elderly, life-long consumers of junk food! | Those of diabetes or of a low blood sugar with episodic weakness and sugar craving | Perhaps a large waistline or sweet wrappers in their pockets! |
| Essential Fatty Acids Omega-3 | Cod liver oil, mackerel, herring | Help control inflammation | Those on a poor diet | None | None |

| NUTRIENT | FOOD SOURCES | WHAT THEY DO | WHO IS AT RISK | SYMPTOMS | VISIBLE SIGNS |
|---|---|---|---|---|---|
| Fish and related oils | Salmon, canola and soya bean oil | Reduce calcium losses in urine | Older people, diabetics, drinkers | None | None |
| Essential Fatty Acids Omega-6, evening primrose and related oils | Sunflower, safflower and corn oils, many nuts (not peanuts) and seeds, green vegetables | Control inflammation, needed for health of nervous system, skin and blood vessels | Those on a poor diet, diabetics and drinkers. Also those with severe eczema and premenstrual breast tenderness | None | Possibly dry skin |

up any health problems you might have by referring to the relevant chapters. If you are in doubt about what you should be doing with your diet then look at The Very Nutritious Diet.

If you are looking for general improvement in your health rather than wishing to address a particular condition, you would be advised to follow the recommendations of The Very Nutritious Diet in order to get a balance of all the essential nutrients. Shop regularly for fresh food, especially for fruit and vegetables, and if you get the opportunity, grow your own fruit and vegetables or buy additive-free or organic produce.

## Judith's Story

Judith, a dedicated forty-five-year-old social worker, regularly worked long hours, and had really neglected her social life. It was thus easy to put her diarrhoea, fatigue and premenstrual problems down to her over-caring and rather nervous disposition. Her self-sacrificing nature meant that she had also sacrificed the quality of her diet. She ate erratically, had a poor intake of fresh foods, and would frequently snack on biscuits. She was reluctant to even mention her problem and it was only because of pressure from a friend that she had consulted us at all.

There was nothing remarkable to find on examination, but certainly the sound of her diet made it likely that she would have some nutritional deficiencies. Tests did reveal somewhat reduced levels of a number of nutrients, including zinc and vitamin B1, but the striking feature was the very low level of vitamin B3. Deficiency of this vitamin in particular can cause diarrhoea and can contribute to depression and possibly menstrual disturbances as well.

She had already begun making changes to her diet to improve its nutrient quality, and to avoid foods that might be aggravating her bowel problems by the time these results returned. There was no immediate improvement from changing her diet, but within a week of beginning high-strength vitamin B her diarrhoea settled completely. Her mood improved, and premenstrual symptoms lessened. She took this opportunity, with the support of her friends, to make changes to her lifestyle, reducing her work commitment and developing some social interests. A new hairstyle and some evening classes were two useful steps forward.

Overall there was a very good reduction in her levels of physical symptoms, Her generous, caring nature continues and doubtless she will have to take care that she does not over-commit herself both physically and emotionally.

# TAKING CARE OF BODY AND SOUL

Pacing ourselves and investing time in our own well-being is not something that comes naturally to most of us. When we are pre-occupied with caring and providing for our family, our home, as well as our workload outside the home, it sometimes requires real discipline to allocate regular time for personal enhancement. Often, with the best will in the world, our New Year resolutions to exercise regularly and make more time for relaxation go out of the window at the first sign of a hiccup in our routine.

There is plenty of hard evidence to suggest that stress under-lies many major health problems, and that regular exercise and relaxation are two sound ways of avoiding these, and of keeping both your mind and body in good shape. Taking time out for yourself is not just a nice idea, it is a necessity, especially if you lead a full and demanding life. As I am a working mother with four children, Alan felt I was probably more qualified to talk about the lifestyle burdens that women have to contend with. So when I refer to *we* in this chapter, I am referring to women as a collective group.

## *The Benefits of Relaxation*

Stress and relaxation are at opposite ends of the spectrum. When you are able to maintain the balance there's a good chance of you remaining healthy. However, when the scales tip and stress out-weighs relaxation, symptoms of ill-health often rear their heads. With our fast pace of life and our heavy commitments, taking time out for ourselves is often a luxury we consider we cannot afford. But in reality can we afford *not* to make time to relax and unwind, for we know the powerful affect stress can have on us. It has been shown to suppress ovulation in menstruating women, to greatly contribute to digestive disorders like irritable bowel syndrome, to play a key part in migraine headaches, and to increase the number of hot flushes at menopause.

The ability to 'switch off' and refresh ourselves is the key to sanity, but it may not be as easy as it sounds. When you are pre-occupied, wound up and tense, it may be hard to lose sight of the benefits of taking time out. Being able to thoroughly relax is actually an acquired skill—which for some of us takes a little practice—but all that is required is some time, and a comfortable space in which to spend that time. Once you have learned the art of relaxation you can practise it at any time, and, best of all, it is free. Even setting aside time to *think* is therapeutic. Sometimes we go headlong into adverse situations simply because we didn't make time to plan tactics, something which is as true for family and social situations as it is for problems at work.

We all deal with the stresses and strains of life in different ways. Some of us bottle them up and then fall apart one rainy day. Others soldier on feeling disgruntled and perhaps comfort eat or take to the bottle as a result. Regardless of how stress affects you, it is important to take some quiet time each day, as little as 15 or 20 minutes is all that is needed.

## Simple Relaxation

You will need a quiet space where you can confidently switch off. If necessary, put the answerphone on, or take the phone off the hook. Let other family members know that you don't want to be disturbed for a while, and put on some comfortable loose clothes. Either lie down on a mat, on a soft carpet or firm bed. Make sure that you are comfortable with the room temperature and lighting. You can play some calming music in the background. Once you feel comfortable, do the following, step-by-step:

1. Place a pillow under your head, and stretch out full length. Relax your arms and your lower jaw.
2. Take a few slow deep breaths before you begin.
3. Then concentrate on relaxing your muscles, starting with the toes on one foot and then the other. Gradually work your way slowly up your body, going through all the muscle groups.
4. As you do so, first tense each group of muscles and then relax them, taking care to breathe deeply as you relax.

5. When you reach your head, and your face feels relaxed, remain in the relaxed position for 10 to 15 minutes.
6. Gradually allow yourself to 'come to'.

## Other Methods of Relaxation

There are many other relaxation methods available, some of which you will be familiar with. Yoga and meditation are both widely practised doctrines which allow you to practise mind over matter. Massage is a useful tool and so too are creative visualisation, biofeedback and autogenic training. Many of the martial arts like tai chi are therapeutic too. If you find it difficult to close your mind down, it may be a good idea to choose a system of relaxation to try and then to get a little tuition in its principles. Here's an idea of what's on offer.

## Yoga

Yoga has been practised throughout the world for thousands of years. It works on the principle of bringing about a harmonious balance between mind, body and soul. It is particularly effective at helping to relieve stress and stress-related conditions. To get started, it's best to attend a yoga class and then to practise the postures at home on a regular basis. There are many good books on yoga (see the suggested reading list in Appendix III), and there are also a few yoga videos which you might find helpful. Yoga poses can be very powerful, so it is important to have some instruction in the early stages.

## Massage

We often subconsciously touch or rub a painful area in an attempt to bring about relief. Massage is a term used to describe a fairly ancient art of healing by touch, which is designed to relieve tension, improve circulation and help the body rid itself of toxins. It can also relieve pain by stimulating the production of brain chemicals called endorphins, the body's own painkillers, and by blocking transmission of pain messages by increasing the sensory input to the brain.

There are now many different massage techniques from which to choose, and lovely relaxing aromatherapy oils to use which aid relaxation. If you haven't had a professional massage before, it is worth asking around to find a local person with a good reputation.

It is a real treat. If your budget does not permit regular visits to the masseuse, then ask your partner or a friend to do the honours. You could enrol on a massage course with a partner and then practise on each other. Most adult evening colleges have classes and there are many good books on this subject (see the suggested reading list in Appendix III).

## Self-massage

It is possible to massage many parts of your own body, your face, head, neck, shoulders, lower back, abdomen, arms and legs. You will need some almond oil, to which you add a few drops of an aromatherapy oil of choice. Geranium, lavender, orange and ylang-ylang are particularly mild and relaxing. It is best to stick to the mild oils as oils are absorbed through the skin and stronger oils can cause other problems if used inappropriately.

Rub yourself in a clockwise direction on your abdomen, with stroking motions on your arms and legs, kneading your shoulders, and smoothing your neck. Give your face and your temples a rub, gently stretching the skin, and with two fingers each side gently massage your temples in a circle. Lastly, rub your ears between your thumb and forefinger, starting at the top and working your way down to the ear lobe, pulling gently at the same time. It feels wonderful and increases circulation to your face and head, as well as easing stress.

## Creative Visualisation

This is a favoured method of distraction from the stresses of everyday life. If you can recall pictures of holidays when you wished time would stand still or other wholesome fantasies, you can have them all. Creative visualisation is simply a structured method of daydreaming.

Get yourself comfortable in a quiet space, preferably warm and darkened, and without a telephone extension. Lie down, close your eyes and then just float off. Look at those lovely mind pictures until your heart is content. As time goes by, you will develop the ability to 'stay' in your daydream without your mind wandering. When you come round, you should feel warm, calm and relaxed.

## Self-hypnosis

This is a self-induced state that makes the mind susceptible to new ideas. When practised regularly it helps to bring about a feeling of calmness and mental agility. It is a system of implanting positive messages which have a therapeutic value, and is thought to be particularly useful in helping to relieve stress, high blood pressure, migraine and insomnia. Some people find that it also helps them to overcome addictive habits. Half an hour each day can leave you feeling refreshed, relaxed and more positive.

## Meditation

Another way of separating you from your body, meditation has a calming and renewing effect on both mind and body. You will need to learn to meditate at a class, but once you have the skill you can use it at any time, and anywhere.

## Autogenic Training

This method of relaxation, designed to tap into the body's own in-built powers of self-healing, consists of repeating six different commands slowly, in sequence, until you reach a semi-hypnotic state. The end result is a much more relaxed and positive you— and requires only half an hour or so three times per week initially, but it does involve taking instruction initially.

## Biofeedback

Another relaxation technique which requires you to link up to a biofeedback machine, or relaxometer. The deep states of relaxation reached through this method have been shown to influence blood pressure levels and brain-wave patterns.

All of these methods and more can be learned at specialist centres throughout the country. It may well be worth investing some time on a few dark winter evenings to learn to outsmart the stresses and strains of daily life.

# The Benefits of Exercise

If you are exercising at least four times per week to the breathlessness stage, and have done so for years, perhaps you should skip this chapter, which is aimed at the 'reluctant exerciser'.

Many of us wish that our bodies were self-exercising. Whilst we acknowledge that we feel saintly after an exercise session, the thought of getting up on a dark morning in order to exercise before the day begins, understandably, doesn't seem that appealing. But, like most bonuses in life, physical fitness has to be worked for. Why do we need to be physically fit, we hear you ask, as you are not planning on entering any competitions? And anyway you lead a busy life, surely that's enough?

As our knee bone is connected to our thigh bone and so on, it follows that if we exert ourselves physically, it will have a positive overall effect on both our body and our mind. Exercising to the point of breathlessness stimulates the release of brain chemicals, called endorphins, which not only raise our mood, but also influence our hormones. Rushing around and leading a busy life may just leave us feeling absolutely exhausted, especially chasing after children from morning till night. We have yet to meet someone who feels 'high' from these activities. But exercise, on the other hand, helps to improve our energy levels and to overcome symptoms of depression, anxiety, insomnia, and it also increases our sense of self-esteem and well-being. In fact exercise has been shown to be more successful in overcoming symptoms of depression and anxiety than psychotherapy. Being in good physical shape is also good for our ego, especially as we age, and shouldn't go unnoticed by our partners.

More good news is that exercise may offset ageing of the central nervous system, as well as being cardio-protective. It also stimulates the heart, which in turn stimulates the flow of blood around the body, which flushes out toxins and keeps our skin glowing. So there are many benefits to be had, and we are not talking Olympics here!

Research shows that we need to exercise three or times per week at least, to the point of breathlessness. But this is not a competition, you need only exercise to gradually increase your fitness level. If you haven't exercised for years, it may take only a few minutes initially before you need the armchair. Each exercise session should be slightly longer than the last one, until you feel 'comfortable' exercising for 40 minutes. It may take a few months to build up to that, and it is worth keeping an exercise diary so that you can monitor your progress. If you are currently under your doctor's supervision, and haven't exercised for a while, it is advisable to get a medical blessing before embarking on your exercise regime.

More good news is that you do not necessarily have to join the gym, or do an hour's aerobics class with a group of stick insects, but you do need to choose the kind of exercise you *like* in order to stick at it. For those who haven't exercised for some time, we usually recommend starting with some brisk walking or gentle skipping, and perhaps a short work-out with an exercise video.

An exercise programme should be for life. It takes months to build stamina and only weeks to lose it if we stop exercising, which is rather infuriating. You are likely to be more successful at sticking to this regime if you make yourself a schedule. It is all too easy to cry off because of other commitments. If you find it hard to stick to your schedule, arrange to meet a friend for a game of tennis or squash, or make a date to have a gentle jog or swim together. That way it will be harder for you to make some sort of excuse.

When you make the decision to exercise regularly, your motivation must be sound in order to maintain the commitment. Whilst most women would not object to having the vital statistics of Pamela Anderson or Cindy Crawford, your reason for exercising is health. You want to protect yourself from heart disease and to keep your bones strong, thus preventing the bone-thinning disease, osteoporosis. Any visible physical improvements are a bonus. You want to develop and improve your *Stamina, Strength and Suppleness*, the three S's.

## Stamina

Stamina refers to the efficiency of the heart and lungs in delivering oxygen to the muscles, and can be measured by the amount of time it takes you to get breathless. We can gradually build our stamina, with regular low-intensity aerobic exercise. Aerobic exercise simply uses large muscle groups like the legs and arms, which then demand more oxygen, making the heart work harder. With regular aerobic exercise the heart and lungs become more efficient, which means they will not have to 'work' so hard in daily life. Increasing your stamina also means that you can achieve more for less effort.You should eventually be aiming for four to five forty-minute sessions of low-impact aerobic exercise per week in order to reap all the benefits that exercise has to offer.

## Strength

The definition of strength is the maximum force needed by a muscle or group of muscles to overcome a resistance. In other words how much effort it takes to push, pull, lift, climb and carry without injuring yourself. Women can increase their strength by as much as 50 per cent without gaining muscle size. Stronger muscles will mean that you can get more out of your day—be it in the garden, in the house, or at leisure. Having strong back and abdominal muscles will also improve your posture and guard you from most lower back pain.

## Suppleness

Joint mobility is something you take for granted early in life, but as you get older joints naturally stiffen through lack of use. It really is a case of 'use it or lose it'. Stretching exercises will help to maintain your mobility, and are easy to practise at home whilst listening to music or in front of the television. Stretch your muscles slowly, holding each position until you feel the strain, but not pain.

Where specific exercises are of value to a particular condition, like heart disease, osteoporosis, fatigue, PMS, pregnancy and so on, you will see that we give specific instructions and a target to aim for in the relevant chapter.

## The Pay-off

If you have always avoided exercise, you are probably grimacing at the thought of what you know should be ahead. Let us assure you that you will reap the benefits of your labour. We have seen so many patients who have not previously exercised begin their exercise programme reluctantly, and then surprisingly come to love it. They feel it improves their energy levels and vitality, and notice improvements in their skin quite quickly. For every hour you spend exercising you will get the equivalent time back in increased stamina, strength and suppleness. Additionally, it is now well accepted that regular exercise helps to protect us against heart disease, arthritis, protects our bones against the bone-thinning disease, osteoporosis, and helps us to avoid depression. So exercising is not just a nice idea, both the long- and short-term benefits are well worth the investment of a few hours each week.

# THE STRENGTHS OF COMPLEMENTARY THERAPIES

Although making dietary changes, exercising, relaxing and taking nutritional supplements are the prime factors in women's health, it is also undoubtedly valuable to explore the world of complementary therapy. Unlike orthodox medicine, holistic medicine looks at the *whole person*—the mind, the body and the spirit, and how they interact.

The years of abusing our bodies eventually take their toll. Strains that are placed upon women over time—not eating the right diet, being pregnant and breast-feeding, generally coping with stressful situations, premenstrual syndrome and symptoms of the menopause—may well be more than we can easily tolerate, and the stresses can affect the smooth running of our bodily processes. If your symptoms are severe, it may well be worth investigating what acupuncture, acupressure, cranial osteopathy, herbal medicine or homoeopathy have to offer. They are powerful tools that can sometimes help to speed up the recovery process.

## *Acupuncture*

Chinese medical thinking is quite different from that in the West in that it considers symptoms rather than named conditions, and the diagnosis and subsequent treatment address the whole person, the mind, body and lifestyle. Acupuncture can be a useful tool in the treatment of female problems and is appropriate for severe symptoms. You should always consult a properly trained and registered practitioner. Contact the Acupuncture Association of Australia (see Appendix V) for a list of accredited members.

### *The Philosophy*

Chinese medicine, which has been in existence for thousands of years, treats the whole person, rather than using the Western method of addressing specific conditions. It works on the premise that a universal energy known as chi, which has two complementary qualities (yin and yang), must be in perfect balance in order for good health to exist. The term yin encompasses the feminine principle (cold and the state of rest) whereas yang includes the male principle (heat and activity). These principles are active to appropriate degrees in both men and women, and when the balance is upset, illness is the result.

Chi flows through the twelve meridians or channels of the body, which are each associated with a particular organ, such as the lungs, liver or spleen. Herbal remedies and acupuncture are used to restore the balance of yin and yang, and thus promote healing.

## What Treatment to Expect

As well as taking an in-depth medical history the Chinese doctor will take your pulse at six different points on each wrist to get the measure of each of the twelve vital organs of the body. Your tongue will also be inspected closely, as its texture reflects the condition of the vital organs.

Acupuncture uses stainless-steel needles, which are inserted into specific points, along meridians or lines, in order to affect the energy flowing to an organ. The needles, which remain in place for approximately 20 minutes, don't actually hurt, but they may cause a tingle, mild ache or heat sensation.

Chinese medicine also encompasses the use of herbs rather than drugs, which are aimed at keeping the yin and yang, which are seen as complementary and interdependent, in constant harmony. Many of the herbal remedies used by Chinese doctors are available in pill form and are relatively inexpensive. They should only be used with the guidance of a qualified practitioner, as taking a yang preparation when a yin medicine is required will further exaggerate the imbalance and may well make your problem worse.

# Acupressure

The Japanese finger pressure method, otherwise known as shiatsu, is more appropriate to minor or occasional problems than acupuncture.

In this system the body is influenced in various ways by the stimulation of key points, found along the course of energy channels circulating near the surface of the skin. These are the same as acupuncture meridians, but the points are stimulated by pressure rather than needles.

In order for shiatsu to be effective it is important to apply the right kind of pressure for an appropriate length of time. Some professional instruction would be useful initially so that you can recognise the correct method. Once you have mastered the art of applying pressure to appropriate points, you can self-administer at home.

# Cranial Osteopathy

Many of us suffer with subtle back or neck problems that occur as a result of general wear and tear. Long-standing headaches can sometimes be totally cured by some good osteopathic treatment. It is certainly worth consulting a cranial osteopath if you feel the tension building up in your back or neck, or if you suffer from regular headaches.

## The Philosophy

Cranial osteopathy, or cranio-sacral therapy as it is known, is a specialised form of osteopathy which is gentle yet potent. The aim is to gently coax the muscles, tendons, joints and connective tissue to establish correct function and release restriction, thus restoring normal circulation, the flow of energy and glandular secretions.

The cranio-sacral mechanism is made up of the cranium (the skull), the sacrum (the bone at the base of the spine), the membranes surrounding the brain, the spinal cord and the fascia, a continuous clingfilm-like sheet that surrounds the muscles, organs, joints and bones. The tension of this fascia is all-important. If you have ever worn an all-in-one pants suit that is too tight or too short, you will have felt somewhat uncomfortable. If the tension in the body's fascia becomes too tight, you can't just take it off, and it is possible that body functions can be affected in the long term.

Cranial osteopathy works on two basic principles: first, that structure can affect function, and second, that impairment in the structure, or reduced mobility, will affect blood flow. Blood flow is of supreme importance in osteopathy, and treatment is aimed at improving local circulation and freeing-up the supply of blood to the nerves.

Everything in the body moves with the cranial rhythm, which is the rhythm of the central nervous system. It's like a breathing rhythm, and is constant, even when we sleep. The movement helps blood flow generally and can help impaired local circulation after trauma.

If there are restrictions to soft tissue (like muscles), to the fascia or to the membranes, then blood, lymph and cerebral spinal fluid is restricted; as a result, nutrition to that area is affected.

## What Treatment to Expect

Cranial osteopaths, like acupuncturists, like to take their time over the initial consultation, in order to take a complete history and to assess the problem fully. The treatment involves lying on the osteopath's consulting bed whilst balancing takes place. It is extremely subtle. It feels like mild finger pressure, but the effect is powerful. Often patients fall 'asleep' and experience a very pleasant sense of well-being. It is important to rest afterwards, and sometimes things feel worse the next day. One treatment takes several days to work, and so you would not be required to attend more than fortnightly or monthly. Courses are usually short, although the course of treatment may be extended for chronic problems.

# Herbal Medicine

Curiously, herbal medicine is older and more ubiquitous than any other type of medication on earth. It is as old as food and people, and there is no place which has been inhabited by people and plants that has not had its own herbal medicine. The great majority of plant medicines in use today were discovered by the hunter-gatherers, and so pre-date history itself. There is very good evidence that in all past and present hunter-gatherer societies, the responsibilities for gathering and learning about plant medicine belonged to women. So perhaps we can take some comfort in knowing that afflicted women discovered their own remedies.

As civilisations emerged, men became involved with agriculture and medicine, and tended to form analytical systems. As China, for example, evolved the polar principles of yin and yang, so European medicine relied on the concepts of love and strife: these resolved into four elements which in turn were thought to be represented in the body by the four bodily fluids or humours. Many of these concepts still inform the best herbal medical practice in the West today, along with naturopathic ideas, many learned from native North Americans. Like Chinese medicine, European herbal medicine places great emphasis upon diet and exercise and other environmental factors.

## The Philosophy

While herbal medicine aims to treat your current condition, it takes into consideration your past history from the time you were born, and the health of your parents at the time of conception. So, even if your symptoms are the same as your neighbour's, your prescriptions are unlikely to be the same. In other words, while we are all subject to the same biophysical laws, each one of us has a unique tissue profile and therefore the treatment (by a once-living plant organism) needs to be unique.

## What Treatment to Expect

The prescription you will receive may consist of a combination of a few or many different herbs. Sometimes you will be given herbs to take at different times of the day; and on occasions, herbs for different times of the month. Herbal medicine has been shown to speed up the healing of broken bones and to aid absorption of minerals from the digestive tract. It can be a very powerful tool. If you would like to consult a trained herbalist, you will find the address of The Herbalists Association of Australia in Appendix V.

# Homoeopathy

The word homoeopathy comes from two Greek words: *homoio* which means 'same' and *pathos* which means 'suffering'. It was developed by Doctor Samuel Hahnemann in the eighteenth century, as a system of treating sick people with safe medicine. Whereas orthodox medicine (or allopathic medicine, as it is referred to) aims to treat symptoms with a drug that will produce an opposite effect, homoeopathy treats 'like with like'.

A homoeopathic remedy is designed to produce the same symptoms as those you are suffering, and in doing so aims to cancel them out. The dosages used are minute and may contain no substantial amount of the original material. In this latter case, it is thought that the medicine, pill or liquid contains an energy, or 'spirit', of the original medicine. Even these extreme dilutions have been shown to be effective in many conditions, including arthritis and hayfever. Many people appear to have benefited by their use for all sorts of conditions.

## The Philosophy

Homoeopathy is an approach to treatment which aims to assist nature with her own process of healing rather than by-passing her altogether. Like other holistic treatments, it treats each person as an individual. A trained homoeopath takes an exceedingly thorough history before suggesting the most suitable remedy. It is very much a gentle, preventative, method of treatment which works best in conjunction with improved dietary and lifestyle measures.

Followers of homoeopathy regularly use remedies to help themselves and their families for anything from coughs and cold to menstrual problems.

## What Treatment to Expect

Once diagnosed you will usually be presented either with little white pills made from lactose, which melt under your tongue, or a tincture, which is a liquid. You will be given instructions about the frequency to use your remedy, and advice about diet and lifestyle. The remedies are widely available and they are reasonably priced. Sometimes it's trial and error until you find the remedy that suits you, but it may be worth persisting.

If you do decide to consult a holistic practitioner, use one that is recommended or find a properly qualified person from the register kept by each association. Sadly, there may be some non-qualified people practising, and these should be avoided. The addresses and telephone numbers of the relevant associations can be found in Appendix V.

# PART TWO

# *The A–Z of Problems*

# ABDOMINAL WIND AND BLOATING

Gas in the bowel is certainly not something we bring up in social conversation, and yet on average we produce 1.5 litres per day, enough to fill a small balloon, which means that in a year we are talking about some 500 litres! Wind is often accompanied by a sluggish and constipated bowel, but fluid retention or lax abdominal muscles can contribute as well. Bloating can occur at any time, and is often worse premenstrually. It is best tackled by addressing the underlying problems of bowel sluggishness and anything that can influence wind production.

The subject of abdominal wind has only been taken seriously in the last decade. A variety of gases are produced by billions of mainly friendly bacteria that inhabit the large colon, the transverse section of the large bowel. (Surprisingly, there are more bacteria in the colon than there are cells in our body.) They are found only in tiny amounts in the small bowel where the majority of digestion and absorption of nutrients takes place. They first appear in our caecum, which is the first part of the large bowel, on the right side of the abdomen at about the point where the appendix is, or was if it has been removed, and are waiting to pounce on the leftovers from the meal you ate several hours before.

These bacteria produce a variety of gases, some of which our own cells are incapable of producing. They include hydrogen, methane and carbon dioxide, all of which have no smell. The gas that smells like bad eggs is hydrogen sulphide, and it is more commonly produced by those living in the West, because of dietary factors.

## *What Are the Symptoms?*

The trapped gases cause bloating, which may be painful or painless, and often results in the sufferer having a lower self-image because frequently clothes don't fit. Some of the wind manages to escape through burping, or to give it its medical term, erucation, or through the back passage when its passing sometimes creates loud noises or an offensive smell. It may be accompanied by social embarrassment, especially if you cannot control its passing and the smell is noticeable by others. Severe sufferers commonly avoid social events because of their symptoms.

## *Who Gets It?*

The degree of wind and bloating is related mainly to the type of diet eaten, and to how food is digested. Those with a poor digestion, especially disease of the pancreas, will find that many foods will aggravate this problem. High-fibre foods are particularly to blame. An excess of fats can make it worse too.

## *What Causes It?*

It is not the result of air we swallow, whilst breathing or eating, as most of this is absorbed during the digestive process or brought back as a burp. The amount and type of wind that any one individual produces is influenced by the following.

◆ The type of food eaten, especially fibre-rich foods.
◆ How well the food is digested in the small bowel.
◆ How quickly food and residues pass through the small bowel to the colon.
◆ The type of bacteria present in the colon, which may also be influenced by the type of diet we eat, presence or absence of illness, use of antibiotics and even the type of bacteria in the colons of those with whom you live.

What causes wind production can and does vary from person to person. Something that encourages wind in one person may well have no effect on another. And what causes you wind at one stage may not cause any problems at another time. So it is really a combination of factors and what goes on in the bowel can influence many aspects of body health. Excessive production of wind is more likely to occur if:

◆ You consume foods to which you are intolerant—and in theory this could be any food depending on your individual sensitivities.
◆ You eat foods that contain sugars that you cannot easily digest, and these are then fermented by the bacteria in the large bowel and converted to gas. The same can occur in fewer cases following the excess consumption of table sugar (found in most sweets and sweetened foods), fruit sugar or fructose (found in most fruits and vegetables), or the artificial sweetener Sorbitol (found in cool-tasting mints and some sugar-free sweets).

◆ You eat foods that are known to be hard to digest, especially if they are not well cooked or are eaten in large amounts. The list is potentially very long, and can certainly consist of any of the following:

◇ wheat, especially wheat bran and wholemeal products
◇ coarse oats, barley and rye
◇ sweetcorn, especially if whole and not chewed well
◇ brown rice
◇ potatoes
◇ dried, beans, lentils and sometimes peas
◇ vegetables of the *Brassica* family (cabbage, cauliflower, broccoli and Brussels sprouts) and Jerusalem artichokes
◇ shells of prawns and other crustacea
◇ mushrooms
◇ onions, garlic and leeks
◇ asparagus

◆ You have a rapid gut transit time—which can be encouraged by drinking coffee and eating large meals. A low-fat, high-carbohydrate, high-fibre diet might make the situation worse too. The combination of rapid passage through the small bowel, especially if the meal was hard to digest, will result in the bacteria of the colon getting their full share.

◆ You have poor digestion. If you have recently lost weight and experience abdominal pain, you should see your doctor without delay.

◆ You are making an excessive use of laxatives.

◆ You have been prescribed some relatively new drugs to control diabetes, as these inhibit the digestion of sugar.

◆ You eat large amounts of caramel, burnt sugar and modified starch. These have all been chemically altered by heat or the cooking process, which makes them harder to digest. Caramel is widely used as a colouring and flavouring agent, so you will need to read labels carefully. There is also a significant amount in beer.

## What Your Doctor Can Do

The answer is probably very little other than investigations for severe wind and bloating which are accompanied by other digestive symptoms. In truth, as our doctors know relatively little about diet, they too are probably suffering in silence. Occasionally preparations based on mint or old-fashioned charcoal preparations can be helpful. If the wind is accompanied by diarrhoea, weight loss or blood in the stool then obviously medical investigations will be necessary.

## *What You Can Do*

- Eat slowly, taking care to chew your food well.
- Avoid the foods that you know upset you.
- Ensure that your vegetables are not undercooked.
- If you enjoy eating dried beans, soak them overnight, shake them to remove the husks and cook them thoroughly. Many, including red kidney beans, need to be cooked for at least 10 minutes at a rolling boil, and then simmered for an hour before they are ready to eat. This reduces the potential wind-producing culprits—two tough carbohydrates called stacchyose and raffinose. Black-eyed beans and red kidney beans are usually the biggest wind producers in the bean family.
- Eat smaller portions and take time to relax after a meal to aid digestion.
- Avoid foods rich in sulphur and sulphites as these chemicals encourage the conversion of hydrogen in the colon to hydrogen sulphide—the bad-eggs gas. The main dietary sources of these chemicals are:
  - ◇ bread
  - ◇ foods preserved with sulphur dioxide, such as dried fruits, and fruit squashes, plus anything else containing a sulphite or metabisulphite compound (where label reading comes in again)
  - ◇ wines, beers and cider, which often contain sulphite as a preservative (this is not required to be mentioned on the label)
  - ◇ eggs and all members of the onion family
- Avoid caramel, burnt sugar and foods containing them.
- Don't smoke heavily during or after a meal as this can inhibit digestive function and for some could result in increased wind production.
- Eat charcoal biscuits, an old-fashioned remedy that might help.
- Have a pot of live yoghurt each day as this is rich in semi-friendly bacteria.
- Be patient, it could take up to six weeks to see stable improvement.

◆ Swallow your embarrassment and consult your doctor if these self-help measures don't work.

## Relaxation

Both relaxation and hypnotherapy genuinely seem to improve the way the bowel functions, and are useful tools for diarrhoea sufferers. It seems that they influence the function of the gut muscles, encouraging them to work in an efficient coordinated fashion. It is also possible that with the regular help of relaxation and some hypnotherapy a person may become more in control of their bowels as they are perhaps less sensitive and more tolerant of the disturbance in function.

Regular massage of at least the abdomen and lower back, with some of the aromatherapy oils mentioned on page 30, is desirable for severe sufferers. Making sure you take time out to relax each day will also bring its benefits.

## Complementary Therapies

Herbal medicine is likely to offer you a mixture that will calm your bowel down and aid digestion, and it is also worth consulting an acupuncturist. Homoeopathy may have a remedy that would bring relief from your symptoms. Any of these systems may help, but it is important to try one at a time, otherwise there will be a very confusing picture.

## Sonya's Story

Sonya was a thirty-three-year-old woman who was married with two children and worked as an administrator. She was admitted to hospital several times as a result of her symptoms, but was offered little effective help from the doctors who examined her.

*Following the birth of my second baby I began suffering with severe bouts of abdominal bloating and pains. One night I had the most terrible attack and thought I was dying. The doctor was called, and by the time he arrived I was hyperventilating. He called an ambulance, and I was taken to casualty, writhing and groaning in pain. The examining doctor was surprised by the amount of pain I was in, and was unable to make a diagnosis. I was kept in overnight for observation and given pain-killers. The following morning I was sent home with a diagnosis of colic, and no follow-up treatment whatsoever. The only suggestion my doctor had was to eat more wholemeal bread and bran, which made my symptoms even worse.*

*My symptoms affected my whole life. When I had them I found it hard to work and could hardly cope with my family duties. I had no choice but to leave the parenting to my husband. I dreaded family holidays and wondered what the future held for me.*

*I was recommended to the WNAS clinic. At my first consultation I was asked about many aspects of my history, diet and lifestyle. I was given a diet, exercise and supplement programmes to follow, which I duly did.*

*Within the first month I noticed a spectacular difference, and within four months the symptoms were gone completely! I am three years on now and can honestly say that I feel better than I have for years. I'm now able to cope with my job and am a competent wife and mother, and I am immensely grateful. I do wish that the doctors that I had seen over the years had been armed with adequate knowledge about diet, which would have saved me a lot of pain and trauma.*

*See also*: Irritable Bowel Syndrome, Premenstrual Syndrome. Plus Recommended Reading List (*Beat IBS Through Diet*), Useful Groups and References.

# ACNE

Acne, or to give it its proper name, *Acne vulgaris* is perhaps the commonest skin complaint in that most of us have had some experience of it during adolescence. Three types of 'spots' make up acne:

- ◆ the redheads or papules
- ◆ the yellowheads or pustules
- ◆ the blackheads or comedones

These usually appear on a background of inflamed red skin. This is most commonly on the face, back or shoulders. These three spots—red-, yellow- and blackheads—are manifestations of the inflammation, infection and resolution that occur in this condition.

Initially there is an increased sensitivity to hormones in the skin. Testosterone, which is present in both men and women, stimulates the production of sebum or grease. The ducts that carry this grease to the surface become blocked, get inflamed, then infected, and then either discharge themselves or resolve, leaving a blackhead behind which is the thickened remains of the infected pus of the yellowhead.

## Who Gets It?

Many do in adolescence. Boys are more often affected than girls and some, due to genetic factors, are not affected at all. Many women in their twenties and thirties are also affected as there may be minor hormonal changes or increased hormonal sensitivity that leads to the persistence of acne. Acne can also be caused by a few drugs: steroids, phenytoin and phenothiazines. Exposure to chemicals containing chlorine can also be a rare cause.

## What Your Doctor Can Do

Therapy is aimed at reducing the bacteria on the skin surface, reducing the production of sebum, or altering the hormonal stimulus to acne especially in older women.

◆ Local applications of antiseptic, especially benzoyl peroxide, help by inhibiting the growth of bacteria and reducing sebum production. A local application of retinoic acid helps to unblock plugged follicles and is used when blackheads dominate.

◆ Prescribe an antibiotic skin application or antibiotics by mouth. There is a variety of preparations with around a 75 per cent success rate. Sometimes the bacteria become resistant to one antibiotic, and a change is needed. A swab may help decide the best sort.

◆ Hormone-based treatment, using either the oral contraceptive pill or a combination of oestrogen with a small dose of an anti-testosterone preparation, is useful for more resistant cases.

◆ A powerful drug derived from vitamin A, 13-cis-retinoic acid, is highly effective as it inhibits the excessive production of sebum. It is only used by medical specialists in those who have failed to respond to other treatments. As its use is associated with foetal abnormalities, women taking it should use contraception.

## *What You Can Do*

◆ Keep your skin clean. Clean your skin thoroughly after using make-up.

◆ Sunbathe. This often helps, though it may increase the number of blackheads.

◆ Squeeze the blackheads. This is worthwhile provided that they are not pushed inward into the deeper layers of the skin.

◆ Change your diet. Despite popular belief, no diet is of proven value in acne! For some, avoiding chocolate seems to help. It is possible that a low-fat diet (weight-reducing if necessary) with high intakes of fruit and vegetables and a reduced intake of wheat might help some sufferers.

## *Nutritional Supplements*

The only one of proven benefit is zinc. It is not as effective as antibiotics. A dose of 30 mg per day is needed. Higher doses should only be taken under supervision. Most useful if there is a lot of inflammation or cystic swellings.

## *Complementary Therapies*

Consider homoeopathy and herbalism.

## *Miranda's Story*

Miranda was a very attractive and petite forty-two-year-old woman. She came to the clinic as she was feeling generally low, and had a chronic skin problem. The PMS symptoms that she had manifested themselves in terrible depression, mood swings and a near-suicidal state of mind.

*I had suffered from acne from the age of sixteen and, despite visiting dermatologists, beauty experts and black magic practitioners, and having swallowed every antibiotic known to man, nothing worked on a permanent basis. I was about to start a hospital-supervised course of treatment that had possible bad side-effects, but again could not be guaranteed to be permanently successful, when I decided to visit the WNAS.*

*I was taken off wheat, rye, barley and oats for a period of three months and I began to notice the improvement in my skin. I was also not eating red meat or dairy products, but was taking supplements of Optivite, zinc and Efamol. After approximately three months I incorporated rye bread into my diet without problems.*

*After six months my skin was clear. Several months later I tried to reintroduce wheat into my diet, with disastrous results. Even small amounts, i.e. in sausages, soup, casseroles, would bring me out in painful cysts. So wheat was completely removed from my diet, along with dairy products. I do eat red meat occasionally without ill effect. I use soya products instead, which is really no hardship these days. I recently paid another visit to the clinic as my menopause has now begun, and was delighted to discover that soya products are a rich source of naturally occurring oestrogen.*

*It is so wonderful to have clear skin and not feel ashamed to be seen without make-up. Even my mother, who suffered along with me for so many years, recently remarked that visiting the WNAS has transformed my life both physically and mentally.*

# ACNE ROSACEA

This is a mainly facial rash that usually develops in middle-aged to elderly people. Like common acne there is a degree of skin redness, with papules (redheads) and occasionally pustules (yellowheads) but never blackheads. Flushing is prominent on the cheeks and nose and is usually made worse by alcohol. Sometimes the eyes become involved with redness of the eyelids and clouding of the vision in severe cases.

## What Your Doctor Can Do
The main treatment is use of long-term, low-dose antibiotics, usually tetracycline, as given for acne vulgaris. Those suffering with eye symptoms as well will need special attention.

## What You Can Do
- Avoid known aggravating factors; most commonly these are alcohol and anything else that may trigger a flush, like spicy foods and hot drinks.
- Try a diet low in amine-rich foods as is used for migraine (see Menu for Migraine). In sensitive individuals this type of chemical can affect the blood vessels in the head, triggering migraine, and the possibility exists that they also affect the

blood vessels of the face too. This means avoiding cheese, chocolate, tea and coffee, and many other foods too.

## Complementary Therapies

Consider homoeopathy and herbalism.

---

## Barbara's Story

Barbara was a thirty-three-year-old woman who developed an increasingly severe facial rash. Her undoubted good looks had been spoiled by a red, pimply-looking rash that was distributed mainly over across her cheeks, down her jaw-line and on to her nose. Over a year ago this had been diagnosed as acne rosacea and had not responded to a course of antibiotics from her own doctor.

Close examination showed that there were possibly two types of rash. The typical acne rosacea was mainly on the cheeks, but also there were some red itchy bumps along the jaw-line. This latter type of rash we have seen in young women in association with a suspected allergy to wheat.

Beverley was asked to follow a diet using the treatment for migraine—avoiding all amine-rich foods, as well as wheat, oats, barley and rye which may all contain gluten.

She was also asked to take supplements of zinc and vitamin B.

Within three weeks there was an over-50 per cent improvement in the appearance of her rash. Interestingly, the itchy bumps had cleared almost completely and her skin felt much more comfortable.

The rate of improvement was probably too quick for it to be anything to do with her supplements, and it seemed that the avoidance of certain foods was the particularly important factor.

She added back in foods that had previously been excluded, on a step-by-step basis, and was able to identify those that had contributed to her rash in particular. It transpired that alcohol was a particular culprit.

# AGEING

We now live for longer and, as time passes, there will be more retired people and less workers in the Western world. Health-care services will be stretched and so it makes sense for us to implement self-help measures to preserve our fitness, health and physical appearance.

It is rapidly becoming obvious that the elderly, those of sixty-five and over, contain a wide variety of individuals with varying levels of health. We are also beginning to identify those factors that determine those who age quickly. Those factors associated with premature death or rapid ageing are:

- cigarette smoking
- excessive alcohol intake
- poor quality diet
- social deprivation, e.g. living alone
- low levels of physical activity
- low levels of mental activity
- genetic factors, identified and unidentified

The genetic factor is interesting as we know that there are genetic predispositions to high blood pressure, heart disease and diabetes. Genetic factors may also play a small part in many other diseases. It is clear that there are interactions between a person's genetic predisposition and the effects of their diet, for example salt intake, and whether it raises blood pressure.

Overall intake of nutrients during the course of a lifetime may be an important factor. Interest is centred upon the anti-oxidants, vitamins, minerals and other non-essential dietary agents that protect tissues against highly reactive chemicals called free radicals. Free radicals are produced during the course of normal metabolic activity in all cells of the body, and can damage tissues, causing chemical change. There are many protective mechanisms which minimise this damage and, as a result, these free radicals only last for minute fractions of a second. Certain nutrients help mop up these potentially damaging free radicals, including:

◆ vitamin C
◆ vitamin E
◆ vitamin A (both beta-carotene and retinol)
◆ B vitamins
◆ zinc
◆ copper
◆ manganese

If left unchecked, free radicals damage the wall of the cell as well as its internal chemistry in a way that is potentially irreversible. The outward signs are deteriorations in skin quality, changes in the eye, such as cataract formation, some of the changes seen in arthritis, and the gradual development of atherosclerosis. Diets rich in foods containing the nutrients listed above seem to protect against cardiovascular disease and cancer, in particular. The simple message, therefore, is eat lots of fruit and vegetables, and limit your exposure to noxious chemicals, especially cigarette smoke.

## Nutritional Deficiencies in the Elderly

It is in the extremes of life that we are particularly vulnerable to nutritional problems. New-born infants, especially premature ones, and ill, elderly patients both have special nutritional needs. These are under-recognised and not easily provided by a healthy diet and simple vitamin and mineral supplements.

In 1993, the CSIRO conducted a detailed nutritional study of elderly Australians which revealed widespread deficiencies. Nutrients that were commonly deficient included iron, vitamin B12 and folic acid, any one of which could cause anaemia, and there were also deficiencies of vitamin A, B complex and C, which could influence mood, muscle function and resistance to infection. Other studies have confirmed these findings and uncovered trace nutrient deficiencies including zinc, which helps resistance to infection, selenium, which is involved in anti-oxidant protection, and chromium, which may influence predisposition to diabetes.

The risk of nutritional deficiencies in this group rises with:

◆ history of poor diet
◆ high alcohol intake
◆ recent weight loss
◆ medical problems

◆ use of drugs, especially diuretics, antibiotics if prolonged use is required, steroids and digoxin, a drug for heart disease

## What Your Doctor Can Do

◆ Be alert to the potential problems of nutritional deficiencies in the elderly.
◆ Look for signs of nutritional deficiency:
   ◇ sore, smooth tongue, cracking at the corners of the mouth
   ◇ peeling of the lips
   ◇ flattened or upturned finger or thumb nails
   ◇ excessively dry skin
   ◇ easy bruising
   ◇ heart failure
   ◇ severe muscle cramps
   ◇ depression
   ◇ loss of appetite
◆ Test nutritional status of ill, elderly patients. Simple blood tests for anaemia, measuring serum zinc, serum and red cell magnesium, tests for the B vitamin deficiencies, especially vitamin B12 and folic acid, should all be on offer at local hospital level. More specialised tests should also be available.
◆ Advise patients about healthy eating, and in particular if help with eating is needed in many older patients, when foods may need to be in semi-liquid form and easy to digest. High-fibre diets are inappropriate for the majority of ill, elderly patients. There should not be an over-reliance on sugar and refined foods, even those that are easy to consume. Good nutritious foods include all dairy products, eggs, ice cream, vegetables (especially if prepared as soup), meat (especially if minced), mashed potatoes with added milk or cream, stewed fruit and fortified drinks which are very useful as meal replacements or between meals when additional kilojoules are required.
◆ Finally, and most importantly, doctors should be prepared to prescribe nutritional supplements. Despite their age, the elderly do very well with the right treatment!

# *Problems of the Elderly, and the Nutritional Answer*

As a general rule, higher doses of supplements may be needed initially, say for two to three months, until nutritional levels are normal, and then pills can be reduced generally to half the amount.

| | |
|---|---|
| Recurrent upper respiratory tract infections | Zinc and high potency multi-vitamins |
| Congestive heart failure | Strong doses of vitamin B complex |
| Osteoporosis | Supplements of marine fish oil, evening primrose oil and calcium daily, or calcium, 1 g daily, and vitamin D, 400 IU daily, for the housebound elderly. |
| Heart rhythm disturbance | Supplements of magnesium, 300 mg daily, and multi-vitamins. |
| Muscle cramps | Supplements of magnesium and multi-vitamins. |
| High blood pressure | Vitamin C, 1 g daily, to reduce stroke risk, and supplements of magnesium, 300 mg, to lower blood pressure, especially in women. |
| High risk of cardiovascular disease | Vitamin E, 600 IU daily, but not if receiving the anti-coagulant Warfarin. |
| Diabetes | Supplements of chromium, 200 µg daily if mildly diabetic, subject to approval by their doctor (see Diabetes). |

## *What You Can Do*

This is given on the basis of the elderly person being a near relative to you, the reader of this book.

◆ Advise your parent's doctor about her recent diet.
◆ Discuss with your parent which types of foods they like to eat, that are nutritious and are easy to prepare.
◆ Make regular use of meal replacements when convalescing.
◆ Be prepared to administer supplements in a number of situations even if they are not prescribed by your parent's doctor.

*See also*: Arthritis and Musculo-skeletal Problems, Cardiovascular Disease, Osteoporosis, Diabetes, Dementia. Plus Recommended Reading List and Standard References.

# ALCOHOLISM

There has been much debate recently about how much alcohol is actually good for us. New research into alcoholism shows that women get drunk faster than men and do more harm to their bodies than men whilst doing so. Women alcoholics are more susceptible than men to liver disease, brain damage and cognitive defects like memory loss and reduced problem-solving ability. A comparison study undertaken recently at Tübingen University in southern Germany found that women with almost six years of alcohol dependency have the same degree of cognitive impairment as men with ten years of dependency.

According to the Australian National Health Survey of 1989–90 three-quarters of all males and one-half of all women drank alcohol during the week of the survey; 5 per cent of women chose wine. High and even moderately raised levels of alcohol consumption are associated with a large number of diverse medical conditions. For this reason there has been careful assessment of what the upper safe levels of consumption are.

There is increasing evidence that women have fewer of the enzymes in the liver and gut wall that break down alcohol before it enters the bloodstream, which means that a woman weighing 60 kg will get drunk more quickly than a man of the same weight. It should be remembered, however, that there is considerable variation in the tolerance to alcohol. This is genetically determined, but may be influenced by intakes of vitamin C and possibly other nutrients. How the alcohol is consumed also determines the degree to which intoxication takes place.

During this century women, like men, have become alcohol consumers. Often alcohol is used as a comfort to soothe away the stress of a hard day. Whilst this may be acceptable in moderation, the temptation to blot out our stresses with alcohol is sometimes great. Alcohol is also used as a social lubricant, perhaps giving confidence to those that otherwise lack it. Nowadays, a higher percentage of women drink excessive amounts of alcohol, which will undoubtedly play a role in the declining quality of their health.

Excessive consumption of alcohol is associated with the following diseases.

- Liver damage and eventually liver failure, especially with very high doses.
- Alcoholic brain damage which is irreversible and causes loss of memory. It can also damage the nerves in the hands and feet, but this is partially reversible.
- Elevated blood pressure which is reversible.
- Increased risk of heart disease at high intake.
- Heart failure and increased risk of serious heart rhythm disturbance.
- Increased risk of stroke especially in combination with obesity and high blood pressure.
- Increased risk of accidents including road traffic accidents, accidents at work and accidents in the home.
- Increased risk of cancer, especially cancer of the oesophagus and stomach.
- Risk of damage to the pancreas.
- Damage to the unborn baby in pregnant women—foetal alcohol syndrome.
- Increased risk of osteoporosis—not necessarily seen with modest to moderate consumption.
- Increased risk of many psychiatric problems, especially depression.
- Increased risk of cataracts.
- Elevation in certain blood fats.
- Aggravation of peptic ulcers, and indigestion.
- Occasionally a cause of blindness, damage at the back of the eye—in association with tobacco.
- Strongly associated with gout.
- Strongly associated with facial flushing and Acne Rosacea.
- Worsening of hot flushes in menopausal women.
- May worsen epilepsy.
- Associated with falls in the elderly.
- Disturbed sleep—insomnia and sleep apnoea.

## What's Good about Alcohol?

Consumption of alcohol may protect against a number of diseases. Part of this may be because many modest drinkers are also healthy eaters. This is often the case with the middle classes in Western countries. So far the evidence supporting the protective effect of modest alcohol consumption includes:

◆ Minimising cardiovascular disease.

◆ Helping minimise the number of colds, but only in non-smokers.

◆ Helping a condition called Benign Familial Tremor—a mild tremor of the hands which affects middle-aged and elderly adults.

◆ Helping poor circulation to the legs—peripheral vascular disease.

◆ Stimulating the appetite.

◆ Relaxing the muscles.

## What Is a Safe Amount to Consume?

Many authorities now recommend that the safe upper limit for women is two units a day and men four units a day. One unit is equivalent to 300 ml (½ pint) of beer, one-sixth of a bottle of wine, one pub measure of spirits. Most home measures of spirits are two units. Wine seems to have particular properties in helping prevent cardiovascular disease, but recent evidence suggests that the benefits are not confined to this beverage alone.

## Alcohol and Nutrition

Moderate drinkers who are consuming either an average or sub-standard diet, often have modest reductions in a number of essential nutrients, including many of the B vitamins, zinc and magnesium. This has a subtle impact upon their health and is likely to influence energy level, nervous system function and possibly hormone function. Consequently the adverse affects of alcohol are going to be influenced by the person's diet. The Very Nutritious Diet may help minimise some of the potentially damaging effects.

It is our recommendation that anyone consuming more than the recommended amount should take multi-vitamins, especially those which provide the vitamin B complex. Serious deficiency of vitamin B1 results in permanent brain damage. This has reached such proportions in young people in Australia, the former USSR and Poland that there has been serious discussion of fortifying alcoholic beverages with vitamin B. This has yet to take place, and the Australian brewery industry turned the option down.

That said, by all means enjoy the odd glass of wine, beer or spirit, whatever your tipple is, but enjoy it as *part* of a healthy diet and lifestyle.

*See also*: Heart Disease, Preconception, Pregnancy, Cancer, Osteoporosis, Menopause, Depression, Insomnia. Plus Recommended Reading List and References.

# ALLERGY AND INTOLERANCE

The word 'allergy' simply means altered reaction, and it is used commonly by doctors and the public, but often with rather different meanings. The term 'intolerance' is also used, to describe an adverse reaction of a similar sort but with a rather different basis.

## *Allergy*
The term is now properly confined to adverse reactions involving the immune system. This means that there are changes in the white cells or the antibodies produced by them. These reactions may be to:

- something that is breathed in, 'an inhalant' such as a pollen
- a food, and this can be almost any food
- a food additive, as in the case of colourings
- a drug given by mouth, injection or as a skin preparation
- an insect, as with housedust mite allergy or wasp sting allergy
- an animal or their secretions, e.g. cat saliva and rodent urine
- chemicals in cosmetics
- dusts, e.g. wood or metals
- metals, like jewellery, particularly earrings

The reaction may be immediate as in the case of hayfever, or delayed as is often the case with allergies to foods.

# Intolerance

The term used to describe all other reactions that do not involve immune mechanisms. They are more common than allergies and can vary substantially in type. They mainly involve foods but can also occur with inhaled chemicals such as sulphites in asthma. The mechanism of intolerance is fascinating and outside the scope of this book.

The main types are:

◆ simple irritants as with asthma and sulphites, e.g. in wine
◆ toxic effects
◆ effects of chemicals found in some foods, e.g. intolerance of amines in migraine
◆ metabolic effects of food as in reactive hypoglycaemia
◆ enzyme deficiencies involved in digestion as in intolerance of milk sugar, lactose, causing diarrhoea
◆ other enzyme deficiencies especially in the liver, as in the intolerance of fruit sugar
◆ metabolic effects of food that is spoiled or fermented
◆ the effects of food on bowel bacteria and flora

All of these are discussed in much more detail in the relevant parts of the book.

## What Causes Them?

Nowadays it would seem that the majority of doctors are prepared to accept that allergies and even intolerances do happen from time to time. What is still not certain, nor indeed widely agreed, is the type of health problems that can be caused and how frequently adverse reactions of one kind or another occur.

## Conditions Caused by Inhalant Allergy

◆ asthma
◆ rhinitis (seasonal, such as hayfever)
◆ rhinitis (non-seasonal)
◆ conjunctivitis—eye irritation

## *Conditions Caused by Food Allergy*

- asthma
- immediate reactions causing mouth, lip or facial swelling (angioedema)
- coeliac disease
- cows' milk protein allergy in children
- colitis in infants and occasionally adults
- Crohn's disease occasionally
- rheumatoid arthritis
- conjunctivitis

## *Conditions Caused by Food Intolerance*

- irritable bowel syndrome
- migraine headaches
- asthma
- rhinitis
- urticaria
- some types of food poisoning
- intolerance of certain carbohydrates, e.g. milk sugar/lactose, ordinary table sugar, fruit sugar
- hyperactive behaviour in children
- possibly mood disturbance in adults

All of these conditions, except coeliac disease, have a variety of other causes and this needs to be considered carefully by the doctor. Each topic is dealt with individually throughout the book. The Simple Exclusion Diet and The Strict Exclusion Diet will be useful.

*See also*: Asthma, Hayfever, Coeliac Disease, Rheumatoid Arthritis, Irritable Bowel Syndrome, Migraine, Crohn's Disease. Plus Recommended Reading List and References.

# ANAEMIA

Anaemia simply means a lack of blood, and there are many causes of this. Iron deficiency, the most usual underlying reason, is one of the commonest medical conditions worldwide, and despite the prosperity of Western society, it is still a problem often experienced by women of child-bearing age. Additionally, there is a large variety of other blood conditions, some nutritional, some moderately common and many rare, that can also cause anaemia.

Because of its importance, all hospital laboratories routinely measure the level of haemoglobin, the blood pigment which carries oxygen around the body.

There have been many attempts to determine exactly what the normal haemoglobin level is in women, men and children. Definitions vary slightly and in practice the normal range for women is between 11.5 and 16.0 grams per decilitre (⅒ litre). Haemoglobin is carried around inside red cells, which in turn are produced from large 'cell factories' in the bone marrow, concentrated at the ends of the long bones, in the ribs and pelvis. The cells that produce red blood cells are also related to those producing our white cells which are involved in resistance to infection, production of antibodies and minute cells called platelets which help in the prevention of bleeding. Occasionally certain blood disorders influence all three types of cell.

Red cells that carry the haemoglobin are actually dying cells. Unlike all other cells of the body they do not contain a nucleus 'brain'; they do not have the ability to renew themselves, and thus have a limited life span of 120 days usually. During this time they carry oxygen from the lungs through the heart and off to the peripheral tissues such as the brain, muscles and skin where, after depositing the oxygen, they collect carbon dioxide, which is also bound to the haemoglobin. On the return journey through the lung they release the haemoglobin and pick up yet more oxygen. Such is the happy lot of the red cell.

The production of haemoglobin requires a number of factors. Iron is essential as this mineral is found in the structure of haemoglobin itself. Vitamin B12 and folic acid are needed for the production of chemicals required for the making of the red cell envelope. Adequate protein intake, potassium, vitamin A and other

B vitamins are also required. Only rarely are deficiencies of these the cause of anaemia.

## What Are the Symptoms?

As anaemia is a condition which comes on gradually, there is time for the body to adapt to it, and a sudden fall in blood pressure or symptoms of shock are rarely seen. The first signs may be:

◆ mild fatigue and slight paleness
◆ shortness of breath on effort
◆ palpitation and worsening of any pre-existing disease of the heart or lungs
◆ light-headedness, giddiness and buzzing in the ears
◆ poor appetite and nausea

Very often these are features of nutritional deficiency, especially of iron, as this is the commonest cause of anaemia. This in turn will result in its own symptoms including:

◆ a sore tongue
◆ recurrent mouth ulcers
◆ cracking at the corner of the mouth
◆ flattening and upturning of the thumb and fingernails
◆ split and brittle nails
◆ poor hair growth
◆ a blue tinge to the white of the eyes

It is also possible that mild iron deficiency with a low or normal haemoglobin can also cause fatigue, but not all doctors are agreed on this.

## What Causes It?

The main causes of anaemia are as follows.

◆ Lack of essential nutrients, especially iron, folic acid and vitamin B12.
◆ Increased blood loss from heavy periods or bleeding from the bowel. The causes of heavy periods include fibroids, hormonal disturbance and other gynaecological problems. The causes of loss of blood from the bowel include cancer of the colon or

stomach, peptic ulcer (especially if aspirin or anti-arthritic drugs are also taken), and bleeding from a hiatus hernia.

◆ Poor absorption of essential nutrients can affect the levels of iron, B12 and folate, either in tandem or with just one of these nutrients being deficient. Disease of the stomach, coeliac disease, pancreatic and small bowel disorders are all possiblities.

◆ Chronic diseases such as liver and kidney problems, severe arthritis, and chronic infection.

◆ Genetic disorders affecting the production of haemoglobin. This is very common in Africa, the Far East and communities where people of these origins have migrated. Conditions such as thalassaemia and sickle cell disease can, in their mild forms, produce a mild anaemia which may cause relatively little ill health, but in severe forms cause major anaemia in childhood.

Fortunately, even from the result of a simple blood test for anaemia the doctor can very rapidly have a good idea of the likely cause. This is because many tests on red cells, measures of white cells, platelets and a test called the ESR (erithrocyte sedimentation rate) that gives a general measure of inflammatory processes throughout the body are also measured.

## What Your Doctor Can Do

Your doctor can do a variety of tests. The first is a full blood count which measures the haemoglobin and looks at the shape and size of red cells. If the haemoglobin is low, then further tests are required. One of these is a measure of serum ferritin or other test of iron adequacy (transferrin saturation), as a low serum ferritin will usually confirm iron deficiency. This is a simple test and is widely available. It is prudent to perform this in most women of child-bearing age presenting with anaemia.

Often tests measure serum vitamin B12 and red cell folate. These widely available tests will need to be performed if a certain pattern of anaemia is present on full blood count. Lack of folic acid is likely to occur during pregnancy, as a result of certain blood disorders, as a result of malabsorption, or if the diet is very poor. Lack of vitamin B12 may occur after several years in strict vegans whose diet is deficient in this vitamin, in some types of malab-sorption or if the stomach is unable to produce the necessary agents that are required to absorb this vitamin from the diet. This lymphatic condition is termed pernicious anaemia.

The doctor may also investigate the cause of the anaemia by assessing the diet, possible blood loss from the gut (stool tests to detect minute quantities of blood may need to be performed), assessment of symptoms that may suggest malabsorption, e.g. diarrhoea and weight loss, and assessment of menstrual flow. Women are notoriously bad at assessing how heavy their periods are. The presence of flooding severe enough to stain underwear, having to go to bed because of flooding, needing to wear a tampon plus towels are all rough but useful pointers to the menstrual flow being excessive.

In older patients, especially women after the menopause (and in most men), some attempt should be made to assess the possibility of gastrointestinal blood loss. This is particularly important for unexpected iron-deficiency anaemia, and may lead to early detection of colon or gastric cancer. Barium meal, barium X-ray and telescopic investigation of the bowel by a gastroenterologist may all be required.

### Initiate treatment

Treatment will often be in the form of iron supplements, as ferrous sulphate taken by mouth. Occasionally iron will need to be given by injection but this should be extremely rare. Vitamin B12 will need to be given by injection if the deficiency is due to malabsorption, or in tablet form in the case of a vegan with poor oral intake. Supplements of folic acid can be prescribed separately, and doses several times the normal daily intake are recommended if there is any degree of malabsorption. Smaller supplements may need to be given in a variety of blood disorders where there is increased production (and destruction) of red blood cells.

### Treat any underlying disorder

This may require a referral to a bowel specialist, dietician or gynaecologist.

### Monitor treatment

If the assessment was correct there should be a rise in haemoglobin level often within two weeks of treatment. Other changes on a blood test should indicate that new red cells are being formed. Blood counts should continue to be monitored until the haemoglobin is normal and it may be prudent for a further check three months later to make sure there has been no subsequent fall.

Despite our knowledge of anaemia, and the ability to investigate patients thoroughly, sometimes the cause is not found. In one recent appraisal of patients with severe iron deficiency anaemia no cause was found in some 36 per cent of them.

## What You Can Do

◆ Go and see your doctor if you have any of the symptoms that are potentially attributable to anaemia, and any features that suggest you may be particularly at risk, such as heavy periods or poor diet. A past history of anaemia is an important risk factor too.

◆ Keep a diet diary for a week and take this along to your appointment. Do this as well if your doctor diagnoses anaemia in you. It will help aid analysis of your dietary intake of iron, vitamin B12 and folic acid.

◆ If you have heavy periods, keep a record of the number of tampons and towels that you use, and the number of days you bleed in the menstrual cycle. Again this will help your doctor make a decision.

◆ If you are taking supplements of iron, never take them with tea, coffee, red grape juice or blackcurrant juice. These all contain tannin which will inhibit the absorption of iron. You normally absorb 10–15 per cent of the amount of iron in your diet, and the same is true of iron supplements, although this rises if you are iron deficient. Taking an iron supplement with tea reduces absorption to a third of these values. Taking it with a supplement of vitamin C (100 mg or more) can double the amount of iron absorbed. A good way of taking your iron pill is with a glass of fruit juice or a piece of fruit.

◆ If your iron supplement is causing indigestion, constipation or diarrhoea, a change in the type, reducing the dose, and taking it with food, may all help minimise side-effects. In our experience side-effects are rare if patients take care in this way.

◆ For most people a simple iron supplement of ferrous sulphate, 200 mg one or two daily, will suffice. A variety of more specialised (and more expensive) iron supplements are available on prescription or through the health-food shop. The over-the-counter preparations are usually much weaker, and larger doses may need to be taken in order to correct severe iron deficiency.

◆ If you are deficient in vitamin B12 and need supplements, do not take supplements of folic acid until the vitamin B12 deficiency is corrected. If in doubt about this speak with your doctor. Large supplements of folic acid in a person with untreated vitamin B12 deficiency may lead to increased vitamin B12 problems, causing nerve damage.

◆ Whatever the cause of your anaemia try and eat The Very Nutritious Diet or, if vegetarian/vegan, see The Vegetarian or Vegan Diet for your appropriate option. As a general guide, foods that are rich in protein, either of animal or vegetable source, tend to be good sources of iron. Animal sources of iron are better absorbed, and may also enhance the absorption from vegetarian foods. So even allowing small amounts of animal products into a vegetarian diet increases the balance of this mineral.

◆ Take your iron and other supplements as recommended. You may well need to take the iron supplements for three months after the haemoglobin has risen to normal in order to build up iron stores and to ensure that energy levels rise to their optimum range.

## Complementary Therapies
There should really be no need of these in patients with anaemia.

## Belinda's Story
Belinda was a thirty-eight-year-old woman who, on many occasions over the last few years, had been found to be mildly anaemic, though this never fully resolved despite taking iron tablets. Her periods were not particularly heavy. She did complain of mild fatigue, as well as poor hair growth, abdominal bloating, constipation and some premenstrual symptoms. In the past she had had breast cysts which were still sometimes a problem, and a few years earlier had had several uterine fibroids removed because of severe anaemia.

At the time she was first seen, she was still mildly anaemic, haemoglobin 10.7 g (the normal range is 11.5 to 16.5). Other tests revealed that she was indeed iron deficient and there was a very low level for serum zinc. Her weight was steady at 48 kg. It wasn't clear quite why she had these problems. We prescribed some iron supplements taken with vitamin C or fruit juice, supplements of zinc and multi-vitamins. This sort of supplement regime could certainly help her fatigue and poor hair growth. There was little clinical improvement in the first two months; she was therefore asked to follow a gluten-free diet. This meant avoiding all wheat, oats, barley and rye which she did most carefully. There was a gradual and gratifying improvement. Abdominal symptoms disappeared, her fatigue lessened, her hair growth improved and, best of all, her haemoglobin rose significantly well into the normal range at 12.5 g. Serum zinc level became normal too.

She felt better than she had for years. I wondered whether she may have been developing coeliac disease, but further tests for this fortunately proved to be negative. She had experienced abdominal symptoms and these increased every time she had tried to introduce wheat into her diet. Hopefully in time she will grow out of her gluten sensitivity.

*See also*: Essential Nutrients, Liver Disease, Coeliac Disease, Pancreatic Disease, Bowel Disorders. Plus Recommended Reading List and References.

# ANXIETY

Anxiety in its mild form is a natural state associated with stressful situations, and is suffered by everyone at some time. The things people get anxious about include exams, interviews, relationships, finances, acts of violence and rabid dogs. Some degree of anxiety, which subsides after the event, would be considered to be appropriate, given the circumstances. However, when the anxiety escalates and in some cases brings on panic attacks and palpitations (rapid or irregular heartbeats), medical intervention is necessary.

When severe anxiety is present the whole body feels 'wired up'. The person finds it difficult to relax or concentrate, over-reacts, feels tense, nervous and agitated. Sleep is likely to be disturbed, with periods of insomnia, and early-morning waking. The person may also experience a dry mouth, muscle tremors and diarrhoea, all of which are very distressing.

## What Are the Symptoms?

| | |
|---|---|
| Heart | Palpitations and awareness of missed heartbeats<br>Discomfort in the chest |
| Chest | Overbreathing<br>Pain in the chest |
| Muscular | Aches and pains |
| Nervous system | Shakes<br>Headaches<br>Dizziness<br>Tinnitus (ringing in the ears)<br>Prickling sensations<br>Poor concentration and memory |
| Digestive | Dry mouth<br>Difficulty in swallowing<br>Indigestion<br>Excessive wind<br>Diarrhoea |
| Bladder | Frequent need to pass water |
| Uterus | Amenorrhoea—lack of periods<br>Period pains |

There are three main types of anxiety which are quite distinctive:

◆ General anxiety, which is continuous.
◆ Phobic anxiety, which occurs from time to time when in certain situations or places.
◆ Panic attacks, which occur from time to time but are not related to a situation or place necessarily; the response is often out of proportion to the situation.

There is also an anxiety which is experienced by some women premenstrually.

# General Anxiety

The causes of general anxiety are not fully understood, but it is thought that it could be attributable to a combination of any of the following:

◆ genetic disorders
◆ insecure relationships in childhood
◆ stressful events in life
◆ nutritional deficiencies
◆ possibly food allergies

## What Your Doctor Can Do

Carry out physical investigations to eliminate the possibility that the anxiety is related to a physical disease or problem. Thyroid problems, hypoglycaemia (low blood sugar), and tumours of the adrenal glands can all be accompanied by symptoms of anxiety, as can psychiatric disorders like depression, dementia or schizophrenia.

Once pure anxiety has been diagnosed the treatment your doctor has to offer is mainly psychological:

◆ Setting your mind at rest is the first step, so that there is a clear understanding that the symptoms are not related to any major illness.
◆ Stress management advice to help you to come to terms with the trigger of your anxiety.
◆ If you are hyperventilating (over-breathing), you should be given instructions about how to breathe, by re-breathing expired air from a paper bag to restore the normal concentrations of carbon dioxide.
◆ You may be offered drug treatment like Valium, which produces rapid relief of anxiety, but should not be prescribed for more than three or four weeks.
◆ Alternatively antidepressants are used to control anxiety, but this is a longer-term treatment and should be considered as a last resort.

# Premenstrual Anxiety

The main symptoms of premenstrual anxiety are nervous tension, irritability and mood swings, beginning as early as two weeks before the period and becoming progressively worse as the period approaches.

There are several possible factors, both hormonal and dietary, that might cause it.

◆ Some doctors think that an excess of the hormone oestrogen or an increased sensitivity to it may trigger changes in brain chemistry, resulting in anxiety. The average diet, high in fat and relatively low in fibre, can increase the levels of this hormone.

◆ Also, high levels of oestrogen slow down the rate at which the stimulant caffeine is broken down by the liver. This is why some women become more sensitive to tea and coffee when they are pregnant or when taking the oral contraceptive pill.

◆ A lack of vitamin B and possibly the mineral magnesium can also cause changes in the chemistry of the nervous system that can aggravate feelings of anxiety and irritability. Interestingly, it seems that some women (and men) who are prone to anxiety and panic attacks are more sensitive to caffeine and genuinely have a more sensitive body metabolism which makes them very susceptible to the effects of a lack of vitamin B or magnesium.

◆ A comparison of caffeine consumption in Chinese nurses and workers in a tea factory revealed a strong association between increased caffeine consumption and the severity of premenstrual symptoms. We conducted our own survey in the United Kingdom with *Fitness* magazine, which was published in 1992. 377 women took part. Caffeine consumption was nearly two and a half times higher in PMS sufferers compared with non-sufferers.

◆ A final and important factor is hyperventilation. This mouthful simply means over-breathing. Often when one becomes anxious it is natural to increase the rate and depth of respiration. This provides more oxygen to the bloodstream but also removes more of the waste gas carbon dioxide. This lack of carbon dioxide causes a change in the body chemistry which can actually aggravate or cause a variety of symptoms, including numbness and tingling in the fingers, hands and around the mouth, muscle cramps, headaches, light-headedness, increased anxiety, physical and mental fatigue, and confusion. The solution is to relax, reduce the rate and depth of breathing, and if symptoms are severe, to breathe in and out of a paper bag for several minutes. When these symptoms chronically occur, formal advice and breathing exercises may need to be given by a physiotherapist or psychologist.

........................................................................................................................

## Celia's Story

Celia, a thirty-one-year-old mother of two young children, had been suffering for years with mood swings that left her feeling frightened and depressed.

*I'd be chugging along fairly normally then, suddenly, I would burst into tears over nothing at all. My mood seemed to change from one hour to the next, and the frightening thing was that I had no warning it was about to happen—it was as if I just snapped. I went from feeling perfectly normal to thoroughly depressed, and my patience threshold was non-existent. The slightest little thing would spark me off and I'd feel like lashing out. I'd been suffering like this, three weeks out of four, for six years, since the birth of our first son, until I reached crisis point one morning whilst hanging out the washing. All I did was drop a sock on the floor, but I burst into tears, it felt like the end of the world and I was sure I was going mad.*

*In desperation I opened up to my husband, who was always supportive. We decided that perhaps I needed to get a part-time job, as I'd hadn't been out of the house whilst the boys were small. Now they were at school it seemed like a good idea, but I didn't manage to get a job and nothing changed.*

*I went to visit my doctor and explained about my wild moods and tearfulness. He was very sympathetic, but said he only had antidepressants to offer me. I hate taking pills, but I was so desperate, I promised to try them for three months. I didn't feel I had any choice; I had reached the point where when I woke up each morning I knew I couldn't face the day.*

*The antidepressants drained me and left me feeling completely zombified. My quality of life was non-existent and I didn't even feel that I was fit to drive the children around. I tried to stop taking them, but my symptoms returned with a vengeance.*

*Finally, I thought that my only hope would be to see a psychiatrist. He asked me all about my sex life, and my marriage. And, as I talked to him, it dawned on me that he wasn't going to be able to help me at all. The only thing wrong with my sex life and my marriage was that I was feeling so ill. Sex hadn't been that great whilst my moods had been so up and down, but I knew it was not the cause of my bad moods. And so I renewed the prescription for the antidepressants, and* carried on taking them, feeling like a washed-out zombie for the following year. If it hadn't been for my husband and the boys I really think I'd have been suicidal. I can't believe that my husband didn't pack his bags and leave, I must have been so awful to live with.

My husband tried to cheer me up and found a dream house for us to move to, hoping it would pull me out of my problems. I thought long and hard about it, and told him I was going to throw the pills away, and somehow help myself. I booked some counselling sessions which helped a bit. But what really changed my life was an article I read in Family Circle magazine about a woman describing her mood swings. I read the article over and over again. I just couldn't believe it. She was describing precisely what I had been going through, and had cured her problem, not with pills, but by changing her diet!

I wrote to the organisation mentioned in the article, the WNAS, and I bought their book. They sent me a questionnaire asking me about my diet, lifestyle and moods. I was then provided with a special programme which involved changing my diet completely. I felt so awful the first week, which they said I would, I actually wondered if it was worth continuing. One morning at the end of that first week, I woke up feeling terrible. I made breakfast and crawled back into bed. I stayed there all day, and when I woke up the next morning I felt fantastic. I hadn't felt that good for ages. I couldn't believe it. It was as if a dark cloud had been lifted from me.

The longer I was on the programme the better I felt. It has been five years now, and I feel wonderful. I'm lively, energetic and those horrendous and unpredictable mood swings have gone completely.

# Phobias

The difference between phobic disorders and general anxiety is that the symptoms are intermittent and relate to specific situations. Phobias like agoraphobia (fear of open spaces) and claustrophobia (fear of closed spaces), can limit the ability of the sufferer to work or socialise easily. Possible phobias are many and varied. Some people are afraid of heights or needles, others are too nervous to socialise or attend a social gathering, and others are afraid to leave home or get into an elevator.

The most common phobias we see at the WNAS are agoraphobia and claustrophobia to a lesser degree. Sufferers feel terrified and threatened at the prospect of going out of the house in the case of the agoraphobic, or being in a confined space in the case of the claustrophobic. The fear is usually characterised by a panic attack with palpitations, with dry mouth, muscle tremors, and in severe cases, fear of a heart attack.

Interestingly, almost 90 per cent of agoraphobic sufferers are women. We had contact some years ago with a marvellous woman running a national group for agoraphobic sufferers. From her research data we discovered that 91 per cent of her sample of ninety-four also suffered premenstrual syndrome.

## What Your Doctor Can Do

Your doctor can refer you for some behaviour therapy. This is the usual treatment, and there is a variety to choose from, including desensitisation and cognitive manipulation.

Essentially there are different methods of getting the sufferer to confront their phobia, either by talking to themselves, or by facing the phobia head on in the company of a therapist, or others who have no such phobia. In addition, he may offer you some of the options listed for general anxiety.

## Harriet's Story

Harriet, forty-two-year-old mother of three, had been taking antidepressants for twenty-four years to ease her agoraphobia and panic attacks.

*I had my first panic attack when I was sixteen following a dental abscess. Looking back, that was the start of my agoraphobia, although I didn't realise it at the time. First of all my doctor put me on iron pills, but when my test came back in the normal range, I was then given tablets for my nerves. I can't remember the name of the first two, but they seemed to make my panic attacks worse. Within a short time I was prescribed Valium, at first 15 mg per day, increasing to 30 mg per day, which I stayed on for twenty-four years. The Valium knocked me out, I was like a zombie. They seemed to ease the panic attacks initially, but gradually I needed more and more pills to keep the symptoms at bay.*

*For the rest of my teenage years my social life was affected. I had a boyfriend for a while, but the symptoms of agoraphobia made me afraid to go out, and he got fed up waiting around for me. I met my husband at a dance when I was nineteen He didn't mind staying in, and we eventually got married when I was twenty-one.*

*I had our first child when I was twenty-three, and the pregnancy was followed by postnatal depression. I had such severe panic attacks after the birth every time*

I went into town, my horizons got smaller until eventually I was housebound and frightened to go through the front door. I couldn't even go out to do the food shopping. When our son was five he developed cancer in his leg, which I obviously found very stressful. He did survive, thank goodness, but the stress of it left me with obsessional neurosis, on top of my agoraphobia. It was a turning point for me. I just sat in a chair all day, didn't bother to cook or clean the house.

I eventually had two more children—but I was so afraid during my pregnancies as I felt the Valium might harm the unborn children. I managed to cut down to 20 mg per day during my pregnancy, but I was too scared to cut down any more as I didn't know how to do without them. I was prescribed a hormone, Duphaston, after the third child, but it did not make any difference.

My husband resorted to working long hours as he couldn't cope with me. Fortunately the children's school was over the road to our house; I could just about manage to get to the pavement, but I couldn't cross the road as I felt so dizzy. The Valium prescriptions just kept coming, I'd be given 100 pills at a time without ever being seen by the doctor.

After twenty-four years, in desperation, as my symptoms had become worse before my period was due, I sent my husband out to find a book on premenstrual syndrome, and he came back with Beat PMS Through Diet. My doctor then offered me beta-blockers and said they weren't habit-forming, but I didn't want to take any more drugs. I decided to make an effort to follow the recommendations in the book and to come off the Valium. I contacted the WNAS and had a telephone consultation.

Coming off Valium was hell. The withdrawal symptoms were like nothing I had ever experienced before. Within six weeks of following the WNAS programme I was feeling human again, and much more like my old self. I even made an appointment to get my hair done. I felt on top of the world. Then I woke up one day feeling really angry and resentful, as I realised I had lost twenty-four years of my life. I can't even remember the children growing up and I feel so sad about that. My doctor was clearly ignorant, which upsets me greatly, as I can never replace those years.

I have been better for three years now. I am still having some counselling to deal with all the traumas in my life, but the end is in sight. I now cope well with my family and my home, and am getting involved with a local medical charity. Today I am catering a party for 100 guests to celebrate my father's ninetieth birthday tomorrow—I couldn't even have dreamt about doing that four years ago!

## Susan's Story

Susan was a twenty-year-old chef. She found it particularly difficult to carry out many of the functions of her job because of her symptoms.

*My health had deteriorated over a period of years. My most frightening symptom was claustrophobia. I was particularly afraid of underground trains, lifts and the walk-in fridges at work which I needed to use on a regular basis as a chef. I also suffered with cravings for sweet food, especially before my period, chocolate-related migraine headaches which meant I felt awful after bingeing, and I also experienced panic attacks and depression.*

*My doctor had prescribed antidepressants over a period of years, the last one being Prozac. He also referred me to a psychiatrist for phobia therapy. I came across the book* Beat PMS Through Diet. *The book suggested the WNAS could help with symptoms similar to mine, so I contacted them. After completing a long questionnaire and diet diary I was told to eat little and often and to cut out all junk food, including chocolate, cakes, biscuits, sweet foods and cola-based drinks. Additionally I cut out caffeine and wheat. I took supplements of Optivite and Normoglycaemia and exercised.*

*Within three months I was off the antidepressants, my phobias had completely gone, and so too had the migraines and the premenstrual cravings for food. Lifts were no longer a problem and I had no trouble going in and out of the fridges at work. I felt so well, better than I ever hoped. I also lost just under 6.25 kg in weight without dieting. I started my treatment four years ago. I must admit I have had a few lapses along the way, particularly when I'm on holiday, but at least I know how to get myself back in to tip-top shape again afterwards.*

# Panic Attacks

These can be very frightening episodes, which come on suddenly, apparently unprovoked by a certain situation, unlike the phobias. The symptoms can be similar to the general anxiety symptoms, but in addition are usually accompanied by palpitations, which often cause additional anxiety about the possibility of heart disease. In the past this disorder was referred to by heart specialists as a heart condition known as 'effort syndrome'.

Prior to the panic attack the brain sends a message to the adrenal glands which causes an adrenaline surge, sometimes known as the 'flight and fight' mechanism. The anxiety that a medical emergency is impending is so severe that it sets up a vicious circle, leading to physical symptoms, which then justify the fear of physical problems, which then leads to more anxiety, which causes the panic attack.

Once again panic attacks are suffered by many women in their premenstrual phase. In a survey the WNAS conducted on 1000 patients it emerged that 91 per cent had previously suffered with anxiety before their periods, and the severe sufferers often had panic attacks leading up to their periods.

## Adrienne's Story

Adrienne was a twenty-two-year-old student nurse, who was very alarmed by the onset of severe anxiety and panic attacks. Her mother brought her to the clinic after seeing a television programme that featured our work.

*My symptoms came on suddenly when I was twenty-one. We had moved house and so I was feeling a bit isolated from my friends, plus I had begun a nursing course during that year which meant living away from home. My Grandad died that year too, which I found upsetting as we are a close family.*

*At times my symptoms were uncontrollable. I became very depressed, withdrawn and anxious. I just felt like hiding in my room. I was verbally aggressive towards my family and refused to eat when I was depressed. My head used to pound so much it felt like it was going to explode. I was very afraid, and dreaded my symptoms which were considerably worse for two weeks before each period.*

*At first my doctor suggested vitamin B6, which didn't help. Then I was put on the Pill, which made me feel bloated and weird in the head. I was also given Duphaston and antidepressants, and eventually Estraderm patches which made my symptoms worse, and I now discover are for menopausal symptoms.*

*I had to give up nursing as I couldn't concentrate or absorb anything. I returned to my family home where I either sat on the sofa all day, on a good day, or hid away in my room. My family were clearly distraught by the situation, but at a loss to know what to do for me. One day whilst sitting on the sofa I happened to see a WNAS patient on a TV chat show. When she described her former symptoms it sounded just like she was describing me!*

*My mum went straight out and got me the book they mentioned, which I read from cover to cover without stopping. I got started on a self-help programme immediately, and made an appointment to attend the WNAS clinic. I stopped all the hormones and antidepressants and was given a diet, exercise and supplement programme to follow, which was very different from my previous way of eating.*

Mum helped with the shopping and the cooking which made it a lot easier for me.

Within a month my depression and anxiety had vanished which was such a surprise. Unfortunately, as I thought I was better I didn't follow the programme strictly for the next month and ended up feeling almost as bad as ever. I realised I had to follow it to the letter and got my act together again. Within two months all the symptoms had disappeared again. I decided not to return to nursing for the time being, but instead got a job with an insurance company, working with lots of other young people in the area.

That was a year ago, and I haven't had a bad day since. I keep to my diet, still take some supplements, regularly exercise, practise relaxation, and every fortnight I have some reflexology. Without my symptoms I felt more like socialising, so I have developed a circle of friends. I feel like a completely different person, with a future, and am so grateful I found the WNAS.

## What Your Doctor Can Do

◆ Offer the options discussed for general anxiety.

◆ Prescribe high doses of benzodiazepines, like Valium. Prolonged treatment is unwise, though, as it leads to dependency, as you will see from Adrienne's experience.

◆ Give Tricyclic antidepressants which control symptoms in the longer term, but it may be given in high doses and then has many side-effects. The problem with this treatment is the relapse rate has been found to be high when the medication ceases.

◆ Refer you to a psychologist or psychiatrist for some cognitive therapy, designed to change the fears and physical symptoms, which predispose you to the panic attack. It involves coming to terms with the irrational basis for your fears over several sessions. Once again the relapse rate is high once therapy has ceased, although lower than for drug therapy.

## What You Can Do

◆ Follow the instructions for The Simple Exclusion Diet. This will keep you busy for at least eight weeks.

◆ Take regular exercise, at least four good sessions per week to the point of breathlessness. If you can't manage to get out of the house use a skipping rope and an exercise video to build up your stamina.

◆ Try to practise relaxation each day, deep breathing, meditation, yoga, or anything you find therapeutic.

- Take a generous dose of multi-vitamins and minerals daily, plus extra B vitamins, and vitamin C.
- Get some help to sort out the stress in your life, either from a friend or a therapist.
- If you suffer with premenstrual syndrome, follow the instructions we give for Premenstrual Syndrome, plus refer to the book *Beat PMS Through Diet*.
- Take some herbal 'tranquillisers' like Quiet Life, or Blackmores Tranquil Night.

## Complementary Therapies

There is a good chance that you will find additional help from many of the complementary therapies, and again it is a matter of choice. There are numerous homoeopathic remedies to try, depending on which type of anxiety you suffer. A medical herbalist will mix a prescription to suit your symptoms if you feel you need more than the herbs mentioned in the self-help section.

Acupuncture is particularly good at slowing down the energy flows in your body, and is undoubtedly worth a try (provided you don't have a phobia about needles!). Other therapies would be cranial osteopathy, to ease the tension within your body, and any sort of gentle massage, preferably with relaxing aromatherapy oils. Yoga, meditation and any of the techniques discussed for stress relief would be useful tools too.

# ARTHRITIS AND MUSCULO-SKELETAL PROBLEMS

There are many different types of arthritis and conditions affecting muscles, ligaments and bones. We do not intend to cover them all but will deal with the common ones and those where nutritional factors seem to play an important part. Historically many arthritic conditions were treated by dietary change from the early part of this century onward. This was true for both conventional medical practitioners and naturopaths. The last fifty years has seen the development of many drugs—anti-inflammatory agents, steroids, immune-altering drugs and others. These are effective but often only partially so, and frequently cause side-effects. Non-toxic effective treatments such as dietary change and nutritional supplements are not only popular but can be highly effective. The last ten years has seen the publication of many studies re-investigating the worth of the older dietary and nutritional treatments which have proved to be surprisingly (to the conventional doctors only) effective.

There are also many rare types of arthritis that are associated with a variety of other illnesses, which include psoriasis, colitis and Crohn's disease, some types of gastroenteritis and other infections. Treatment, both medical and nutritional, is very much as for rheumatoid arthritis. Exclusion diets are an unknown quantity in such patients.

## Rheumatoid Arthritis

This is a common type of chronic arthritis where there is much swelling and pain in both small and large joints. The hands, especially the large knuckle joints, are most commonly affected and this usually involves both sides in a symmetrical pattern. Stiffness of these or other joints, which is worse in the morning, is a typical feature. Sometimes one or more larger joints are involved, such as an elbow, wrist, knee or ankle joint.

The joint swelling, which is often warm to the touch, is due to considerable inflammation of the synovium. This is a thin layer of tissue that surrounds many joints and is responsible for the production of the lubricating synovial fluid. Thus in rheumatoid arthritis much of the swelling is due to an increase in this fluid. Sometimes other parts of the body such as the lungs, eyes and skin are involved in this. The inflammatory process involves a mixture of white cells and proteins called immunoglobulins. These are antibodies which, instead of being directed at infecting organisms, are actually directed at each other. A sort of immune mutiny. The 'fight', as it were, takes place mainly in the joints and involves many other inflammatory chemicals: the equivalent of the body's police. The real question is what triggered this fracas in the first place, and why it becomes so chronic. Tests for rheumatoid arthritis check for the presence of these 'self-directed' immune proteins.

Possible triggers are infections, food allergies and genetic factors.

## *Who Gets It?*

About 1 per cent of the population worldwide suffer from this arthritis, with women being three times more likely than men to suffer. The commonest age of onset is in the forties, with it being more likely to start in the winter months. The onset is often gradual, with stiffness present for several months before the arthritis is obvious. Sometimes there is a sudden and severe onset.

There can be a strong family element, especially for the more aggressive forms of this arthritis. Some groups are especially vulnerable, e.g. some American Indians probably because of genetic factors. As a rule the cause remains an enigma.

## *What Your Doctor Can Do*

Investigations to determine the type of arthritis, the presence of any associated anaemia or other problems are all important and are easily assessed by the use of blood tests and X-rays. Treatment is usually considered on a step-wise basis, with simple treatments being used first and the more powerful drugs being reserved for aggressive disease. Often the side-effects of these drugs limit their long-term use.

♦ Painkillers such as paracetamol and codeine are used for mild disease.

♦ Anti-inflammatory drugs called NSAIDs (non-steroidal anti-inflammatory drugs). There are many types, including simple aspirin, all of which are of similar efficacy. Delayed release preparations and suppositories are useful. The most serious side-effect is bleeding from the stomach which is much more likely in older patients. This type of medication does not stop the progress of the disease, however, and it is worth noticing that aspirin may increase the need for vitamin C.

♦ Gold, D-penicillamine, hydroxychloroquine and sulphasalazine are all termed second-line drugs used when NSAIDs are not effective enough and if many joints are involved. D-penicillamine may cause deficiencies of zinc and vitamin B6.

♦ Steroids are very effective but high doses produce many unwanted effects, especially osteoporosis or bone thinning. Low doses, 10 mg or less per day of prednisolone, are effective and much less risky. Eating The Very Nutritious Diet that is low in salt and high in calcium, possibly with supplements, may reduce the side-effects of long-term steroid use.

◆ Other drugs include immune-altering and anti-cancer drugs. These are real heavyweights, but if used in small doses and carefully monitored, they have the potential to alter the excessive activity of the immune system that is a part of this disease.

◆ Surgery is sometimes needed to repair or replace damaged joints and tendons.

◆ Antibiotics are perhaps worth a final note as recent scientific research has lent support to the old idea that tetracycline antibiotics are sometimes helpful in this condition. The original theory put forward over thirty years ago was that the arthritis was due to an infection. Further research will hopefully tell us more.

## What You Can Do

A lot, so don't give up. Rheumatoid arthritis is often a long-term condition and usually a conventional or complementary treatment will work. The real difficulty is knowing which is right for a particular individual. There is much merit in combining approaches, especially use of a NSAID with either a low-dose steroid or a second-line drug and dietary manipulation and use of nutritional supplements, especially fish oils.

In approximate order of importance consider the following:

◆ Lose weight if you are obese. Very few dietary treatments will work if you are significantly overweight, and nothing will help your knees and hips as much.

◆ Consider an exclusion diet. Allergy to some foods is now widely accepted as occurring in rheumatoid arthritis. Reactions to milk, cheese, wheat, other grains and artificial colourings are all documented. You could follow The Simple Exclusion Diet yourself for three weeks, or go through The Strict Exclusion Diet with supervision. If there is a good response, then the careful re-introduction of foods at possibly weekly intervals is needed to determine which, if any, contribute to the disease process.

◆ Supplements of fish oils have been shown to be effective in several trials. Large doses need to be taken for three or four months. They should provide 1.3 g of DHA (Docosahexaenoic acid) and 1.3 g of EPA (Eicosapentaenoic acid) per day. This approach is best combined with either The Very Nutritious Diet or The High Essential Fatty Acid Diet.

◆ Supplements of zinc (30 mg per day) or selenium (100–200 µg per day) have shown some benefit in some but not all studies. Again, they are most likely to help if you are deficient in these nutrients and are best combined with a multi-vitamin supplement and a good diet.

◆ A vegan diet can be helpful, possibly because it reduces the intake of saturated fats. One of the reported successful vegan diets also excludes wheat which may explain some of its benefit.

◆ Other supplements might benefit. They include calcium pantothenate, 2 g daily, New Zealand green-lipped mussel extract, and possibly some plant extracts with anti-inflammatory effects, such as pine bark extract, pycnogenol.

Most of these treatments will take several weeks if not two or three months to be effective.

## Juliet's Story

Juliet, a thirty-five-year-old professional woman, had begun to suffer from psoriasis several years earlier. The arthritis had only begun in the last year, but she remembers that her joints had often been stiff as a child. Now she had painful swelling of the small joints in her hands and pain in her feet that had limited her social activities, but had not stopped her from working. She had to take an anti-arthritis drug every night to help get a good night's sleep and to minimise the degree of stiffness in the morning. The psoriasis was relatively mild, and she only used occasional ointments to control it.

She had observed that a number of foods appeared to aggravate the arthritis, including red wine and cheese. She was advised to begin an exclusion diet, taking care that she had a good overall nutrient intake as her weight was low at under 50 kg. There was further improvement with these measures in her joint pains, and careful re-introduction of foods identified several that worsened her symptoms, including beef and dairy products.

She had to avoid these long term and therefore took a calcium supplement, which was vital in view of her low body weight and her impending intention to become pregnant.

She was further helped by taking regular supplements of high strength fish oils. Tests had shown that her blood levels of these anti-inflammatory agents were low. She took them in conjunction with supplements of multi-vitamins and selenium. These needed to be modified later on when she became pregnant. She also took a supplement of folic acid before conceiving.

Her arthritis was very well controlled by her changes in diet together with nutritional supplements. Eventually she had a very successful pregnancy. She continued to take supplements of vitamin B, fish oil and calcium during pregnancy and when breast-feeding to ensure a good balance of these nutrients.

## Osteoarthritis

This is a common type of arthritis where there is loss of the protective surface of cartilage over the ends of bones, with subsequent changes to the underlying bone. This usually involves an increase in the amount of bone leading to swelling and distortion of the joint, most easily seen in the joints at the ends of the fingers and in the knees. As well as these joints, the hips, base of the thumbs and the spine are commonly affected.

Pain and swelling are the most noticeable complaints and in the hands stiffness is usually less of a problem than with rheumatoid arthritis. The arthritis is often mild and limited to the fingers where despite a degree of deformity there may be little disability. When a hip or knee are affected the loss of mobility may be considerable, especially if the sufferer is overweight.

### Who Gets It?

Age is the main risk factor with some 10 per cent of the over-sixties being affected. Osteoarthritis of the fingers is more common in women, and is particularly likely to run in families. Damage to a joint at any time in the past, excessive sporting activity or repetitive occupational use can all increase the risk of this type of arthritis, though this only applies to a minority of cases. Obesity is strongly linked to osteoarthritis of the knee and to a lesser extent of the hip. This type of arthritis is thus often considered as a degenerative disease which slowly evolves over many years rather than one where there is a clear-cut trigger to the inflammatory process.

## What Your Doctor Can Do

There is no cure for osteoarthritis. There are, however, many ways to control or lessen the pain and reduce the degree of disability.

♦ Assessing the disease and disability normally involves a few simple blood tests to exclude other types of arthritis and X-rays to assess the damage to the most problematic joints.

♦ Pain control using NSAIDs (non-steroidal anti-inflammatory drugs) can be highly effective. Their use is often limited by the gastrointestinal irritation and internal bleeding that they may cause. Paracetamol is a less effective alternative.

♦ Physiotherapy, use of a walking stick, adapting shoes, and a splint to support a joint such as the knee are all useful measures.

♦ Surgery is needed for those with advanced disease of the knees and hips where joint replacement can be highly successful. It should be remembered that the success rate is not 100 per cent. Other surgical measures are useful for deformed joints.

♦ Other measures to control pain are important especially when there is widespread joint involvement. Sometimes the pain comes from the muscles around the joints, especially in the spine and lower limb. In spinal arthritis, use of a Trans-Dermal Electrical Nerve Stimulator (TENS) machine may help reduce the pain, in much the same way that acupuncture does.

## What You Can Do

♦ Lose weight if you are overweight and especially if the knees or hips are involved. The improvement from this can literally be (un)staggering.

♦ Exclusion diets are not as a rule helpful in the way they are with rheumatoid arthritis. Occasionally they are worth considering in younger people with recent onset of their disease, and where there is a lot of swelling around the joint. This picture would suggest a high degree of inflammation rather than degeneration. The authors have seen both sensitivity to wheat and dairy products in such patients.

♦ Improve muscle strength and reduce muscle pain. This is an under-emphasised aspect of care, and applies especially to those patients where the hip and spine are affected. The pain of the arthritis leads to inactivity, which results in more muscle weakness leading to increased disability and pain. The solution involves increasing physical activity (despite the pain) and improved nutritional state to help muscle function and strength. The most important nutrients in regard to this latter are magnesium and potassium, lack of which leads to muscle weakness and spasms, and vitamin D, deficiency of which is most likely in those aged over seventy-five and the house-bound. To improve the balance of these nutrients try eating The Very Nutritious Diet, and take supplements of a multi-vitamin and 250 mg of magnesium per day.

◆ Other supplements could be beneficial for some but there are few studies. As in rheumatoid arthritis, correcting a deficiency of zinc or selenium, and providing a supply of fish oils and anti-oxidants such as vitamin E and beta-carotene could have anti-inflammatory effects.

## Noreen's Story

Noreen had had to give up her work as a cleaning lady at the tender age of sixty-four because of increasingly severe pain and swelling in the small joints of her hands. This had begun over the last year and investigations by her own doctor had not shown any gout or rheumatoid arthritis. The picture of change was typical for rheumatoid arthritis for which she had been pre-scribed a NSAID drug. This had helped, but had not controlled her pain and discomfort.

She ate an excellent diet, was a non-smoker and a non-drinker and the only abnormality was that she was a little overweight at 76 kg. I asked her to begin a weight-reducing diet and take cod liver oil supplements whilst she awaited the results of some nutritional investigations. This showed a sur-prisingly low level of zinc, 7.6 mmols per litre (11.5–20). Supplements of zinc and multi-vitamins were added and within three months her zinc level had returned to normal. There was a surprisingly good degree of improvement in her pain, eventually to a point where she was able to stop her anti-arthritis drugs completely. She continued on a small dose of zinc, multi-vitamins and fish oils, as well as keeping her weight below 70 kg.

# *Gout*

Though less common than rheumatoid arthritis and osteoarthritis, gout is still an important cause of joint pain and swelling. It affects both men and women, though usually only relatively older women. It is highly responsive to treatment. Gout is due to an accumulation of crystals of sodium urate or uric acid, which is derived from the breakdown of certain foods and chemicals in the body called purines. The level of uric acid rises in the blood and then precipitates out around various joints, often as a result of relatively minor trauma, and sets up an inflammatory reaction. Typically it is the big toe joint that is first affected and the ankle, wrist, elbow, knee and hands are often involved later on.

## *Who Gets It?*

It is more common in men who may be affected at a relatively young age. Obesity and alcohol consumption playing a large part in its development. In older people, deteriorating kidney function and use of diuretics (water tablets) increase the risk. Accumulation of the toxic mineral lead and certain chronic blood and other diseases are also known predisposing factors.

## *What Your Doctor Can Do*

Firstly treat the acute attack, which can be severe.

- Drugs such as NSAIDs (non-steroidal anti-inflammatory drugs) in large amounts or colchicine, a drug derived from the crocus, are very effective.
- Aspirin, except in high doses, can actually make matters worse!
- In the long term, after the acute attack is over, use of the drug Allopurinol (Zyloric), which prevents the build-up of uric acid, is needed especially when the attacks are recurrent and there is an inadequate response to self-help measures. Occasionally damage to the kidney also occurs and more specialised treatment is needed.

## What You Can Do

◆ Drink plenty of liquid, preferably water, during an acute attack.

◆ Lose weight if you need to. Take care, as crash or starvation diets can raise the level of uric acid.

◆ Cut down on alcohol, especially beer, as this is rich in the purines that are converted into uric acid.

◆ Avoid purine-rich foods: liver, kidneys, sweetbreads, fish roe (including caviar).

◆ Supplements of vitamin C, at a dose of 4 g per day, helps lower blood levels of uric acid and increases its loss in the urine.

◆ Supplements of zinc and magnesium should in theory help, but their effect is probably not great.

◆ For some, further dietary advice and restriction of fructose, fruit sugar, might be needed.

# Ankylosing Spondylitis

This is a type of chronic arthritis that mainly affects the spine and low-back area. The sacro-iliac joints where the spinal column joins the pelvis are frequently affected. The illness may be accompanied by inflammation in other parts of the body, notably the eyes and the bowel.

## Who Gets It?

Mainly men, but a few women do too. It usually first affects patients between the ages of twenty and forty. Symptoms of low-back pain and increasing stiffness may be present for several years before a diagnosis is made.

## What Causes It?

The cause is unknown, but there is a strong association between this type of arthritis and several genetically determined markers that are present on white cells. The chemical nature of these particular markers called HLA-B27 (Human Lymphocyte Antigen-B27) is similar to chemicals produced by a certain bacterium called *Klebsiella* which can be present in the normal human gut.

## What Your Doctor Can Do

There is no cure. Usually treatment centres upon anti-inflammatory drugs, and physiotherapy and exercises to maintain mobility of the spine.

## What You Can Do

This is at present uncertain. There has been a suggestion that dietary changes that would discourage the growth of the *Klebsiella* organism in the gut could be helpful. Such a diet was low in certain carbohydrate-rich foods, but more work is needed before we know if it is effective.

Anti-inflammatory supplements and a diet rich in essential fatty acids would seem to be a reasonable and not too arduous approach. Try multi-vitamins with zinc and selenium. Supplements of fish oils might help as they do for rheumatoid arthritis.

# Fibromyalgia

Fibromyalgia is a relatively new term which replaces the old term fibrositis. It is a common condition characterised by tender painful muscles, most usually those around the shoulders and neck. Tender nodules or lumps can sometimes be felt in the affected muscles. Examination of these nodules reveals muscles whose regular anatomy is distorted with a mild degree of inflammation. Part of the problem appears to be a failure of the muscles to relax properly. This results in increased tension and pain in the muscles.

## Who Gets It?

It most commonly affects young to middle-aged women. It does not follow trauma, nor is it related to excessive use or arthritis.

## What Your Doctor Can Do

- Prescribe simple painkillers; not very effective.
- Prescribe a small dose of an antidepressant called amitryptiline (Lentizol, Tryptizol) a type of tricyclic antidepressant. This has pain-killing properties and is reasonably effective. Worth considering if sleep is disturbed by pain as it can help sleep if taken in the evening.
- Test to exclude other types of muscle inflammation or arthritis.

## What You Can Do

A massage often helps; try using aromatherapy oils as well. Some are very relaxing.

◆ Heat is also helpful, such as hot water bottle, a hot towel or a hot pad which can be easily applied to the painful area, or sunbathing.

◆ Supplements of magnesium can be very useful. We think of muscles as being able to do work by contracting. Every time a muscle contracts it then needs to relax before it can contract again. Muscles are not like pieces of elastic, as the process of relaxation is an active one needing energy and the mineral magnesium. Low levels of this mineral are known to occur in those with fibromyalgia. So you can try supplements of magnesium, about 300 mg per day, in combination with The Very Nutritious Diet, low in salt and reduced in kilojoules if you need to lose weight.

◆ Exercise helps. It may not feel like it initially, but provided your symptoms are not too severe, gentle exercise, especially swimming, can be very helpful. In the long term, those who do exercise regularly suffer less from this painful condition.

◆ Osteopathic or chiropractic treatment can be helpful to correct any displacement in the spine that may be triggering the problem.

These treatments often take several months to work. You can combine the self-help measures with painkillers if necessary.

## Jacqueline's Story

Jacqueline was not old, but within the two years before her fortieth birthday she was diagnosed as having an early menopause needing HRT, and as having a low bone density and a tendency to develop osteoporosis. She had also experienced excessive weight gain with fluid retention, but none of these were bothering her so much as her feeling of fatigue and muscular aches and pains. Eventually an under-active thyroid was diagnosed, and was treated, but the level of fatigue and muscle pain continued unchanged. Indeed her HRT was well managed, her osteoporosis treated and though on paper she should be doing well, still her symptoms of fatigue and muscle pains continued.

Her weight blossomed to 79 kg from previously having been below 70 kg. Some nutritional tests showed that she had a very low red cell magnesium value of 1.82 mmols per litre (2.08–3.00). Her levels for a number of other minerals, including zinc and potassium, were borderline. It appeared she was not just having difficulty hanging on to calcium, which is important for her bones, but the low magnesium almost certainly would be affecting her muscle function and fatigue.

A weight-reducing, low-salt, high-calcium and high-magnesium nutritious diet was followed, together with substantial supplements of calcium, magnesium and multi-vitamins. There was no quick improvement. However, over four months there was a gradual increase in her energy level, and the muscle aches and pains diminished significantly.

She was still predisposed towards fluid retention whenever she consumed any salt. Her need for thyroid hormone and HRT continued, and probably will for many years. Now, however, she experiences the full benefit from them, perhaps because some of these nutrients interact with the action of these hormones. It does however, appear that she will need calcium, magnesium and vitamin supplements long term in order to maintain her health.

# Muscle Cramps

These are simply episodes where a muscle, most often in the leg or hand, contracts and fails to relax. The sustained contraction causes a build-up of lactic acid which results in pain. Unlike fibromyalgia there is no change in the structure of the muscle or associated inflammation.

## What Causes Them?

A lack of sodium, potassium or magnesium can lead to muscle cramps. Those who work in very hot environments and sweat a lot, the elderly, those on diuretics (water tablets) and women during pregnancy may suffer in particular. Those who do not have good amounts of potassium and magnesium in the diet from fresh fruit and vegetables are at risk too.

## What Your Doctor Can Do

◆ Check the blood levels of sodium, potassium and magnesium (a red cell level of this latter is perhaps the most useful).
◆ Occasionally disturbances in calcium level, too low or high, can be a cause.

- Prescribe quinine sulphate which is an old-fashioned but effective remedy.

## What You Can Do

- Eat The Very Nutritious Diet.
- Drink plenty and ensure a good intake of sodium salt if you are in a very hot climate.
- Try supplements of magnesium, 300–400 mg per day, and a multi-vitamin supplement. Magnesium is a very safe supplement to try and has been used successfully to reduce muscle cramps in pregnancy.
- Gentle massage for painful muscle groups.

## Complementary Therapies

Acupuncture is worth considering. Homoeopathy too has some remedies, and a popular one is Cuprum Met., a homoeopathic preparation of the mineral copper.

# ASTHMA

Asthma is a common condition characterised by shortness of breath and wheezing due to narrowing of the airways in the lung. This narrowing is to a large degree reversible, particularly in the early stages of the condition, and can be triggered by a variety of factors including allergies and irritants. Many of these are identical to those factors that cause or trigger rhinitis (see Hayfever and Allergic Rhinitis).

The airways are narrowed because of swelling of the tissues that line them, because of an increase in the production of mucus which may be hard to clear and because the ring of muscle around the medium-sized airway contracts, reducing the internal size of the airway. All this means that it is harder for air to pass in and out of the lung. A key feature is an increased lung sensitivity to many non-specific irritants which in normal individuals do not cause breathing difficulties: cold air, dusts, exercise and even laughter can all trigger wheezing in the asthmatic. There is almost always a noticeable reduction in the ease of breathing in the early morning or during the night in the untreated asthmatic. On top of these, there are three major triggers which often lie behind the more serious episodes: they include infection, allergy and pollution.

## What Are the Symptoms?

Wheezing and a feeling of shortness of breath are the main, but not the only, symptoms of asthma. These are almost always improved by the use of drugs that open up the airways (called bronchodilators). A cough may be the sole complaint in children or mildly affected adults, and is often the reason for a sufferer seeking advice. White sticky phlegm may be produced too, and this may be discoloured if there is infection. Characteristically these symptoms vary. They are almost always worse in the morning and at times during the day when the individual may have been exposed to a triggering factor. The easiest way to observe this is by asking the person to record their 'peak flow measurement' several times each day. This is done using a simple light-weight peak flow meter, and recording three or four measures per day for a week or longer.

## Who Gets It?

More and more people, over the course of the last twenty years, with the latest figures showing a doubling of asthma prevalence, especially in younger sufferers. This increase in prevalence has occurred in Europe, North America and Australasia. Asthma affects about 20 per cent of children, 15 per cent of teenagers and 10 per cent of adults in Australia and NZ. It is not the dangerous illness today that it once was as there are many effective treatments and it is simple to manage for most people. It is the third most common problem managed by general practitioners in Australia. Asthma and bronchial hyper-responsiveness seem to be more likely in:

◆ urban dwellers, in middle-class families
◆ in some polluted environments
◆ in non-breast-fed infants
◆ in the children of smoking parents
◆ in those who consume a lot of salt and salty foods

Genetic factors are also relevant for both allergic and non-allergic asthma. In childhood-onset asthma there is often an allergic component, with an association with eczema, and often sensitivity to grass pollen, housedust and cats. If one parent is atopic (has allergic tendencies), the risk of a child developing inhalant allergies nearly doubles, compared with children of non-atopic parents, and nearly doubles if both parents are atopic. The risk of developing these allergies is also greater for boys and if the child was born underweight.

## What Causes It?

In addition to the factors that contribute to bronchial hyper-responsiveness, the three main categories to consider are those already mentioned: allergies, infection and pollution. Recent research suggests that there are interactions between these whereby pollutants and viruses increase the magnitude of the allergic response.

### Allergic causes

These are very similar to those that cause rhinitis. They can cause both an immediate reaction with a peak effect at 5–15 minutes, and a delayed reaction peaking at 4–6 hours, and which can last for 24 hours. Thus daily exposure to an allergen may mean that there are nearly continuous symptoms with no discernible aggravations that would allow you to easily connect a possible allergen with the asthma. Possible allergens include the following:

◆ Housedust mite.
◆ Animals. Cats, and to a lesser extent dogs, birds (and feather-filled furnishings) and laboratory animals.
◆ Grass pollen. An allergy can cause asthma as well as hayfever. Sensitivity to tree and weed pollen and rarely flower pollen may be minor triggers.
◆ Mould sensitivity. *Aspergillus fumigatus* is a common garden and household mould which releases its spores in autumn and winter, and can produce chronic asthma in which the fungus actually infects the lung. Other mould spores are present in the atmosphere in the late summer and early autumn. They are more likely to be present in rural areas and some are released after rainstorms.

Allergy to fungi that commonly cause skin infections such as athlete's foot or nail infections is another, albeit rare, cause of asthma.

◆ Foods. Some of these may be obvious because they produce reactions within a few minutes or an hour or two of consumption. This probably applies to less than 10 per cent of asthmatics, and common culprit foods are nuts, eggs, milk, wheat, soya, fish and shellfish.

Very delayed reactions to foods are notoriously hard to assess. Cows' milk products and wheat are possibilities. A reason that the role of these or other foods is unclear is that sensitivity to them may result only in an increase in catarrh, or produce biochemical changes in the lung that then require the presence of other more potent trigger factors before there is a discernible effect.

◆ Health-food supplements. These are a rare possible cause, with asthmatic reactions and even death following consumption of royal jelly.

◆ Artificial colourings. Notably Tartrazine E 102 and Sunset Yellow E 110 in approximately four per cent of asthmatics.

◆ Preservatives in food. Sulphites (E 220–E 227) in approximately 5–10 per cent of asthmatics. Sulphites are also found in many wines, and this beverage may occasionally trigger attacks.

◆ Dust. From woods, wheat, other grains, tea, coffee, soya beans, and other foods.

◆ Fumes. From soldering of metal and the soldering flux rosin.

◆ Dust or fumes. From chemicals, medicines and enzymes in occupational exposure.

◆ Chemicals. Those used in paint sprays.

*Infective causes*

These are an important possibility, and though antibiotics are often given during an acute episode, it is often more to cover the possibility than the actuality of infection.

◆ Viral infections seem especially common in children.

◆ Bacterial infections should be suspected if yellow or green phlegm is present. This is very relevant to older patients with a history of long-standing lung problems.

◆ Parasitic infection, not in the lung, but elsewhere, may sometimes be a trigger due to the development of an allergy to the parasite's proteins which then cause a reaction in the lung. Only suspect if there are other symptoms of parasite infection or a history of foreign travel.

As a rule infections may be more likely if the diet is inadequate and there are deficiencies of certain key nutrients. Vitamins A, B complex and zinc may be especially relevant but there are no studies of their levels in asthmatic patients.

### Pollution as a cause

◆ Smoking is the most obvious triggering factor, and this is nowadays very often another's smoke from passive exposure.
◆ Outdoor air pollutants include sulphur dioxide, nitrogen dioxide, chlorine and ozone. These chemicals are either released from industrial processes, are present in car exhaust fumes, are formed naturally by the action of lightning, or form in the photochemical smog that sits like a blanket over many large cities.

   A combination of bright sunlight and the right atmospheric conditions can create a chemical soup containing these potent lung irritants. Ozone seems often to be the most important, and levels of this chemical typically peak around midday. Some weather forecasts now include warnings about poor air quality.
◆ Very fine smoke particles from fires of coal or wood, diesel engines and some industrial sources were once thought to be relatively harmless, but they do seem to cause problems. They may combine with allergens such as pollen and enhance their triggering effects.
◆ Indoor pollutants—is nowhere safe!—include paint strippers, oven cleaners, spray polishes and others. Sunlight may contribute to an indoor photochemical smog effect.

### Other possible causes

◆ The most serious are a group of drugs called beta-blockers used in the treatment of high blood pressure and angina, and in the form of eye drops in the treatment of glaucoma. No-one with asthma or a history of asthma should use these drugs.
◆ Aspirin and occasionally other analgesics may trigger an attack.

There may be some association with nasal polyps or a family history of aspirin sensitivity. This may affect 2 per cent of asthmatics.

◆ Rarely, asthma is much worse premenstrually. The exact cause for this is not clear. It may respond to either the use of steroids or hormonal treatment. Treatment of associated premenstrual symptoms might be beneficial (see Premenstrual Syndrome).

◆ A certain amount of asthma at night and in the early morning is due to the near silent regurgitation of acid secretions from the stomach and their passage in small amounts into the lung. This happens most easily at night when the person is lying down and the reflux of acid from the stomach into the oesophagus or gullet goes unnoticed. Coughing episodes at night with a burning sensation in the central chest would suggest this possible situation. Treatment involves dietary measures to help reduce acid reflux, and use of drugs to suppress excessive acid production. They can be highly effective.

## *What Your Doctor Can Do*

The management of asthma has undergone a substantial review in the United Kingdom, Australia and New Zealand and elsewhere, all in the last decade. This came about because of a continuing high mortality rate which is now beginning to fall, and the realisation that a high percentage of these deaths was preventable.

Management depends upon:

◆ Adequate treatment of acute attacks.
◆ Detection of precipitating cause(s). In some instances this may mean either skin or blood tests for possible allergies.
◆ Assessment of the degree of lung impairment. Most often regular use of a simple 'peak flow meter' will give good information about the severity of the asthma and its variation at different times. More detailed lung function tests are used by chest disease specialists.
◆ Drawing up a treatment action plan based upon the above information and the patient's needs.

Most treatment centres upon the use of drugs most commonly given by inhalers. The main types are:

◆ Bronchodilators such as Salbutamol (Ventolin); these produce a very quick response but need to be given several times per day. Mild asthmatics may not need any other therapy. Excessive use of these inhalers has in the past resulted in an increased risk of death. It is important that the recommended intake and prescribed pattern of use are followed.

◆ Steroid inhalers which come in a variety of strengths. They are useful when the asthma is not controlled by simple bronchodilators. They reduce the swelling and inflammation that narrows the airways, and are most usefully combined with a bronchodilator. Very potent inhaled steroid preparations are now available, and are used for more severe cases. Side-effects such as oral thrush may develop, and continued use may reduce growth rates in children.

◆ Sodium cromoglycate (Nalcrom) is a drug, again given by inhaler, that has a unique action, blocking the allergic reactions that take place in the lung. They are most successful in young children and often should be tried before long-term steroid inhalers are used. They are less effective in adults, but are worth considering when allergy plays a major role.

◆ Oral steroids are used initially as a short high-dose course for severe attacks in either children or adults. Courses lasting seven days or so are relatively free of side-effects, are life-saving, and frequently reduce the time spent in hospital. For those with severe asthma that requires maximal doses of inhaled steroids or repeated short courses of high-dose steroids, then long-term use of daily doses of steroids are worth considering. These are not without side-effects, most usually if the dose of Prednisolone exceeds 10 mg daily. Weight gain, high blood pressure, muscle loss, osteoporosis and development of diabetes may all occur, but are perhaps less likely if the patient is encouraged to eat very healthily and has no associated nutritional deficiencies.

◆ Other drugs are sometimes used by specialists, and include long-acting bronchodilators salmeterol (Serevent) and Oxitropium (Oxivent) given by inhaler, preparations of aminophylline, antihistamines and immune-altering drugs. All of these except the last category are usually tried before long-term steroid tablets are used.

When any of these treatments are first started it is a good policy for the patient's response to be carefully monitored. Recording the peak flow readings in the morning and at a further time later in the day, as well as the level of symptoms, can help decide on the best type of treatment and its dosage. This is important, as many treatments will potentially be given for years.

The drugs for inhalation can be given by a number of devices including metered dose inhalers which use chlorofluorocarbon propellant, dry powder devices and nebulisers for the severe attack. Large spacer devices attached to the inhaler may improve performance and reduce side-effects in the mouth.

◆ Desensitising was once a popular treatment, though it is now rarely used because of occasional deaths. Patients who were strongly reacting to housedust mite or pollen could be made less sensitive after being given a series of injections. Each injection contained a very small but increasing dose of the allergen which, instead of causing an allergic reaction, stimulated the body to produce other antibodies that blocked the action of those antibodies involved in the asthmatic reaction. Thus the allergy was side-tracked. Such treatments may return in the future and be used at specialised centres.

## What You Can Do

The importance of involving the sufferer in the care of their asthma is becoming increasingly recognised. The variable nature of this condition means that the asthmatic needs to know which changes can be made to their treatment and be familiar with what the possible triggering factors are for any acute episode. Avoidance of these triggers is important, especially if escalating doses of drugs are to be avoided.

◆ Take your medication regularly. It sounds simple and it is. Regular use of the agreed medication should mean better lung function, fewer severe attacks and less disability.
◆ Avoid known inhalant allergens. This applies particularly to those who need to use steroids in any form. The need for avoidance of housedust and other inhalant allergens will depend on documentation of the allergy, usually by use of skin prick tests, and recognition that the asthma is to a substantial

degree influenced by them. The measures detailed under Hay-fever and Allergic Rhinitis for the avoidance of the appropriate allergen should be followed. Prolonged avoidance of the allergen can, after a number of months, lead to a reduction in the individual's degree of sensitivity.

◆ Avoid pollutants. Firstly do not smoke. Try not to use wood and coal fires in the home unless they are very well enclosed. You may need to avoid going outside during the time of the day when air quality is at its worst.

◆ Reduce the chances of chest infection. Damp in the home is still a major risk factor for chest infections, and this is in turn related to social class. Treating damp areas and providing adequate heat and ventilation are important. These measures will help limit housedust mites and some moulds.

◆ Improve your nutritional state. Mild nutritional deficiencies and a poor diet certainly influence resistance to infection and the rate of chest infections and possibly the development and severity of asthma. Eat The Very Nutritious Diet. Certain nutrients may be especially important, and they include vitamins A and B complex and zinc.

◆ Eat certain protective foods. A high intake of fresh fruit and vegetables may be desirable. They are rich in magnesium and potassium, and low in sodium. Onions have been shown to have anti-asthmatic properties. Certain chemicals called thiosulphinates and cepaenes, which are formed when the onion is crushed or chopped, seem to inhibit the production of pro-inflammatory chemicals involved in asthma. Apparently you'll need to eat one medium-sized onion per day. Perhaps a bowl of steaming hot onion soup for the acute attack?

◆ Avoid common food additives. These include artificial colourings and sulphites. Watch out for the latter in squashes and wines which do not list them on the label within the EEC. Australians are better informed, as these additives are detailed on the label.

◆ Cut down on salt in the diet. High normal intakes might enhance the bronchial hyper-responsiveness that develops.

◆ Take regular exercise. Provided that necessary care is taken, the asthma is stable, and medication is taken regularly, this can improve the situation over time. Many sports people with asthma take a squirt of their bronchodilator just before exercise.

◆ Protect yourself from cold air. This commonly triggers wheezing. Do so by wearing a scarf and even placing this over your mouth. Alternatively you can wear a face mask, especially if you are cycling in a city and are exposed to traffic fumes.

## Nutritional Supplements

◆ Vitamin C, 1 g twice daily, has an antihistamine effect. Try it for six to eight weeks.

◆ Magnesium is a mineral that has mild anti-allergy and bronchodilating effects. It is not as strong as the drugs. Two recent pieces of research have revealed that the white cells of asthmatics are low in this mineral, and that a poor dietary intake in adults is associated with an increased chance of wheezing. The effect of supplements are awaited, but are unlikely to be very strong. A supplement of 300–400 mg per day for at least four months, together with a high-protein, low-salt diet, is suggested.

◆ Vitamin B6, pyridoxine, was shown in one small trial to help reduce the dependency of asthmatics upon steroids. This supplement has been shown to enhance magnesium balance in women with premenstrual syndrome.

◆ Multi-vitamins and anti-oxidants such as beta-carotene, vitamin E and selenium might protect the lung from chemical assault. Lowered blood levels of this latter mineral have been linked with asthma and sensitivity to aspirin and salicylates.

◆ Fish oil supplements have been tried in asthma with the expectation that their anti-inflammatory effects would reduce the degree of wheezing. In fact some of those who took part experienced a deterioration, and this type of supplement, including cod liver oil, should not be taken by the severe asthmatic without medical supervision.

As before with drug medication, evaluation of benefit is important. Monitoring the response to self-help measures, dietary treatment and use of supplements is best achieved by recording the peak flow daily. Other measures of improvement include general well-being, need for medication, dosage of steroids or bronchodilators, and use of antibiotics. For many of these non-drug measures, improvement is likely to take three to six months, so be patient.

## Complementary Therapies

◆ Acupuncture can help with feelings of shortness of breath, and thus might be of benefit to some sufferers.

◆ Relaxation therapies such as massage and aromatherapy could help, especially where stressful incidents are a frequent asthma trigger.

◆ Herbal medicine is worth consideration, as there appear to be a number of plant extracts with the power to alter lung chemistry. Sanitised extracts of these may appear or pharmacological equivalents may be developed in the near future.

*See also*: Allergy, PMS, Indigestion, High Blood Pressure, What's Wrong with Present-day Diet and Lifestyle?, Nutrition Is the Key to Health, The Simple Exclusion Diet. Plus Recommended Reading List and References.

# BACK PAIN

Back pain is a common complaint with a variety of causes. The pain may vary from intermittent discomfort to severe pain that requires complete bed rest. At one end of the spectrum continuous pain may be caused by a disease in the back itself or as referred pain from some other part of the body that is diseased or infected, and at the other extreme the pain may be related only to pulled muscles or ligaments, and may only be a short-term problem. The sensations can vary from a dull aching feeling to sharp, shooting sensations.

## What Causes It?

There is an almost endless list of causes for common back and neck problems, and they include:

◆ muscular strain from moving awkwardly or lifting heavy items
◆ tearing of a ligament or tendon, or inflammation of the synovial fluid which surrounds the joints
◆ long-standing displacement or curvature of the spine

- arthritis of the spine
- prolapsed (slipped) disc
- vertebral collapse from osteoporosis
- infections such as viral infections
- kidney stones
- pressure on the nerves as in sciatica
- bad posture when sitting or standing
- a gynaecological disorder, like fibroids or cysts
- menstrual period pains
- ill-fitting or high-heeled shoes
- obesity or pregnancy placing strain on the spine
- injuries or accident
- bowel or intestinal problems
- depression and fatigue
- occasionally disease of the internal abdominal organs

## What Your Doctor Can Do

Severe back pain lasting for more than a few days will require assessment by a doctor. All patients with weight loss or severe persistent pain should be looked at particularly carefully, and this may well involve blood tests and X-rays. When underlying medical conditions have been eliminated, your doctor may refer you to an osteopath or a physiotherapist for a course of treatment. Osteopaths are particularly adept at treating pain of musculo-skeletal origin (derived from muscles, tendons, ligaments or bones). They are also trained to detect more common serious disorders that may present with back pain and often they, in turn, can refer you to your GP. Cranial osteopathy is a particularly effective and gentle form of treatment that is well worth investigating if you suffer with back problems.

## What You Can Do

The simplest and most important message for those with back pain is that much of the pain is actually due to muscle spasm. Sometimes this is the only problem or it is secondary to painful skeletal conditions such as vertebral collapse or displacement. Muscle spasm can be relieved by a number of self-help measures, including:

- rest
- local heat or cold application

- gentle massage when the acute episode is over
- ordinary painkillers
- small amounts of alcohol
- supplements of magnesium, a simple cheap and at times surprisingly effective treatment (but which is unlikely to be effective for the control of severe back pain associated with arthritis). Supplements of between 200 and 400 mg of magnesium taken with multi-vitamins will help raise magnesium levels, in blood and muscle, over a two-week to two-month period.
- The Very Nutritious Diet, low in salt and sugar, as this helps magnesium retention.
- Alexander Technique is particularly good at re-training us to hold our bodies in an optimum way, thus preventing future back or neck problems.

Many back problems could be prevented by improving posture and by taking adequate exercise. The following points are worth implementing for long-term back health.

- Make sure you have a comfortable mattress to sleep on which is turned regularly. So many back problems occur gradually as an ageing mattress fails to support your back in the optimum way.
- Ensure that you have a comfortable working chair that supports your back fully, and that your desk or table is the appropriate height.
- When you walk be aware of your posture, keeping your shoulders down and your head high. Imagine you have a piece of string coming out the top of your head which is being gently pulled from above.
- When bending, bend from the knees, rather than stooping over.
- Take regular exercise, but be careful not to cause any further back problems.

## Complementary Therapies

Osteopathy and chiropractic are now of established value. It is helpful to have a local therapist with whom you have good rapport, especially if you have repeated needs for their services. Vigorous manipulative techniques are inappropriate for many older patients, and you may need to enquire of the therapist what type of approaches they use before seeking their advice. Cranial osteopathy is our preference because it is effective and non-invasive.

Homoeopathic remedies for pain relief are a useful tool, and Magnesium Phosphoricum is particularly helpful.

*See also*: Recommended Reading List and References.

# BREAST PAIN

Up to 60 per cent of working women have experienced breast pain at some time which is, surprisingly, a good sign, as pain is not usually associated with anything sinister. Breast cancer is a great concern to us all, though, especially as it is on the increase. Despite the fact that breast examinations and special X-rays, mammography, are now available to detect early breast cancer, there are still some 20 000 new cases diagnosed each year in the United Kingdom. England and Wales come top of the league for breast cancer, followed by Denmark and Scotland. New Zealand comes in eighth, the USA in eleventh place and Australia fourteenth. Having begun in such an alarmist fashion, it should be said that for every patient with breast cancer, ten other women will have a non-sinister breast lump or breast tenderness.

## What Are the Symptoms?
There are various conditions that cause breast tenderness, pain (otherwise known as mastalgia) and lumps, and they are generally covered by the term 'benign breast disease'. This may sound unduly frightening, but non-cancerous lumps, bumps and cysts are quite normal and should not be regarded as disease. The word 'benign' means non-cancerous, and indicates that lumps will not spread and grow to invade other tissue, or affect other parts of the body. Even so, they can be very uncomfortable and a continuing source of worry.

Breast pain can be broadly divided into two categories. In approximately a third of cases, breast tenderness and discomfort occur throughout the month, whilst in the remaining two-thirds, breast tenderness and pain tend to worsen before the onset of a period. The premenstrual pattern of breast tenderness that occurs for up to two weeks before the period, tends to occur in younger patients in their twenties to forties, and can usually be alleviated by natural means.

All women with breast tenderness or a breast lump should have a physical examination to determine the nature of the problem. Mild breast tenderness that occurs premenstrually, and clears completely without the presence of any breast lump, is rarely indicative of anything more sinister. Persistent pain, alteration in the shape of the breast, or a discharge from the nipple, are all symptoms that should make you seek an early appointment with your doctor.

## What Causes It?

◆ In recent years, there has been some evidence to link breast disease with the type of diets we eat. Breast cancer, for example, is more common in countries with a high animal fat intake. Countries such as Japan, where fat intake is extremely low and the diet is composed mainly of vegetables, fish and rice, there is a low incidence of breast cancer and benign breast problems.

◆ Other scientists in the field have suggested that cigarette smoking and caffeine intakes from tea and coffee, chocolate and cola, may be linked with breast discomfort. This is not absolutely proven, but it may be helpful to reduce your consumption of these if breast tenderness is a problem.

◆ Hormonal factors are also important. The oral contraceptive pill, with its content of progesterone, may help to reduce some types of benign breast disease. Giving birth to a first child prior to the age of thirty is associated with a slight reduction in breast cancer risk.

## What Your Doctor Can Do

◆ Examine your breasts and take a history of the problem. If you feel it is a recurring cyclic problem, in that it occurs monthly before your period is due, you should make this known.

◆ If your doctor is not unduly concerned, the next step is to prescribe evening primrose oil, Efamast, at a dose of 3000–4000 g for at least four months. This has been shown to help with benign breast problems.

◆ Your doctor should tell you to eat a low animal fat diet, but may be unaware of the research published in this area.

◆ If your symptoms are not sinister or cyclic, then your doctor may prescribe either painkillers or an anti-inflammatory preparation.

◆ Should the pain or tenderness persist, your doctor may then prescribe powerful hormones, like danazol (Danol), which will stop you ovulating or, as a last resort, bromocriptine (Parlodel), another powerful drug which blocks the hormone prolactin from the pituitary gland. Both of these drugs have a long list of side-effects which may be unacceptable and should be carefully considered.

## What You Can Do

A carefully conducted study published in the leading medical journal, the *Lancet*, in 1988, showed that women with premenstrual breast tenderness, could benefit from a low-fat, high-fibre, high-protein diet. The diet required a substantial reduction in overall fat intake to a level that would mean most of us reducing our fat intake by nearly 50 per cent. To achieve this, the following changes would need to be made.

◆ Eat leaner cuts of meat and trim all visible fat from meat.

◆ Don't eat meat products, such as pies, sausages, and pâté, which are high in fat.

◆ Don't eat the skin from fish, chicken or other poultry.

◆ All meat and fish should be grilled, steamed or baked, and not fried, or prepared with rich creamy sauces.

◆ Dairy intake should be limited, replacing full cream milk with reduced fat or skimmed and using low-fat polyunsaturated spreads, instead of ordinary margarines or butter. Cream is to be avoided too, and low-fat yoghurts or fromage frais are good alternatives.

Other dietary guidelines that are also of benefit in helping to reduce premenstrual breast tenderness include the following.

◆ Eat plenty of vegetables and fruit, which are low in fat.

◆ Aim to consume one portion of green vegetables, a portion of root vegetables and some salad every day.

◆ All green leafy vegetables, potatoes and other root vegetables should be consumed without butter or margarine.

◆ Eat at least two to three portions of fruit daily.
◆ Alcohol, sugar, confectionery and other foods rich in sugar and honey, should be severely limited. They provide empty kilojoules, with no essential nutrients or fibre.

All these measures are particularly important if you are overweight. It has been shown that such diets may help bring down excessive levels of the hormone, oestrogen, which may stimulate breast tissue. A high-fibre diet may help combat a tendency to constipation, which itself has been associated with hormonal abnormalities and even some breast conditions. Overall, the effects of this diet in the study group were very gratifying, but the benefits took some six months to become fully apparent. There was a substantial reduction in both premenstrual breast swelling, tenderness and discomfort, and it may be that these beneficial changes could eventually lead to a reduction in breast cancer risk.

Other potentially beneficial measures include:

◆ Reducing consumption of cigarettes and alcohol, as well as caffeine from tea, coffee, chocolate and cola-based drinks.
◆ Taking the supplement evening primrose oil, Efamol. This is widely available in chemists and health-food shops. The full dosage is 6–8 500 IU capsules taken daily through the menstrual cycle. It is best combined with the above dietary measures.
◆ Taking natural vitamin E, 400 IU per day, has also been shown to help with breast tenderness in one trial.
◆ Wearing a firm, supportive bra. Some women find a sports bra particularly comforting and helpful during the night.

### Self-examination
It is important to have regular breast examinations, especially if you are prone to tender, lumpy breasts. Make sure you examine your breasts yourself on a regular basis to check for any lumps or changes in shape. Many women will notice that their breasts become lumpy and tender in the two weeks before their period, and that this disappears when the period has begun. These symptoms are not a cause for alarm, but should be treated.

### When to self-examine
Some doctors recommend examining your own breasts thoroughly

at a regular time each month, after your period has finished. However, if you happen to be one of the 10 per cent of women who do self-examine, you will know that your breasts may sometimes alter in density and texture at different times of your cycle. It is important to get to know your breasts, and get in tune with your cycle, especially if you are of child-bearing age. It is probably a good idea to examine your breasts on a fortnightly basis—preferably at a regular time. If there is a set time, perhaps at the weekend, when you have a leisurely soak in the bath, maybe that would be the best opportunity, and one that you would not forget.

### How to self-examine

1. First have a good look at yourself undressed in the mirror. Check to make sure there are no changes in shape or colour.
2. Next take each segment of your breast, like the segments of an orange, and with one hand supporting the breast, probe and massage the section to check for lumps and bumps.
3. Finally lie down, with one arm above your head, and check the circumference of the breast, including the section that merges with your underarm. Sometimes glands under the arm may be tender and swollen, indicating that there is some extra activity occurring in the area for some reason.
4. If you have any concerns or confusion, it is best to get your doctor to examine the breast for you.

Most women who self-examine never find a lump, and the vast majority of lumps that *are* found are normal and harmless. Cysts, solid lumps, and discharge from the nipple are all things that occur from time to time, and which are usually hormonally related and with no sinister underlying cause. Be positive about examining your breasts on a regular basis. A lump detected early, which did turn out to be cancerous, would not be life-threatening if treated quickly. The medical profession is extremely efficient when it comes to breast cancer.

Never forget, if you have a pain or lump in your breast, you should be examined by your doctor. If neither the doctor nor the specialist can find anything wrong, then taking care with your diet and using Efamol or Efamast helps many women with benign breast disease. You would also be advised to follow the suggested Menu for Breast Tenderness on page 485.

## Complementary Therapies

Homoeopathy, herbal medicine and massage would be the preferred choices of complementary therapies for breast problems, once it had been established that there was no underlying sinister cause. There are a number of homoeopathic remedies worth trying, such as Natrum mur, Nux, Kali carb or Silica. Herbal preparations are also worth a try.

## Geraldine's Story

Geraldine, a forty-two-year-old mother of two grown children, worked as a secretary and suffered from painful breasts to the point where even walking hurt.

*My problem began when I was thirty-three and would occur every three months. Within three years the frequency and the pain had increased so that for three weeks out of four I was in agony. My GP suggested vitamin B6 which helped for the first few months, but then the symptoms returned. I was instructed to increase the dose, and ended up taking seven pills per day, which I thought might be dangerous. He then suggested I try some evening primrose oil which helped ease the pain a bit, but not completely.*

*That year my husband was killed in a road accident. My children were fourteen and ten at the time, and life was extremely stressful. My breast pain grew worse until, by 1984, I was in pain for the majority of the time. My breast regularly swelled from 34B to 36B, and the skin was tight and shiny. I even wore a maternity bra in bed because I felt so heavy and uncomfortable. I went to see several doctors, one of whom suggested that perhaps I had strained my muscles driving a car!*

*Eventually I was treated with several powerful hormonal drugs. The medical theory was that the shock and stress of my bereavement had brought on an early menopause. I didn't believe this because I knew my symptoms had been just as severe, although less frequent, before I was widowed. When the drugs lost their effect I was prescribed new ones. I gradually put on 4.5 kg and developed severe back pain. When the doctor eventually told me that my back pain was a side effect of the drugs I went home and threw them all down the toilet. Within a week my back was as right as rain.*

*It was at this point I saw a magazine article about a woman with symptoms similar to mine who had been cured by changes to her diet. I really didn't have much faith in this, but I was so desperate I was ready to try anything. I phoned the WNAS and made an appointment. My first consultation was long and probing. I was given a strict diet to follow with no dairy produce, tea or coffee or added salt, no more than two slices of bread per day, and lots of fruit and vegetables. I was also given supplements of Optivite, vitamin C and Efamol, and told to follow an exercise programme.*

*Within a week I was a different woman. I felt so much better I could hardly believe it. It took just four months for the breast pain to completely disappear. I've been pain free for six years now, I still follow my programme and feel completely in control. Being free of breast pain has changed my life. I've been able to take swimming lessons and judo classes which would have been out of the question before. I feel like socialising and am thrilled about finding an answer to the problem that made my life a total misery for so many years.*

*See also*: Breast-feeding Mastitis, Cancer, Premenstrual Syndrome. Plus Recommended Reading List and References.

# CANCER

Cancer is one of the commonest diseases, and it is likely to become even more widespread with our increasingly ageing population. It accounts for the second highest number of deaths—24 per cent for women and 27 per cent for men. In many people's minds, cancer is viewed as a twentieth-century illness, but in fact many types of cancer were observed in ancient times. Practically all of us has known someone, possibly a family member, who had cancer of one kind or another. We all need to know more about cancer, its causes, possible prevention, and in particular how early detection and early treatment may lead to an improved outcome. Self-help and dietary measures have their part to play alongside conventional treatments, and neither avenue should be considered exclusively.

A cancerous growth is simply a growth that may have derived from perhaps one or just a few cells. This may have happened many months, if not years, before the person is aware of the problem. Cancerous cells have two particular qualities: firstly, a rapid rate of growth, faster than that of the surrounding tissues, and secondly, the ability to spread not only through local tissues but to distant sites. Thus patients with breast cancer may find it has spread to the local lymph nodes under the armpit, and from there to perhaps the liver or the spine. It is often the widespread nature of the cancer which results in death.

## What Are the Symptoms?

◆ A lump. This may be the initial growth itself or a secondary deposit. New lumps or bumps anywhere should be taken seriously by your doctor. They do not have to be painful to be cancerous.

◆ Pain. This is not usually an early symptom. Cancer in the bones or where the lump presses on the nerve where it is in a confined space may lead to pain.

◆ Weight loss. This is often the feature of an advanced cancer, but may also occur in the early stages of cancers affecting the stomach or other digestive organs.

◆ Fatigue. This has many causes, but in patients with cancer this can be due to the associated anaemia or other effects on general metabolism.

◆ Fever. Although usually caused by an infection, even in patients with cancer, this may sometimes be a feature of certain blood and glandular growths.

## What Causes It?

◆ Surprisingly, increasing age is about the greatest risk for cancer. Of course some cancers occur in childhood, especially leukaemia and those related to certain rare genetic disorders. For the majority of common cancers, increase in age, especially over the age of forty, is the greatest risk factor. The good news is that in some very old populations the risk seems to fall, but from middle age onwards the risk is rising. This is perhaps because it takes time for some of the other causative factors to have an influence upon cells in a way that will make them change into cancerous ones. A few cancers do occur at a younger age and these include carcinoma of the cervix, some types of breast cancer and cancer of the lymph glands, Hodgkin's disease.

◆ Cigarette smoking is probably the next most easily identifiable factor in cancer. Its association with lung cancer is well known. What is not widely appreciated is that it is also associated with an increased risk of many other cancers, including the mouth, throat, oesophagus, the pancreas, the bladder and others. It is estimated that approximately one-third of all cancers are linked with smoking.

◆ Poor diet is a distinct causative factor. High intakes of fat, especially saturated fats, seems also to be associated with increased risk of breast cancer as well as cancer of the colon, endometrium (lining of the womb), pancreas and prostate. Lack of fibre may also increase risk of colon cancer. A diet high in fruit and vegetables offers some protection against cancer. The amount we eat, and not being overweight may be important factors, especially with regard to breast cancer in women and testicular cancer in men.

◆ Certain viral infections are associated with change in cells that may lead to cancer. This is true in a variety of situations, including cancer of the cervix, in some blood cancers and in patients with the HIV virus. Stomach cancer is associated with chronic infection with the bacteria *Helicobacter pylori*. These forms of cancer are potentially avoidable or preventable. Reducing the number of sexual partners a woman has, if her partner is circumcised or perhaps uses a condom, may all be associated with a lower risk of cervical cancer. Eradication of the *Helicobacter* germ associated with peptic ulcers may lead to a lower risk of stomach cancer.

◆ Environmental pollution probably plays a relatively small part, except in certain situations where there may be high exposure to a variety of industrial chemicals in either air or water.

◆ In certain parts of the world, there are significant amounts of natural radiation. This powerful invisible force can disrupt the structure of cells, precipitating cancerous change. There is a small contribution from the radiation involved in medical procedures. Local areas of pollution from nuclear reactors and more widespread radiation exposure following the Chernobyl disaster will continue to be the subject of medical research, though they are only of small relevance to the majority of us.

◆ A variety of chemicals used in industry are associated with increased cancer risks, and these include rubber, industrial dyes, asbestos, glues and varnishes, cadmium, nickel, and some rare metals.

◆ Exposure to sunlight or ultra-violet light in white, especially fair-skinned, individuals is associated with an increased risk of melanoma and other skin cancers. Melanoma has become one of the commonest causes of cancerous death in young adults in Australia and South Africa as well as in the United Kingdom. The recent increase in line with the desire for increased sun exposure has prompted campaigns such as Slip Slop Slap (Slip on a T-shirt, Slop on high-factor sun cream, Slap on a hat). Heavy sun exposure before puberty in children with ginger hair, seems to be a particularly unwise combination. In older people, other types of less malignant skin cancer, especially rodent ulcers, also develop. These are influenced by sunlight exposure, especially on the face and hands.

## What Your Doctor Can Do

◆ Take your symptoms seriously. Because of the many different types of cancer, and the different ways in which it may present, early diagnosis is not always easy. This must, however, still remain an important goal as only early diagnosis will lead to a better outcome.
◆ Investigate for cancer, which includes:
  ◇ a thorough physical examination
  ◇ blood tests
  ◇ X-rays
  ◇ specialist investigations, especially CT (Computerised Tomography) and MRI (Magnetic Resonance Imaging) scans. These are specialised X-rays which allow visualisation of internal abdominal organs and the nervous system. Specialist blood tests are also being evolved to allow the early detection of what are termed 'tumour markers'. This will tell us there is a cancer somewhere but won't tell us where it is
  ◇ a biopsy or a small sample of the suspected cancerous tissue is taken and usually allows identification of the cancer type by examination under the microscope. This then leads to decisions about treatment
◆ Treat the cancer. This essentially involves the use of anti-cancer drugs, radiotherapy and surgery. These treatments require special medical skill and indeed many types of cancer are now referred to specialist centres. Further treatment for the control of individual symptoms such as pain with painkillers,

removing fluid that may have built up in the abdomen, and nutritional support as well as psychological support should all be part of standard cancer care. Greater awareness is now mindful of the broader needs of the cancer patient and this may involve her in a number of self-help approaches.

## What You Can Do

Gone are the days when the patient was just simply a passive recipient of therapy. There is much that you can do.

- Learn about your type of cancer and how it affects your body. This you can do either from your own specialist or from a number of support organisations.
- Make adjustments to your diet. This will depend upon the type of cancer, the type of treatment you are receiving and whether you are likely to have developed nutritional deficiencies. You may well need further advice and support from your doctor or the dietician attached to the hospital treating you. Some of the likely dietary changes that may be worthwhile are as follows:
  - ◇ The Very Nutritious Diet would be suitable for the majority of patients who have not lost weight as a result of their cancer, and who are not experiencing complications of therapy—chemotherapy, radiotherapy or surgery. This is suitable for long-term use.
  - ◇ A high-protein, high-kilojoule and easy-to-digest diet is suitable for those who have experienced significant weight loss and have difficulty maintaining kilojoule intake. Supplemental feeds, high in protein, based on milk or soya, may be required. For those with swallowing or digestive difficulties, especially in older patients, putting main meals through a liquidiser may be useful. Particularly good foods in this situation include all diary products, eggs, meat, stewed fruit, ice cream, and nuts and seeds if these latter two can be digested.
  - ◇ Vegetarian and vegan diet regimes are recommended by some complementary therapists, and in theory they could be effective. Only recently have there been one or two reports of benefit after many years of unsubstantiated or poorly substantiated claims. At present, they cannot be broadly recommended for the general patient with cancer.

In theory a high fruit and vegetable diet with a limited amount of protein might retard the growth of some cancers. However, in a patient who is seriously ill and rapidly losing weight, this could be a disastrous choice. The skill required to match these sorts of diets to a patient's individual needs will be as great as that required to determine effective chemotherapeutic regimes. This is a situation where expert medical and dietetic research needs to address some of the ideas of complementary therapists.

◇ Specialised diets for specific types of cancer (see Breast Cancer and Cancer of the Colon and Rectum).

◆ Take nutritional supplements. This is as contentious as recommending a diet for cancer. Routine supplementation of cancer patients cannot be recommended. In theory high doses of certain supplements, especially the anti-oxidant vitamins C, E and beta-carotene, selenium and others could minimise the killing effect of radiotherapy and possibly chemotherapy. On the other hand, those who have lost weight because of their cancer, who have digestive difficulties or have recently completed a course of radiotherapy or chemotherapy, are likely to have a number of nutritional deficiencies that need correcting with a better diet and nutritional supplements. Thus there is a dilemma.

A reasonable mid-way course might be only to give nutritional supplements to those who have, or are likely to have, deficiencies, and not to give them to relatively well patients who are receiving anti-cancer treatments, especially if they are likely to have a high degree of success as in Hodgkin's disease, leukaemia and others. Often chemotherapy regimes are pulsed, that is, given every few days or at weekly or monthly intervals. If nutritional supplements need to be taken, then they could be stopped while the chemotherapy or radiotherapy is actually being given.

At the end of treatment there may be need for 'a nutritional rescue programme'. Equally some patients may be too unwell to tolerate the full course of radiotherapy or chemotherapy, and nutritional support before or during therapy may be necessary. Again this situation may require expert advice.

A further situation is in patients who have been 'cured' of a cancer. This now occurs with a variety of childhood cancers and happens more and more in the early treatment of adult cancers such as stomach, colon and breast. There is evidence that such patients, having survived one cancer, may be more at risk of a second type of cancer, either because of a cancer predisposition or because some of the anti-cancer drugs themselves may increase the risk of developing cancer in later life. For them, eating The Very Nutritious Diet and perhaps taking supplements of strong multi-vitamins containing vitamins C, E, beta-carotene and selenium, would be advisable, but no firm recommendation can be made.

◆ Vitamin A as retinol and beta-carotene, the vegetable form of vitamin A, have been put forward as being cancer protective. Diets rich in beta-carotene derived from bread and red, green and yellow fruits and vegetables are associated with lower risks of cancer. The protective agent may not be just beta-carotene but may be other agents such as vitamin C, vitamin E and selenium. This group is known as anti-oxidants because they may protect tissues from noxious chemicals which may 'oxidise' them, reducing damage and cancerous change. High dietary intakes of calcium may well be associated with a reduced risk of cancer of the large bowel.

◆ Physical exercise sounds improbable but, if possible to take, it would improve fitness and well-being. This is only suitable for patients with very minimal forms of cancer or who have recovered from their anti-cancer treatment.

◆ Maintain outside interests. There is increasing evidence that those who have a positive attitude, are socially active and continue a normal life, do better with their cancer. We have personally seen this with a number of patients. This does not just involve diet, supplements and exercise, but making the most of your time on a number of fronts. This may mean spending more time with your family, revitalising old interests and hobbies, beginning evening classes, or taking up outdoor activities such as walking or gardening. Just think back over the last years of your life and try and recall those things that you have enjoyed or have made you feel good. These are the sorts of things that you should now concentrate on. Think also of the sorts of things that you really wanted to do but never did. Perhaps some of these are suitable for you to take up now. Pleasure obtained from personal achievement is good medicine.

## Complementary Therapies

A number of these may appeal to you and are well worth considering. Acupuncture may be helpful for pain and as a general tonic. Herbal medicine may help with a variety of persistent symptoms, massage and aromatherapy are a good way of relaxing, and homoeopathy has a variety of specific anti-cancer remedies. These are prescribable and can be administered by qualified medical homoeopaths. Again, there is some evidence that they may be helpful but no large-scale recommendations can be made. You should consult a medically qualified homoeopath specialising in cancer treatment.

A word of warning on some complementary therapies. Beware of excessive or false claims. These are easily made, not necessarily with intent to deceive or defraud, but out of a desire of the therapist to help. The fact that one or two patients have done well following a particular line does not mean that all will. In the end it is only good-quality research of the type performed by medical practitioners that will prove the case for or against a particular line of therapy. Fortunately, a number of conventional physicians are looking seriously at the benefits of complementary medicine in cancer care.

The main cancers affecting women are described in the following pages in the hope that greater knowledge about risk factors and presenting symptoms brings earlier recognition, earlier and better treatment. This seems to be the most likely way of helping people in the short term.

# Breast Cancer

Historically this has been the commonest fatal cancer in women, though this may now be overtaken by lung cancer because smoking is still very popular among young women. The risk of breast cancer is associated with:

◆ High-fat, low-fibre diets as found in many Western countries.
◆ Absence of pregnancy or pregnancies after the age of the woman's thirty-fifth birthday. The risk is less likely with increasing numbers of pregnancies, and if the woman breast-feeds (only a small additional effect).
◆ Obesity, but only in women after menopause.

- Early onset of menstruation—menarche—and to a lesser extent a late menopause. This means more hormonal cycles with a seemingly greater opportunity of cancer.
- Family history of cancer, especially in a first-degree relative (mother or sister at a young age).
- Fibrocystic disease of the breast perhaps in association with constipation, which may be because of the influence of bowel habit on hormone metabolism.
- The oral contraceptive pill, a small increase in risk after prolonged use.
- Hormone Replacement Therapy, HRT, an increase in risk of up to 25 per cent during and for a few years after use. Again this risk may only be noticeable for after five to ten years' use, and the risk may not be so great with short-term use.

Dietary factors might also influence the rate of growth of the tumour. Obesity is associated with a worse outcome, possibly because of the mild oestrogen-like effect of fat tissue on the female metabolism. Weight reduction, a low saturated fat diet, a good intake of Omega-3 series fish oils and possibly a compound related to beta-carotene, lycopene (found in tomatoes and spinach), may reduce the rate of growth. But we will have to wait many years before we know if this is true.

## Cancer of the Cervix

This cancer is closely connected with sexual activity. There is now clear evidence that cervical cancer is associated with certain viruses that cause change in the cells covering the neck of the womb. These changes gradually occur and may be detected at a relatively early stage as a result of using cervical smears. Regular smears are an important part of care of women of reproductive age as cancer of the cervix may produce relatively few symptoms in its early stages. Irregular vaginal bleeding or bleeding after intercourse are two important symptoms. The risk factors for cervical cancer include:

- Number of sexual partners particularly at a young age.
- Smoking.
- Use of oral contraceptives.
- Possibly diet.

The more prosperous individuals within a community who probably eat better with high intakes of fruit and vegetables do seem
to be at less risk of developing this type of cancer. Disturbed levels
of a number of nutrients have been associated with cervical cancer
but it is not clear whether supplements of these or multi-vitamins
would have any genuine protective effect. Early detection and
treatment have greatly changed the likely outcome from this type
of cancer.

## Cancer of the Womb (Endometrium)

The lining of the womb, the endometrium, may become cancerous. This tissue is particularly sensitive to oestrogens, and some
of the risk factors for its development are shared with those of
breast cancer. They include:

- An early start to periods and late menopause.
- Use of hormone replacement therapy (HRT) where unopposed
  oestrogens (oestrogen without progesterone) are given to
  women with a womb. This no longer happens as progestogens
  are prescribed to induce endometrial shedding and prevent the
  development of this type of cancer.
- Number of pregnancies. The more pregnancies the lower the
  risk.
- Rarely, oestrogen-secreting tumours.
- Obesity in post-menopausal women.

## Cancer of the Ovary

Although relatively rare, cancer of the ovary is increasingly important. Its early detection is difficult, the treatment is not very successful, and consequently it causes an undue number of cancer
deaths. The next decade will see the emphasis on the early detection of this type of cancer, in particular. There are in fact several
types of ovarian cancer, and the risk in developing it is the greatest
in countries with a high standard of living. Other risk factors are:

- An early start to periods or late menopause.
- Lack of pregnancies.
- Family history of ovarian cancer. This may be particularly
  important in detecting those who should be screened regularly
  for its development.

◆ Lack of using oral contraceptives. Like pregnancy, this inhibits ovulation and seems to minimise the risk of its development.

Early detection using ultrasound and blood tests for some tumour markers may prove to be a practical way of identifying this cancer, either in the general population or in those at high risk. The results of various trials are awaited.

## Cancer of the Colon and Rectum

The rectum is the end of the large bowel just before the anus and the colon extends from the end of the small bowel to the rectum. Cancer of the colon, especially on the right side, is more common in women than in men, whereas rectal cancer is more common in men. The risk factors for these cancers appear to be:

◆ High consumptions of meat and fats.
◆ Low consumptions of fibre-rich and starch-rich foods.
◆ A family member with colon cancer especially at a young age— under the age of forty-five. This may also be associated with cancer of the ovary, the womb or bladder.
◆ Colitis and possibly Crohn's disease.
◆ Possibly poor dietary intake of calcium.

There is some suggestion that the rate of growth of large bowel cancer may be influenced by dietary intake of calcium, with low intakes being associated with a higher risk of cancer or more rapid growth. The results of large calcium supplementation trials are awaited.

Early detection by colonoscopy examination, X-rays and testing the stool for the presence of minute quantities of blood are all important. Blood tests for detecting markers of tumour presence or activity are also being developed.

## Cancer Prevention—General Advice

For over a decade expert committees and Government agencies have tried to give advice on diet and lifestyle for the prevention of cancer. This may prove to be one of the most important public-health messages of all. There are a number of guidelines that have been put forward which fit in with the majority of healthy-eating campaigns. Where possible, the majority of the population should follow the following recommendations:

◆ Do not smoke, and minimise your exposure to cigarette smoke.
◆ Limit your total intake of fats, especially that of saturated animal fat.
◆ Ensure a good intake of fruits and vegetables. The recommended intake is five servings of fresh fruit and green vegetables daily. A large salad portion counts as a green vegetable. Yellow, green and red fruits and vegetables are particularly rich in carotene and related compounds which may be cancer protective.
◆ Minimise consumption of pickled and smoked foods.

## Abigail's Story

Abigail was a forty-one-year-old teacher who was experiencing menopausal symptoms following chemotherapy.

*I was diagnosed as having Hodgkin's disease ten years ago, and had both radio- and chemotherapy. I have been clear ever since, but I really wanted to avoid HRT because of my history. When my menopausal symptoms began, I was aware I had to sort out an alternative. I was having a flush an hour at least, and so I went off in search of a solution.*

*I managed to find the book* Beat the Menopause Without HRT *at my local bookshop which I was delighted to discover outlined a scientifically based alternative. I made an appointment to visit the WNAS clinic and was given a tailor-made programme to follow, avoiding certain grains, alcohol, tea and coffee, and asked to concentrate on foods that contain naturally occurring oestrogens, oily fish and plenty of fresh fruit, salad and vegetables.*

*Apart from my menopausal symptoms, I was very tired for much of the time and constipated. I had been living in the Middle East where my husband was working but felt that the hot flushes were so bad there that I came back to the UK. I followed the WNAS programme avidly and within just a few weeks the night sweats had stopped, the flushes were greatly reduced and my constipation had gone completely. I found the exercise difficult initially as I felt so tired, but persisted with my YMCA video and my tai chi which I feel helped enormously.*

*I have been following the programme for three months now, and all my symptoms have calmed down. I feel so much better and I am confident that I can manage quite happily without HRT. I feel years younger than when I began the programme. I have been able to re-join my husband in the Middle East, which was formerly too hot for me, and I am really looking forward to the future.*

*See also*: Recommended Reading List and Standard References

# CANDIDA AND THRUSH

Candida is one of several types of yeast-like organisms that cause infections in humans. There are a number of different varieties of candida, the commonest being *Candida albicans* which can cause infection in the vagina, mouth and skin. Infection with candida is commonly called 'thrush'. It is also the organism that plays a part in the development of nappy rash in infants. The organism grows best in warm, dark conditions and in the presence of sugar. Under these circumstances candida changes from small round dormant spores to a branching spores to a branching structure called a mycelium with the ability to invade and irritate tissues.

Candida is a very common organism we have all had some contact with, and the majority of infections resolve themselves spontaneously. That said, some women experience repeated episodes of vaginal thrush, and there are usually a number of reasons for this (see below). In the last few years some doctors and complementary practitioners have put forward the idea that a number of health problems including chronic fatigue can be caused by infection with candida. The evidence for this is not strong.

## *What Are the Symptoms?*
This depends where the infection is. For women, vaginal thrush causes irritation and a thick, white, sticky discharge. This must be differentiated from the normal vaginal moisture that naturally increases at mid-cycle and is not associated with local irritation. Severe infections in women can cause swelling of the genital tissues and a rash can spread out into the groin.

In men soreness or redness of the penis, sometimes with a

sticky white discharge, may develop. However, many men and women may carry small amounts of candida in the vagina or on the penis without any ill effects.

Candida is often kept in check by the presence of healthy non-disease-causing bacteria in both the vagina and the bowel. Surveys reveal that about 20 per cent of the normal population carry candida in the digestive tract without it causing problems.

Thrush in the mouth, which mainly affects the ill, elderly or those using steroid inhalers for asthma, produces a very sore mouth and a white sticky deposit on the tongue and elsewhere. A slightly furred tongue without soreness is unlikely to be due to candida.

The skin can be infected too and this is usually in warm moist areas such as the groin, armpits or under the breasts. A red sore rash with spreading little red spots or 'satellites' at the edge of the rash is the usual appearance.

## Who Gets It?

In short, we all do once or twice, but for those who get repeated attacks of vaginal thrush there are often one or more predisposing factors. They include:

- Being pregnant. Hormonal changes encourage thrush.
- The combined oral contraceptive pill. Those with a high oestrogen content may increase the risk; this is rarely a problem with newer low-dose ones.
- Steroid drugs. These, whether taken as tablets or as an inhaler, can encourage the growth of candida.
- Antibiotics. By killing off the 'good' bacteria, antibiotics make it easier for candida to obtain a foothold.
- Diabetes. The increased levels of sugar in diabetes make it easy for the thrush organism to grow.
- Anaemia and lack of iron. These can reduce resistance to infection and lead to cracking at the corners of the mouth making it easy for the infection to get started—one to think of in women with heavy periods.
- Other nutritional deficiencies. Lack of zinc, vitamin B and even vitamin A have all been documented as reducing resistance to infection and leading to thrush.
- A poor diet. A diet high in sugar and low in protein can probably make matters worse, though there is no direct proof of this.

◆ Reduced resistance to infection. Anything that reduces your resistance to infection from stress, genetic and blood conditions to cancer, can be significant.

◆ Hormonal disturbances. Thyroid, other hormone problems and low blood calcium can all (rarely) lead to episodes of thrush.

## What Causes It?

As you can imagine, anyone with one or more of the above pre-disposing factors is likely to experience thrush at some time.

A common situation involves a sexually active woman, possibly on the Pill, who may have a mild iron deficiency, and for whom treatment using over-the-counter creams has been only partially successful. Research suggests that, in recurrent cases, candida organisms on the skin or possibly from the bowel provide a source of re-infection. Sometimes this comes from the male partner, and intercourse or use of a tampon may be factors in causing a break in the delicate tissues lining the vagina and allowing infection to develop.

Wearing trousers, tights, and nylon underwear may all promote the conditions that encourage the growth of candida. Local irritation can be aggravated by use of some chemicals found in many toiletries, bath products, soaps and shampoos so it may be necessary to avoid these. Occasionally it appears that some sufferers are actually allergic to or react strongly against candida itself! In these cases, even a minor degree of infection can result in severe symptoms.

There is also evidence that reactions to foods or yeast in the diet may cause a vaginal discharge. This might cause symptoms similar to thrush without candida being present, or the reaction may encourage the growth of candida already present. So for some a change to a healthier diet that excludes some foods can help symptoms of thrush.

## What Your Doctor Can Do

◆ Examine you and take a swab from the vagina to assess the type of infection.

◆ Prescribe an antifungal treatment as a cream, pessary or tablet by mouth.

◆ Perform some tests to see why you have thrush. A urine test for diabetes and a blood test for anaemia and iron deficiency would be the most common and useful.

There is a wide choice of different preparations available that your doctor may prescribe. They can be creams, pessaries or tablets and they all have similar success rates. The main choices are:

◆ Nystatin (Nystan) as cream or pessaries. Once the most popular treatment, now largely replaced by other preparations. It is safe for use in pregnancy.
◆ Clotrimazole (Canesten) is available as a cream or pessary, and is often the first-line treatment. It can be used as a one- or three-day treatment with similar high success rates of over 90 per cent.
◆ Miconazole (Daktarin) and Econazole (Ecostatin and Gyno-Pevaryl), also available as pessary and cream.
◆ Fluconazole (Diflucan) is a new powerful anti-candida drug which is active by mouth and is highly effective after one single dose of 150 mg. It is very effective against *Candida albicans* but not other types of candida.
◆ Itraconazole (Sporanox) is another new anti-fungal agent which comes in tablet form. Two 100 mg tablets twice a day for one day only will usually clear thrush and it has the advantage of being effective against different types of candida—not just albicans.
◆ Nystatin can also be given by mouth but as it is not absorbed this is only useful in clearing candida from the bowel. It is very useful for helping clear thrush in the mouth.

The key point to remember is that all these treatments have a small failure rate and that if one treatment is not successful then another probably will be.

## What You Can Do

Many women do not go to their doctor but get treatment themselves from the chemist using a number of over-the-counter preparations. This is acceptable if you are reasonably certain that you do not have any other infection, and provided that your symptoms clear within three or four days. If not, see your GP.

It is probably useful for you to know that some 50 per cent of women who think that they have thrush may have a different type of infection, and that the success rate for most standard antifungal treatments is 90 per cent. Consequently there will always be a significant number of women whose 'thrush' did not clear with the first treatment they try. In cases like these there is no substitute for an internal examination, a swab to identify the type of infection(s), and tests in the laboratory to find which antifungal agent is the most effective.

In addition to infection itself, the irritation may be due to some degree of allergy to candida itself, to local irritation from toiletries or occasionally to food allergy. There is no easy way of the sufferer determining which of these might apply to them without expert assessment, so the advice given below is relevant for all eventualities.

- Avoid wearing restrictive clothing such as trousers, tights and synthetic underwear. Choose natural fabrics such as cotton or silk.
- Shower rather than bathe, and do not use perfumed soaps and other toiletries that might come into contact with your tail end. If you do have a bath, do not wash your hair at the same time.
- Dry yourself thoroughly after a bath or swimming.
- Do wash and change your underwear every day.
- When washing your clothes and underwear it may be preferable to use a non-biological washing liquid just in case traces of soap remain in and contribute to the irritation.
- Use sanitary pads rather than tampons.
- Always wipe yourself from the front to the back so as to reduce the chance of infection from the bowel. If you are very sensitive, white unbleached toilet tissue may be a good idea.
- The diet should be low in sugar or sucrose, which means not adding sugar to tea and coffee, avoiding sweets, cakes, biscuits, chocolates and non-low-kilojoule soft drinks. For some a diet low in foods that are rich in yeast can help. Yeasty foods include alcoholic beverages (except gin and vodka), vinegar, pickled foods, yeast extract such as Marmite and many stock cubes, most packaged savoury foods including convenience meals and soups, and bread and buns and anything made from baker's or brewer's yeast. Occasionally it may be necessary for the diet to

be even more restricted than this, but fruit restriction is rarely needed.

◆ Supplements may also be necessary. Consider a yeast-free multi-vitamin if you have recurrent thrush. A supplement of zinc, 20 mg per day, can help, as can a supplement of iron such as ferrous sulphate, 200 mg once or twice a day, especially if heavy periods or anaemia are or have been problems.

◆ Capsules containing preparations of the healthy bacteria *Lactobacillus acidophilus* and related species are available and might help clear thrush from the gut (but not the vagina). Eating live yoghurt might also be helpful, and applying plain live yoghurt *to* the vagina is possibly beneficial but would be no substitute for antifungal medication.

◆ A variety of mild naturally antifungal preparations exist and include those derived from coconut capryllic acid and also one from grapefruit. Alas, their comparative efficacy with standard medications is unknown. Consider if all else fails.

## Sally's Story

Sally was a forty-three-year-old headmistress who also had two young children of her own. She had been diagnosed as having thrush in her oesophagus, which was causing her great pain in the chest, particularly on waking.

*I had continued digestive problems which became progressively worse, so my doctor sent me for investigations. I had an endoscopy, where a telescope is passed into the stomach, and a gall bladder scan, and both were clear, except for the thrush found in my gullet. My worst problem was the extreme pain I experienced on waking each day, and the indigestion. I also had an itchy bottom, so I presumed the thrush went right through my gut. Premenstrually I felt angry and clumsy, and had experienced very sore breasts.*

*My job had become very stressful, I couldn't get on top of it somehow. To make matters worse I developed panic attacks which I thought would subside during the school holidays, but they didn't. My libido had also disappeared and sexual intercourse had become painful as my muscles seemed so tight. A friend recommended I consult a cranial osteopath for my back problem, and as luck would have it he referred me to the WNAS for help with my other problems.*

*I was quite sceptical about diet being the solution to what seemed to be extreme symptoms. I was so desperate that I was willing to try anything, so I went along for an initial consultation, which was very probing. I came away with a programme to start on which involved following an exclusion diet, particularly wheat, foods that contain yeast, caffeine and alcohol. I was asked to exercise and take some nutritional supplements.*

*At my second consultation, which was six weeks later, I was able to report that the pain on waking was only minor and had only occurred once in the last month. My itchy tail had cleared up, my period arrived unannounced with no symptoms or bloating, and I felt that I was on the right track. I continued to make progress on all fronts, until Christmas. I was feeling so much better that I went for the dried fruit, chocolate, orange juice and wine. The symptoms flared up and it took a couple of weeks to calm down again, but it really brought home to me how sensitive my body was to these foods and drinks.*

*I have taken up jogging again, which I used to love, and I feel wonderful. All my gut symptoms have disappeared, I no longer feel like I have thrush, my PMS has gone, and I am coping really well with situations at work and at home. We have been juggling with my diet for the last six months, and I have gradually been able to add things back without seeing a return of symptoms. I feel very confident that I can manage my health myself now with my new knowledge, and be there for all those who depend upon me.*

*See also*: The Yeast-free Diet, The Very Nutritious Diet. Plus References.

# CARPAL TUNNEL SYNDROME

This is a common condition where there is pressure on the nerves in the wrist, causing numbness and tingling in the hands, and typically affects the dominant hand of women. Symptoms are worse at night, or on waking in the morning, and the sufferer may have to get out of bed and shake their hands to achieve relief. The pain may also travel back up the arm. The times when it is more likely to occur are during pregnancy, around the time of the menopause and in old age.

## What Causes It?

The common causes include:
- fluid retention
- underactive thyroid
- in pregnancy, hormonal changes
- in obesity, additional strain on the joints
- arthritis of the wrist, particularly rheumatoid arthritis
- over-use during sports, such as tennis or squash

The nerves that carry signals from the brain to the hand pass through a tunnel constructed by the carpals, wrist bones, on the way to the fingers. Sometimes when there is excess fluid in the area, or a change in the shape of the joints as seen in arthritis, then additional pressure may be placed on the nerves running through the tunnel, causing pins and needles, and numbness in the fingers and the arms. When the body is warm the blood vessels swell a little, which accounts for the fact that carpal tunnel syndrome is often worse during the night.

## What Your Doctor Can Do

- Give injections of steroids at the wrist to reduce swelling.
- Prescribe splints to be worn at night—these can be surprisingly effective.
- Diuretics are sometimes recommended.
- If all else fails, recommend an operation to relieve the pressure on the nerves.

## What You Can Do

- Lose weight if you need to.
- Follow a low-salt diet to reduce fluid retention.
- Don't drink alcohol.
- Take supplements of vitamin B complex and B6. Several studies have shown that relatively high doses of vitamin B6, 100 mg daily, may help relieve symptoms. Not all studies have been positive. This is best taken as B complex, 50–100 mg once daily for three months.
- Visit your osteopath for an assessment.
- As a temporary measure, at night, raise your arms above your head to allow the fluid to drain away from the carpal tunnel.

◆ Use ice packs on the wrists to reduce the heat, and subsequently the swelling.

The numbness and tingling very often disappear of their own accord after pregnancy, so it is unlikely that you will have to take any further action after the baby has been born.

### Complementary Therapies

Acupuncture is well worth a try, as are homeopathic remedies, but remember to follow The Low-salt Diet as well. Cranial osteopathy probably has more to offer than any other complementary therapy for this condition.

*See also*: Fluid Retention, Obesity and Thyroid Disease. Plus References.

# CEREBROVASCULAR DISEASE

Cerebrovascular disease is a furring up and sometimes blockage of, or bleeding from, the major blood vessels that supply the brain. Commonly this causes what is termed a stroke or cerebrovascular accident where there is a sudden development of weakness, loss of sensation, loss of balance, vision or consciousness.

### Who Gets It?

The same people who are predisposed to ischaemic heart disease and peripheral vascular disease. The main risk factors seen in practice are:

◆ very high blood pressure
◆ excess alcohol consumption
◆ obesity
◆ smoking

If all four are present, then it is simply a matter of time. Other important risk factors are:

◆ a family history of strokes
◆ the presence of any heart abnormality that may lead to a blood clot forming in the heart chambers which can then break off and travel to the brain
◆ a wide variety of blood-clotting problems and other rare conditions
◆ rarely, but worthy of mention—migraine headaches. Occasionally if these are very severe they may result in a small stroke with residual numbness or tingling in a limb as a consequence. The risk of this is greater if the woman is on the oral contraceptive pill and a smoker. One suspected event like this means that oral contraceptives are to be avoided for ever more

Prevention is the key, as damage to the nervous system from a stroke often leads to a degree of permanent disability. Large strokes and repeated small ones are frequently fatal. Warnings, however, do occur. Small strokes called transient ischaemic attacks, TIAs, commonly precede an impending major cerebrovascular accident. Warning symptoms include symptoms indicating a loss of neurological function which lasts for several minutes or hours and is followed by full or nearly full recovery. These warning episodes include loss of vision, loss of speech, weakness in a limb, loss of feeling in one side of the face, in a hand or a limb, transitory mental confusion or other unusual transitory feelings or disturbed sensations. Combinations of these may occur often with a headache.

## What Your Doctor Can Do
◆ Examine you and quickly assess the main risk factors. The blood pressure, the health of the heart, the presence of diabetes can all be checked quickly.
◆ Prescribe a daily dose of aspirin. This simple drug at a dose of up to 300 mg per day significantly reduces the risk of these warning episodes developing into a stroke.
◆ Treat any high blood pressure. This is probably the next priority.
◆ Assess the likelihood of a major narrowing of the carotid artery—the main artery in the neck. Listening with a stethoscope in the neck gives an idea of this possibility. Further

specialist referral may lead to defurring of the artery by operation—worth it for severely narrowed arteries.

◆ Consider other treatments and assessments. Many of these, which are needed for young patients, those with a strong family history of strokes or high risk predisposing blood disorders, will mean specialist referral.

◆ For those who have had a stroke, hospital treatment is the rule for anything other than the very elderly. Specialised X-rays help decide if the stroke is due to a bleed, the formation of a clot or an embolism—a blood clot from a distant site, usually the heart—which has travelled to the brain.

## What You Can Do

◆ See your doctor at the first sign of trouble.
◆ Do as your doctor says and take any recommended medicines.
◆ Change your diet. Reducing weight, cholesterol and blood pressure by dietary change is very important. High intakes of fresh fruit has been known for years to be associated with a lower risk, and vegetables are protective too. Visit your fruit shop on the way home from the doctor and before you see your solicitor.
◆ Drink alcohol only very moderately.
◆ Do not smoke.
◆ Take some supplements. In theory there should be a substantial role for some supplements but large trials have yet to be performed. Poor dietary intakes of vitamin C, a low blood level of retinol—vitamin A—are risk factors for having a stroke or making a poor recovery from one. A reasonable suggestion might be a stronger multi-vitamin containing 200 mg of vitamin C and 200 IU of vitamin E. Other supplements of fish oils, magnesium and vitamin B might also be worth considering on an individual basis.

## Complementary Therapies

One exciting development is acupuncture. A London-based trial involving conventional doctors and traditional acupuncturists has apparently shown, at least initially, an improvement in the degree of recovery after a stroke in those patients who have received acupuncture. The full report will undoubtedly merit much study and attention. If this proves to be the case, then a long overdue role for the acupuncturist in the district hospital will come into being.

# Coeliac Disease

Coeliac disease is a condition where there is marked sensitivity to a protein found in wheat and other grains. As a result there is damage to the lining of the small bowel, resulting in difficulty absorbing a number of essential nutrients. There may also be a wide variety of other symptoms seemingly unrelated to the digestive system.

## What Are the Symptoms?

Typical features of coeliac disease are weight loss, muscle wasting, diarrhoea, abdominal bloating, fatigue and anaemia. Other not infrequent problems include poor growth in children, delayed puberty, mouth ulcers, fatigue without other features, absent periods, infertility in the male or female and, rarely, heart or arthritic problems.

Under the microscope the lining of the small bowel is made up of tiny finger-like projections called villi. These become shrunken and finally disappear, with malabsorption resulting. This whole process takes many months, even years, and equally recovery on a specialised gluten-free diet can also take several months.

## Who Gets It?

- Coeliac disease is a disease of Caucasians. In Australia, between 1 in 500 and 1 in 1000 people are believed to be affected and many are still undiagnosed.
- There is a strong genetic tendency, with a high risk, if you have an identical twin who is affected. Lesser degrees of sensitivity and change in the bowel may be present in many first-degree relatives of those who have this disease.
- A possible predisposing factor is the early introduction of wheat and other grains into the infant's diet. Now, the recommendation is that wheat is not introduced before four months of age. This may have resulted in a fall in the incidence of childhood coeliac disease.
- Infection with a virus may also be a trigger, perhaps only in predisposed individuals.
- Coeliac disease is also associated with diabetes, thyroid disease and some types of arthritis.

## What Your Doctor Can Do

◆ Investigate suspected cases with:
  ◇ Biopsy of the small bowel taken via a telescope. This usually gives a definite or near definite answer. Subsequent avoidance of gluten should result in marked improvement in the bowel appearance as seen on a second biopsy.
  ◇ Perform blood tests to look for anaemia, nutritional deficiencies and patterns of antibodies that would support the diagnosis of coeliac disease.
  ◇ Perform a barium meal X-ray of the small bowel, which doesn't confirm the diagnosis but may help exclude other conditions.
  ◇ Sometimes challenge with a gluten preparation and repeating the bowel biopsy are necessary to confirm the diagnosis.
◆ Treat with a gluten-free diet which means not consuming wheat, oats, barley and rye, and any food made from them. The degree of sensitivity may be remarkable with even modified starch, communion wafers and some beers causing problems. The advice of an experienced dietician is invaluable, especially for those whose illness does not recover promptly.
◆ Correct nutritional deficiencies. Supplements of iron, folic acid and zinc may be needed. Those with severe malabsorption may also need calcium, vitamin D and multi-vitamins. Eventually long-term supplements should not be required. However there may be a slight relative lack of calcium, selenium and possibly other nutrients. Whether these are important is not certain.
◆ Very rarely patients do not improve with a gluten-free diet, and other treatments are needed: these include steroids and immune system altering drugs.
◆ In the long term other bowel problems may develop despite careful adherence to a gluten-free diet. Life-long follow-up is recommended and re-investigation of those with a return of symptoms is needed.

## What You Can Do

◆ Follow The Gluten-free Diet carefully. Keeping a diet diary for four weeks, which is then reviewed by the dietician, is a useful exercise. It allows assessment of nutrient intake, and may allow early identification of foods that may not be gluten-free.
◆ Other foods may sometimes need to be avoided. Sometimes

milk products contribute to the diarrhoea, possibly because of their lactose (milk sugar) content. When recovery is complete, some of the eliminated foods may be able to be re-introduced into the diet. Sometimes other food sensitivities exist; soya is a particular possibility.

◆ If your bowel has recovered completely, there is recent evidence that some coeliacs are able to tolerate oats. This cereal is lower in gluten than the others. Discuss this possibility with your specialist or dietician.

◆ Take supplements of zinc if appetite is poor, there is poor resistance to infection or a poor response to a gluten-free diet.

### Special Note for Mothers

It would seem prudent for all new mothers who are coeliac not to introduce gluten-containing cereals, including oats, into their children's diet until at least after their first birthday, possibly even later. Refer to the Weaning Section in *Healthy Parents, Healthy Baby*.

# CONSTIPATION

Constipation is a common affliction of those living in industrialised countries. It is a result of the bowel becoming sluggish and therefore not doing its job properly, usually due to a lazy bowel muscle which does not contract regularly and strongly, or bowel muscles that do contract, but in a poorly coordinated fashion.

There are two layers of muscle throughout the gut which extend from the throat. They are involved in swallowing, the passage of food through the gut, and the expulsion of waste from the rectum and anus. They all work to propel food through the gut while it is being broken down, digested, and absorbed into the body, and while the waste residues are formed. The whole process normally takes between one to two days in most men and up to three days in women.

In order for food and digestive material to pass smoothly along the bowel, both muscle layers must work together in a carefully coordinated fashion. First, the ring muscles, which are found at the entrance or exit to the stomach, must relax. This relaxation is then followed by a wave of muscular contraction which pushes a ball of food along the gut and slowly down its length. Each muscle contraction is preceded by an area of muscle relaxation before it. The high pressure generated by the bowel contraction pushes the bowel contents forwards into the low-pressure area of the relaxed bowel. This is what would happen in a healthy gut.

## What Are the Symptoms?

Apart from resulting in much attention being placed on the bowel, constipation can result in a most uncomfortable feeling in the lower abdomen, sometimes accompanied by wind and pain. Straining on the toilet can result in haemorrhoids.

When the bowels are working normally they are usually emptied daily, with perhaps one or two motions. Those who are constipated cannot seem to empty their bowels more than once or twice each week, at even longer intervals in severe cases, and usually with the use of laxatives.

What is not widely appreciated is that other disturbing health problems are also associated with severe constipation in young women. These include:

- hormonal abnormalities, such as a low oestrogen level
- more painful and irregular periods
- breast lumps and pre-cancerous changes in breast tissue
- a greater chance of hysterectomy or operation for a cyst on the ovary
- pain on intercourse and difficulty achieving orgasm
- infertility
- hesitancy in starting to pass water
- cold hands and a tendency to faint

## Who Gets It?

Women are more prone to constipation than men. Firstly the gut transit time is faster in men than women (the time it takes for food to be processed from one end of the gut to the other). Secondly, the bowel seems to be slowed by the presence of oestrogen, the female sex hormone.

In some women with constipation the muscles of the pelvic

floor are tense and not able to relax properly. These muscles support our urethra, allowing water to pass from the bladder to the outside world, and the walls of the vagina as well as the bowel. You can feel these muscles by pulling in your tummy and drawing your buttocks together, as if you were trying to stop the flow of urine in mid-stream. If these muscles are tense and do not relax then the motions cannot easily pass through.

Approximately 50 per cent of the women we see in our clinics each year suffer with constipation to some degree, and in many cases have done so for years.

## What Causes It?

### Lack of fibre

A number of experts have recommended that Australians and New Zealanders should increase their fibre intake. This means that everyone, in theory, should eat more fruit, vegetables and cereals (bread and other foods containing wheat, oats, barley, rye and sweetcorn/maize). The theory is the increased amount of fibre (and, if you remember, fibre is the food that does not get digested) would increase the stool output and reduce the gut transit time. But it doesn't work like that for all of us, unfortunately. In fact it is now acknowledged that some cereals can actually *worsen* constipation.

### Wheat and other grains

Although bran has been heralded as the best remedy for constipation, and is still recommended by many doctors today, more recent evidence suggests that it may serve to worsen symptoms in some people. Early studies in the *Lancet* medical journal showed the benefits of bran in some of a small sample. (Interestingly, these doctors used Allinson's bran; Dr Allinson was a nineteenth-century doctor struck off the medical register for advocating the health benefits of wholemeal as opposed to white bread.)

More recently the *Lancet* carried a report from a group of specialists at Addenbrookes's Hospital in Cambridge, led by Dr John Hunter, which told a rather different story. Their observation was that the avoidance of certain foods helped two-thirds of their patients who had erratic bowel habit including constipation. Wheat was reported as the most common aggravating food, and subsequent work has confirmed this initial observation. Wheat and its associated grains—oat, barley and rye—which all contain the protein gluten, can cause either constipation or diarrhoea.

### Tea

It seems that tea slows down gut-transit time for 50 per cent of people, according to a Scandinavian study. It can then aggravate constipation, having the opposite effect to coffee.

### Dehydration

Lack of fluid is sometimes a cause of constipation, particularly in hot climates. If you take fibre supplements you will need to drink an extra two glasses of fluid per day.

### Periods

It is now widely known that many women become constipated in the week before their period is due. The normal rate at which food moves through the gut slows down, and may well contribute to the abdominal bloating that many women experience premenstrually.

### Magnesium deficiency

Magnesium is needed for smooth muscle control. As the lining of the gut is made up of smooth muscle, when levels of magnesium are low, as seems to be the case in over 50 per cent of women with PMS, the muscle groups do not contract and relax in their usual sequence, and constipation results. Taking supplements of magnesium, to correct levels, seems also to ease constipation.

### Stress

Stress affects the movement of food through the gut. Studies have shown that any stress can inhibit the normal regular contractions that occur spontaneously as part of the digestive system, and might aggravate constipation.

### Pain

Understandably, any painful pelvic condition, including ovarian cysts, endometriosis, period pains, or post-childbirth pains, can easily inhibit the urge to go to the toilet. In addition to these sources of discomfort, piles, or a tear in the margin of the anus or an anal fissure, are almost always associated with a powerful spasm of the muscles in the anus also, making it very difficult for motions to pass through.

### Drugs

A number of drugs can cause constipation as a side-effect, the most common of which include antidepressants and painkillers.

Antidepressants are frequently accompanied by constipation, a dry mouth and sometimes blurred vision, especially at the start of therapy or if high doses are used. This effect is most noticeable with older types of antidepressants such as amitryptiline (Lentizol, Triptizol) and desipramine (Pertofan).

Strong painkillers which are derived from morphine, such as codeine, will invariably cause constipation. This means that when taking any painkiller that contains codeine or dihydrocodeine you can expect to become constipated.

### Lack of exercise

As we get lazier as a nation, the incidence of heart disease, stroke and obesity increases. There is nothing like a good workout to get the bowels moving, so if you have a sluggish bowel and you are not exercising, turn to page 31 and get started!

## What Your Doctor Can Do

- ◆ Recommend a diet rich in fruit and vegetable fibre, rather than bran or wheat fibre.
- ◆ Offer laxatives or a fibre supplement.
- ◆ If the onset of constipation is sudden in an older patient, and accompanied by bleeding or pain, your doctor should test for an underlying reason, like colon cancer. This may mean performing tests for hidden traces of blood in the stools, X-rays or arranging a specialist examination.

## What You Can Do

- ◆ Eat plenty of fibre-rich foods. These include fruit, vegetables, nuts and seeds, some cereals like brown rice, sweetcorn (maize), buckwheat, sago and tapioca. Take care, as some of these foods might make other symptoms worse, especially if you have bloating and wind.

◆ Take a fibre supplement. This can be from your doctor or from a health-food shop. Good supplements include those containing sterculia (Normacol), linseeds (Linusit Gold) and, when tolerated, coarse oats. These are all highly water retentive and can be very effective, especially when combined with other measures to stimulate movement through the gut.

◆ Ensure a good intake of fluid. This is very important if you are elderly or when taking a fibre supplement.

◆ Avoid wheat, oats, barley and rye. Avoid too all foods containing them. This is a major change to your diet, and you will need to refer to the suggested menus given in the Exclusion Diets in Part Three.

◆ Cut down or stop your tea consumption. Limit yourself to two cups of weak tea per day, or drink a herbal alternative.

◆ Drink one or two cups of coffee instead of tea. This may act as a laxative for some. The stimulating effect appears to take about 60 minutes before it is noticeable.

◆ Have a cigarette! Yes, if you are already a smoker, you may be aware that a few puffs—especially first thing in the morning or after your main meal—can stimulate your bowels. This is no recommendation to start smoking and no excuse not to give up, but if you do smoke you can sometimes help your bowels along.

◆ Take some magnesium. This is particularly effective if you don't suffer with intermittent diarrhoea as well, and have premenstrual problems or suffer fatigue. Some women find that it is better for them to take magnesium last thing at night, gradually increasing the dose to what is called 'gut tolerance level'. This means that you will reach a level when the magnesium *causes* diarrhoea, and you will then need to cut back. A safe starting dose is between 200 and 400 mg per day. We frequently have patients who take a combination of linseeds with their morning cereal and up to 800 mg magnesium at night in order to control their constipation. We use magnesium amino acid chelate because it is gentle on the gut, but magnesium phosphate will do. Magnesium hydroxide, in the form of a white liquid and sulphate, in the form of crystals are available from some chemists, and are much more dramatic in their effect.

◆ Take regular exercise. Try exercising three or four times each week. Choose a form of exercise that you have enjoyed in the past so that you continue on a regular basis.

◆ Avoid stressful situations whenever possible. Stress can cause muscles to go into spasm. Yoga is an excellent way of helping your body to relax and improve tolerance of stress. Listening to music, going for a walk, eating a good meal or just enjoying the company of family and friends, are all useful and effective ways of reducing tension.

◆ Set aside time for your bowels. Some of us need peace and quiet and plenty of time to relax our muscles so that the bowels work properly. If you prefer to be undisturbed, choose a time when you can be alone, take the phone off the hook if necessary, and make a hot drink. A morning exercise session may stimulate the bowels too. Try to open your bowels at a regular time each day, like after breakfast or after your main meal— our bodies like habits.

◆ Take a laxative. If the other methods have failed, try a herbal laxative or ask your pharmacist to recommend a preparation that you can buy over the counter.

## Complementary Therapies

There are numerous treatment approaches to try to help relieve the symptoms of constipation. Massage is a favourite one, as it encourages peristalsis, which is the coordinated wave-like muscle contractions that take place in the gut, and will also release tension in those muscles. You should have a regular professional massage, and do some self-massage of the tummy and lower back in between.

Colonic irrigation is said to be effective at flushing out the toxins in the bowel and some people swear by it. Although it is a good idea to flush out the bowel and start again as it were, colonic irrigation is aiming at symptom relief rather than addressing the root cause. But it may be worth a try.

Both acupuncture and herbal medicine are likely to be useful tools, helping to get your whole body functioning optimally. A herbal practitioner can also prepare a special cream for you to insert into your back passage to soothe piles and help to heal cracks and tears.

Taking time to relax formerly each day, perhaps combining relaxation with some self-massage is one way that you can help to speed up the recovery process.

## Nicole's Story

Nicole, a thirty-seven-year-old doctor and mother of two children, had been suffering with constipation for many years.

*I'd had constipation for so long that I thought it was normal for me. I remember a representative from a pharmaceutical company raving about a product for constipation called Regulan which I subsequently tried. It did make a bit of difference to start with, but not a great deal. I remember being constipated during pregnancy. I also developed haemorrhoids after my first pregnancy which were made worse by the constipation. I usually open my bowels every few days and my motions were very hard and pellety.*

*After the birth of my second child I sought advice, as I thought I had a prolapse. However surgery was not practical at the time, as I would have to avoid lifting for two months—impossible with a toddler. Because of the prolapse, in order to pass a motion, I had to actually stick my fingers into my vagina as otherwise everything just sat in my rectum and would not come out naturally. At the end of the day I nearly always felt as if 'everything was falling out' particularly after a large meal. However, I decided I would at least try and get help with my haemorrhoids, and was told they were due to a weak pelvic floor and that I must avoid being constipated at all costs!*

*I heard an interview with the WNAS on the radio and decided to get some advice about my diet, as I was also suffering from PMS which had worsened after my second child. Even though I'm medically qualified I had had so little education on the subject of nutrition as part of my training. The WNAS was brilliant—my constipation and PMS are now a thing of the past. I was recommended supplements of magnesium and organic linseeds to help combat the constipation, and in addition I eliminated certain foods such as wheat, rye and oats from my diet. I must say I have not been constipated since the week after I began the programme.*

*I have to watch my diet, and when I eat foods I should not be eating I can feel some of the symptoms starting up again, but this time I know how to put it right. I don't have that 'falling out' feeling any more, and I have no problems actually passing a motion any more. My bowels feel normal and the prolapse is much better now that I don't get constipated. My severe PMS has gone and I feel comfortable physically and mentally. I feel that I have had my eyes opened.*

*See also*: Irritable Bowel Syndrome. Plus Suggested Reading List (*Beat IBS Through Diet*).

# CROHN'S DISEASE

Crohn's disease is named after an American physician who, over sixty years ago, described, with others, this chronic inflammatory disease of the bowel whose cause remains as elusive as it was then. This condition can affect any part of the bowel from the mouth to the anus. Young adults are those who are most commonly affected, and it seems to affect equal numbers of men and women. Typical features are diarrhoea, abdominal pain and weight loss. The affected parts of the bowel become swollen and inflamed, with large numbers of white cells being present, though what has stimulated this reaction is unclear. Most usually the small bowel, which is primarily involved in digestion and absorption, and the large bowel, are the main targets for this disease.

At times the inflammatory process extends to other distant parts of the body, namely the eyes, joints and skin.

## What Causes It?
This is a much debated subject, with a mixture of genetic and environmental factors at work.

◆ It tends to run in families. In identical twins, if one has the disease, there is nearly a 66 per cent chance that the other will develop it. However, it is rare for both husband and wife to suffer.

◆ Dietary factors are a possibility. Recovery from Crohn's disease can be achieved by the exclusion from the diet of a variety of foods. Whether this is due to an actual allergy or the influence of some foods upon the type of bacteria present in the bowel is uncertain.

◆ Infection with either the measles virus, or a bacteria that is a distant relative of that which causes tuberculosis, are two possibilities.

◆ Immune system overactivity is a possible factor, causing the body to over-react to the presence of bacteria, or even to attack the body's own tissues.

◆ Smoking, antibodies against baker's yeast, the swallowing of toothpaste, and not being breast-fed as an infant, are all possible contributing factors.

## What Your Doctor Can Do

- Assess the extent of the disease. Barium X-rays, examination of the lower or upper bowel with a flexible telescope called an endoscope, and use of radioactive white cells are all used for this.
- Perform blood tests. These will assess disease activity, anaemia and nutritional deficiencies, especially iron, vitamin B12 and zinc.
- Give advice on diet. Any one of the following types of diet may be appropriate. This is best determined on the basis of specialist recommendation:
  - ◇ A high-kilojoule, high-protein diet for those with weight loss and nutritional deficiencies.
  - ◇ A low-fibre diet for those in whom the bowel is very inflamed.
  - ◇ A diet that avoids milk and milk sugar (lactose) for those who are sensitive to it/them.
  - ◇ An exclusion diet if multiple food sensitivities are suspected.
  - ◇ A diet using only specialised pre-digested foods—an elemental diet—used in a hospital setting.
- Prescribe drug therapy. Steroids are the mainstay of treatment, and high doses are required if the illness is severe. Other anti-inflammatory and immune system altering drugs are used, especially if the patient repeatedly needs high doses of steroids. Antibiotics are used for infective complications and sometimes to help with the bowel disease.
- Consider surgery. This would be to remove severely affected parts of the bowel or to tackle the inflammation if it has spread to neighbouring areas.

## What You Can Do

- Take your medicine regularly.
- Staying in regular and good contact with your specialist is very important. Crohn's disease is never cured, and the quality of care will depend on a good two-way flow of information.
- Stop smoking if you are a smoker.
- Avoid foods that aggravate your symptoms. This will for the majority of patients require some expert advice along the lines given above. It seems that the commonest foods to aggravate Crohn's disease are the same that aggravate irritable bowel disease. These are:

◇ wheat and other grains and all foods such as bread, cakes and pasta

◇ milk and cheese

◇ coffee, and possibly tea

◇ some fruits, especially raw, with orange and tomato the most likely

◇ foods that contain baker's yeast, e.g. bread and some buns

◇ other yeast-rich foods, e.g. alcohol, vinegar, pickled foods and yeast extract

◇ foods that are hard to digest, e.g. sweetcorn and beans.

Many of these can be easily avoided without recourse to expert advice. You will need to avoid the foods for three or four weeks to see if there is any improvement.

◆ Take supplements. Probably the simplest supplement to take for those who are not receiving specific advice on this from their doctor is a high potency multi-vitamin multi-mineral preparation. This may need amending if the following situations are present:

◇ severe diarrhoea—a soluble vitamin supplement may be better absorbed

◇ blood loss or anaemia—iron supplements may be needed

◇ poor wound healing or reduced resistance to infection—supplements of zinc

◇ prolonged bleeding in those with severe disease or receiving antibiotics—supplements of vitamin K

◇ long-standing disease with osteoporosis—calcium supplements

◇ sulphasalazine therapy—folic acid supplements

◇ severe or long-standing diarrhoea and muscle cramps—extra magnesium or potassium supplements

◇ severe disease and a restricted diet or special feeding regime—supplements of the mineral selenium

◇ damage to the terminal ileum or its surgical removal—vitamin B12 by injection

◇ severe or long-standing disease and poor night vision—vitamin A

If any of these situations apply, you should discuss the need for such supplements with your specialists. All of these nutrients can be tested for, though some require the use of a specialised laboratory. Correcting any nutritional deficiency can only help, and it is possible that doing so may positively influence the degree of inflammation, the rate of wound healing, resistance to infection, appetite, general well-being and possibly the future risk of cancer.

## Complementary Therapies
None are likely to be effective enough to control the disease.

# CYSTITIS

Cystitis is an inflammation of the bladder caused by a bacterial infection or a mechanical disturbance in the area. Vigorous sexual intercourse can be a trigger, which is why it became known as 'the honeymoon syndrome'. Consequently it should come as no surprise to the reader to discover that cystitis is nearly thirteen times commoner in the general female population than in nuns. Studies estimate that one woman in five will have had a recent episode of cystitis. It is the fifth most common problem managed in general practice.

## What Causes It?
- In approximately 50 per cent of cases the organism *E. coli*, which sometimes travels from the anus area. The bacteria penetrate the urethra, via the perineum, and work their way into the bladder. There is a clear association between diaphragm users and cystitis, again because of the *E. coli*.
- Vigorous sexual intercourse can bring on symptoms.
- Tight clothing, which can put unacceptable pressure on the urethra.
- Vaginal deodorants and disinfectants can also bring on symptoms.
- A prolapse may restrict the urinary flow and predispose an infection.
- Caffeine affects the muscles of the bladder and aggravates symptoms of urgency.

## What Your Doctor Can Do

- ◆ Test your urine to determine which sort of bacteria are present and whether they are sensitive to any particular types of antibiotics.
- ◆ Prescribing antibiotics is the usual method of treatment. However, studies have shown that approximately two-thirds of female sufferers recover naturally without antibiotics, and even after treatment with antibiotics symptoms can return.

## Penny's Story

Penny was a thirty-seven-year-old researcher who had been suffering with bouts of recurrent cystitis. These were becoming almost constant by the time she approached the WNAS.

*I had my first episode of cystitis three years ago. It was painful and unpleasant, but it came and went and I didn't give it much thought. The following year I had three separate bouts which I found alarming. I consulted my doctor and researched self-help methods to overcome the symptoms, but nothing really seemed to help. This last year, I reckon I had cystitis every month, at period time. I really lived in dread of the symptoms as the month progressed.*

*I approached the WNAS for advice after reading one of their books as I was suffering with diarrhoea, and horrendous period pains. I completed their question-naire and diet diary, and then made an appointment for a telephone consultation. I was given a programme to follow which involved changing my diet, taking regular exercise and some nutritional supplements. I also started being meticulous about my hygiene, and began using baby wipes after going to the toilet.*

*To my absolute delight I haven't had any cystitis since I began the programme, the diarrhoea has cleared up and I have now had several pain-free periods. I am amazed and relieved as I am due to get married in a few months' time and we are hoping to start a family straightaway.*

## What You Can Do

- ◆ Drink plenty of liquids, particularly water, throughout the day. Aim to have the equivalent of a glass of water every hour whilst the symptoms are acute to flush your system through.
- ◆ Drink a few glasses of cranberry juice each day as this affects the lining of the bladder and reduces the growth of pus cells.
- ◆ After sex and after a bowel movement wash yourself carefully

with warm, unperfumed soapy water, wiping yourself from front to back to wash the germs away. Sit so that your anus is at a lower point than your urethra, and let the water run down to wash away any faecal bacteria.

◆ Choose unperfumed bath products, as allergies can develop, and the urethra may become inflamed as a result.

◆ Add a small amount of bicarbonate of soda to the water you drink; this can help to ease the symptoms by making your urine more alkaline.

◆ Avoid drinking caffeine, and use alternative drinks, as coffee can make the bladder irritation worse.

◆ If you use a diaphragm, and your symptoms are recurrent, try switching to an alternative method of contraception for a while.

## Complementary Therapies

Homoeopathic remedies like Cantharis, Staphisagria or Apis may well bring relief. Herbal remedies may also be helpful as an adjunct to the conventional methods of overcoming symptoms of cystitis. Aromatherapy can be useful and juniper oil can be used as part of a lower abdominal massage.

*See also*: Recommended Reading List and References.

# DEMENTIA

Dementia is the subject of many jokes, has numerous terms to casually define it, and is something we often casually admit to suffering ourselves. But true dementia is really no joke. It is characterised by a loss of cognition, which means a loss of the ability to use one's mind in a variety of ways; this includes memory, use of language, visual awareness of space, perception, thinking and problem-solving and personality. Significant loss of two or more of these functions in someone would qualify for a diagnosis of dementia. Underlying psychiatric problems such as depression or a physical illness that reduces the level of consciousness (e.g. heart disease) must first be excluded. One in five of elderly people aged eighty years or more will develop dementia. There are in fact many causes, a few are treatable and there may be some with a nutritional element. Alzheimer's disease accounts for approximately two-thirds of cases.

## How to Recognise Early Dementia

This information is presented as an aid to relatives and friends of those who might be developing a problem. The majority of such cases present slowly, almost insidiously, and it is not usually until there have been several events that real suspicion should arise. Then only assessment by an experienced doctor will lead to a proper diagnosis. There are a number of questions to be asked, such as, 'Is the problem really dementia, or is there some other illness?', 'What is the likely cause?' and 'Is it treatable?'

The most useful information comes from a close relative or similar witness. They should be asked to describe suspicious events where the person's mental functions may have failed them. Then the following checklist should be answered:

- memory, both for recent events and for distant ones
- use of language, finding and using words correctly, understanding what is said or written, reading and writing ability
- numeracy, especially with money when shopping
- perception: of self as in appearance and dressing; of nearby objects; and of where they are and ability to find their way around
- thinking, planning and problem-solving
- personality and conduct toward others
- features of depression
- delusions or hallucinations

Many other details are important to assess the general level of health including:

- consumption of alcohol and tobacco
- use of drugs
- past health, especially heart disease, and if there is a history of a stroke
- a recent fall or injury

- the presence of a severe headache
- loss of control of the bowels or bladder
- recent weight loss or fever
- type of diet consumed
- the cause of death or state of health of all first-degree relatives.

## What Your Doctor Can Do

After assessing the problem the next step is to examine and then investigate the patient. This will mean a number of tests including those for:

- anaemia and infection
- kidney and liver function
- calcium, sodium and potassium
- vitamin B12, folic acid and possibly vitamin B1
- thyroid function
- chest X-ray
- X-ray of the brain—CT scan

The purpose of these tests are to exclude causes of dementia other than Alzheimer's disease, and identify those few that are treatable. Particular thoroughness should be shown if the patient is young, the deterioration is rapid, there is an unsteady gait, loss of control of eye movement, a loss of bowel or bladder control, a tremor or features to suggest repeated small strokes, infection or a disturbance in metabolism.

Treatment may involve drugs, surgery and occasionally correction of nutritional deficiencies or treatment of an infection or a metabolic problem.

Very often the diagnosis is one of Alzheimer's disease which can only be made by the exclusion of other conditions as there is no test for it. The theories behind the causation of Alzheimer's disease include genetic predisposition, aluminium accumulation, and past head injury. The greatest risk factor is by far and away age. Treatment is very unsatisfactory. Only one drug has had any real success and that is Tacrine which is of very limited benefit. It helps maintain the level of chemicals involved in the transmission of signals from one nerve cell to another.

## What You Can Do

The information here tells you how you may help someone with dementia.

- Don't give up hope. The rate of decline is very variable. Join an appropriate patient group.
- Get them to eat as well as possible.
- Cut down on alcohol if this is excessive (more than 2 units per day).
- Get their doctor to check their drugs if they are taking some and decide whether they are all really necessary.
- Maintain a daily routine. This helps them to remember what they need to do.
- Label things and rooms if they are forgetful.
- Help keep them physically active. A 30–40 minute walk per day is ideal.
- Help them keep mentally active. This may help them preserve their faculties. Reading, watching TV (and discussing it), keeping up hobbies and socialising are all important.
- Supplements of vitamins may be appropriate. Vitamins B and C if deficient can have a small influence on concentration. There is no harm in giving a modest supplement of these especially if the diet is less than perfect. Expect no miracles.
- Inform the driving licence authorities.
- Make arrangement for the management of the person's financial affairs.

## Complementary Therapies

Complementary therapy is unable to reverse the process of dementia.

*See also*: References.

# DEPRESSION AND MOOD SWINGS

We all experience mood changes from time to time, which is a perfectly natural phenomenon. Bad news, the loss of a dear one, prolonged dull weather, financial problems and lack of sleep are a few examples of changes that may depress our mood. The majority of us bounce back relatively quickly, but for approximately one in ten women symptoms of depression become chronic, even when the apparent stimulus is long gone.

Mood swings are a lower harmonic of depression, and affect us at different times in our lives. As women we experience numerous hormonal events which can leave us feeling drained. Childbirth is a good example. Before a period or during the menopause are other key times when extra nutrient demands are placed upon us. When we are unable to meet the demand, symptoms of depression and mood swings can result. From a survey we conducted at the WNAS on 1000 patients with premenstrual syndrome, we discovered that 96 per cent of them suffered with mood swings in their premenstrual phase, 62 per cent severely; 94 per cent of the women also suffered from premenstrual depression, 83.8 per cent severe to moderately. This, we felt, was a frighteningly high number, and in view of the possible consequences of depression, not something that should be taken lightly. As premenstrual depression is such a common condition, we will deal with the cyclic aspects of depression, before going on to examine the more chronic symptoms.

## *Premenstrual Mood Swings*

Depression is a common premenstrual symptom, and usually presents with other symptoms such as anxiety and breast tenderness. In 1959 Dr Katharina Dalton published a study in the *British Medical Journal* which showed that the time of admission to hospital of depressed patients coincided with the menstrual period, the premenstrual phase, and ovulation. Our research also showed that those most likely to suffer from premenstrual depression are more often overweight and do less exercise than non-sufferers.

The balance of certain nutrients has an important influence on both hormone and brain chemistry. Magnesium, for example, influences how the ovaries respond in the normal menstrual cycles, and many other nutrients are also important in this respect. It is also known that in people with severe depression the chance of finding some degree of B vitamin deficiency is much higher than would be expected in the general population. These nutrients have been used successfully in treating both PMS and depression.

The balance of hormones—or whatever determines their balance—seems to be crucial in controlling mood, and as the years pass by it becomes even more apparent that our diet and lifestyle can influence our hormones and our moods.

## What Your Doctor Can Do

The average woman who complains to her doctor about fluctuating moods and depression in her premenstrual phase, or at the time of the menopause, will probably not have any physical symptoms. As the majority of family doctors lack information about nutrient levels, they will have a limited number of options on offer.

- First you would be given a physical examination, with routine blood screening to eliminate the possibility of an underlying problem.
- If nothing tangible is found, your doctor is likely to either offer hormone treatment or tranquillisers.
- An enlightened doctor would ask you about your eating and exercise habits, and about your stress levels.
- You may be referred for some counselling.
- Alternatively, you may be simply told to pull yourself together.

## What You Can Do

- Follow the recommendations in Premenstrual Syndrome, and the dietary recommendations.
- Use the Supplement Chart on page 410 to work out which supplements you should be taking, and ensure that you take them regularly, at least until your symptoms have abated.
- Get some help to sort out any stressful situations that face you, including your current commitments, if you find them overwhelming.
- Never underestimate the value of exercise—it has been scientifically proven to influence your mood and helps to lift depression. You need to exercise for at least four good sessions each week.

◆ Make some time for yourself, no matter what your schedule, and don't be afraid to indulge yourself in the odd treat now and then, most of us more than deserve them!

◆ Spend time with friends who like to laugh, and watch some comedy films.

◆ Hum in the bath, and at other convenient times. Sound therapists have discovered that humming alters our breathing pattern and as a result increases our energy levels and raises our mood.

## Complementary Therapies

Our recommendations are pretty good at sorting out premenstrual mood swings and depression, but it may take a few cycles before you feel the benefit. In the meantime, it is worth trying some herbal preparations, or a homoeopathic remedy or two.

# Chronic Depression

Unlike premenstrual depression, a true depressive disorder persists, and the symptoms are not linked to the menstrual cycle. True depression can accompany a physical illness or can be an illness in its own right. So the first thing a doctor has to do is eliminate an underlying physical cause before assuming that you are suffering with pure depression. One to two men per thousand suffer with depressive disorders, three times as many women.

## What Are the Symptoms?

The main features of a depressive disorder are low mood, lack of enjoyment and loss of interest in usual pastimes, and becoming generally withdrawn. Often people suffering with depression also have disturbed sleep and wake early in the morning, lack energy and find that their appetites for both food and sex are reduced. They seem to see life through dark grey glasses, and are pessimistic, regard most endeavours as hopeless and often display suicidal tendencies. Even their physical appearance may be affected with a downturned mouth, frown lines on their forehead and a stooped posture.

In rarer cases people suffer hallucinations and delusions, which are thought to centre around guilt, feelings of worthlessness, illness and poverty, and this is termed psychotic depression. When these symptoms are present the risk of suicide is usually at its peak.

Most depressive illness, when untreated, lasts for between three and nine months, although it can drag on for years, and is recurrent. So unless you address the root cause of the symptoms you can expect future episodes.

## Key Features of Depression
- depressed mood, or mood swings
- lack of energy
- lethargy and despondency
- unable to experience enjoyment
- pessimistic attitude
- suicidal thoughts
- regretful and guilty recollections
- disturbed sleep with early morning waking
- insomnia or somnolence
- reduced appetite for food
- loss of libido
- constipation
- weight loss or weight gain
- amenorrhoea (absent periods)

## What Causes It?
There can be many underlying causes of depression:

- Marital problems, bereavement, redundancy, financial stress and so on. Very often symptoms of depression can arrive as the result of an accumulation of stresses and strains.
- An under-active thyroid gland can produce symptoms of depression, and so too can other serious illness, like cancer, kidney, liver or heart disease, anaemia and diabetes.
- Serious infections.
- Alcoholism—prolonged consumption of excessive amounts of alcohol.
- Repeated lack of food.
- Chronic pain.
- A drug side-effect.
- Deficiencies of B vitamins, calcium, magnesium, copper, iron potassium, folic acid or essential fatty acids. Numerous studies have shown that patients with depression commonly have low levels of one or more of these nutrients.

◆ Excessive consumption of caffeine, as heavy caffeine users have a tendency to be more depressed and have a lower academic performance.
◆ Food sensitivities.

## What Your Doctor Can Do

◆ Determine whether you are suffering with pure depression and that there is no underlying physical cause for your change in mood. This would be done by physical examination and routine blood tests, to check for anaemia, infection, thyroid function, and kidney and liver disease. There would also be a urine test to check for diabetes.
◆ Decide whether you need help from a psychiatrist, or whether you should be treated in the surgery. As a rule of thumb, those who are suicidal, not eating, or who are hallucinating should be given specialist help without delay.
◆ Advise counselling that would help you deal with immediate problems, and come to terms with past traumas.
◆ Encourage you to take each day as it comes, and to temporarily relinquish some of your responsibilities.
◆ Prescribe antidepressants. There is now a bewildering choice. Remember that there is a lot of individual variation in response and several may need to be tried before one is found to be effective. A psychiatrist may use stronger drugs like Lithium, a mood regulator, or ECT, electro-convulsive therapy, which is not common these days because it causes irreversible brain damage.

## What You Can Do

◆ Eat wholesome food regularly, and in particular avoid sweets and chocolate as these can worsen symptoms, especially when they are eaten in the place of nutritious food.
◆ Follow the recommendations for The Very Nutritious Diet.
◆ Spend some time in a stress-free environment with a companion who is willing to listen to you.
◆ Get some help to sort out the immediate stress or trauma you are facing.
◆ Ensure you get plenty of fresh air and sunlight, when available, each day.
◆ Exercise six days per week to the point of breathlessness, as

this will induce an endorphin release, which helps to lift you out of your depression.

◆ If possible, arrange to have your nutrient levels measured so that you can determine whether you have any deficiencies.

◆ Take supplements of high-potency multi-vitamins, B vitamins, vitamin C, magnesium and anything else that may be indicated following your tests.

◆ Spend 15–20 minutes each day relaxing to soothing music, or a relaxation tape, or perhaps try some yoga or meditation. Follow the recommendations in Part One re relaxation.

Essentially, what you need is good food, nutritional supplements, plenty of exercise, good company, a break from your routine, and time to reflect and reorganise.

## Complementary Therapies

The medical herbalist will undoubtedly have a potion for you. Basil and St John's Wort, amongst other herbs, may be helpful. Likewise, the homoeopath will choose a remedy to suit your individual set of symptoms. Aromatherapy massage might help to ease the blues also.

## Justine's Story

It was clear from the outset that thirty-six-year-old Justine was an unusual patient. She was intelligent, and although significantly depressed, had very clear insight into her problems after twenty years of depression. In particular she had observed that throughout her large family virtually all the female members were miserable. She had coped with her depression well, only rarely making use of antidepressants. She had managed to develop a career in administration which she continued with full time, even though she had a young child.

The pattern of her depression made her feel that there was some chemical basis and she thought that, at least in part, this might have a nutritional component. She was a non-smoker and ate a reasonably good diet, although occasionally convenience meals had to be used because of her busy lifestyle. She drank 15 to 20 units of alcohol a week when she first saw us.

Indeed there is research to support her suspicions. Sometimes depression does run in families and subtle changes in brain chemistry are known to occur with certain patterns of depression. The accepted treatment however involves antidepressants.

In Justine's case nutritional investigations revealed markedly abnormal results. The levels for vitamin B1 and vitamin B6 were extremely abnormal, putting her easily into the worst 1 per cent of results for patients we see. There was a reduced level for magnesium and a borderline level for vitamin C. Low levels of these nutrients are associated with depression, fatigue and increased risk of suicide. The severity could not be explained by her diet and thus it is possible that there was some genetically determined metabolic factor contributing to these abnormalities. Without investigating other members of the family it would be impossible to be certain about this.

She began an improved diet, together with supplements of high-strength vitamin D, multi-vitamins and magnesium. Her day-to-day depressive symptoms lessened and in the following month her premenstrual mood changes were also diminished. She chose not to continue with the antidepressant which had been prescribed by her psychiatrist. Episodes of stress and arguing with her husband became less. She was careful to limit her alcohol intake to 14 units a week as levels greater than this may indeed increase a demand for vitamin B.

She may well prove to be the sort of person who needs to take vitamin supplements long term in order to maintain good physical and mental health.

## Depression, Postnatal

This brand of depression occurs after the birth of a baby, and can vary from the 'baby blues', which may arrive in the first seven to ten days after giving birth, to a full-blown psychotic disorder, with total rejection of the baby. The baby blues is very common and, in a well-nourished mum, should pass almost as quickly as it arrived. Severe postnatal depression is far less common, and needs immediate attention.

The most common symptoms of the baby blues include depressed mood, crying, insomnia and irritability, and are experienced to some degree by at between 66–85 per cent of women, depending on the criteria used to define it. It is thought to occur in women who have a history of premenstrual syndrome. Postnatal depression is less common, affecting some 10 per cent of women, and it has been noted that there is often a previous history of depression in this group of sufferers.

## What Are the Symptoms?

- mood changes that vary from depression to elation
- lack of interest in the baby
- withdrawn and tearful
- irritable
- extreme fatigue
- insomnia
- anxiety
- thoughts of suicide
- thoughts of harming the baby

## What Causes It?

- It is thought that fluctuating levels of the hormones progesterone and oestradiol shortly after the birth of a baby may be an underlying cause. However, there are differing opinions amongst the medical fraternity.
- Thyroid insufficiency occurs in approximately 5 per cent of women.
- Low levels of nutrients, particularly vitamin B6, calcium, magnesium and essential fatty acids, may be factors.
- An unsatisfactory relationship or lack of support from family members.
- Disrupted lifestyle or status as a result of the birth.
- A difficult labour that did not fulfil a woman's hopes.

## What Your Doctor Can Do

- Check your thyroid function, including a check for thyroid antibodies.
- Check your iron levels, and in an ideal world your blood levels of calcium, B6 and magnesium, all of which have been shown to be low in some women in clinical studies.
- Arrange for some counselling to help you talk through your emotions.
- If the symptoms persist, prescribe antidepressants.
- In a minority of cases of extreme postnatal depression the help of a psychiatrist and hospital treatment will be necessary.
- There are ways in which the family can be more supportive. A home help for two weeks is often a good idea.

## *What You (and Your Family) Can Do*

◆ Communicate. You should never feel ashamed of feeling low after the birth of a baby. Your family and friends will want to support you, so you must let them know how you feel.

◆ Offload any responsibilities you can. In those first few weeks after having a baby Mother Nature prefers you to be supported, in a calm environment, and to take time to get to know your baby, whilst getting your strength back. Not so many years ago, women were expected to 'lie-in' for four weeks after having a baby. Translated, this meant that everyone else rallied round to do the household chores and the new mum was left to feed, sleep and get to explore her new relationship with the baby.

◆ Eat well. If possible, get your partner, friend or relative to prepare wholesome meals for you. If you are breast-feeding you will have increased nutrient demands which you need to bear in mind. Follow the recommendations for The Very Nutritious Diet, and refer to the Nutritional Content of Foods lists in Appendix I. The nutrient demands that are placed on you during pregnancy and breast-feeding are greater than at any other time in your life—so make sure the cook knows that!

◆ Take supplements. Research shows that many nutrients, including essential fatty acids can be in short supply after the birth. Take a good strong multi-vitamin and multi-mineral supplement, and evening primrose oil combined with marine fish oil.

◆ Get out regularly. Walk out with the pram in the fresh air every day, even short distances will make a difference.

◆ Have time for yourself. Get your partner, friend or mum to look after the baby for a few hours on a regular basis, so that you can have some time for yourself. You may choose to sleep initially, especially if you are having disturbed nights. Take advantage of the time, get your hair done, buy some new clothes, or meet up with a friend for a bit of reassurance.

◆ Take regular exercise. Six weeks after the birth you should be able to do a gentle workout. Stretching exercises will help to restore your muscle tone, and will make you feel better about yourself. Gradually, over the months, ease into low-impact aerobics, as this will encourage the release of the brain chemicals, endorphins, which help to raise your mood.

◆ Try to socialise. Make every effort to attend social gatherings in your area, particularly those run by Early Childhood Development Centre. It will be good for you to meet other new mums, many of whom will be experiencing the same problems as you. You could support each other.

A healthy diet, vitamin and mineral supplements, plenty of rest, adequate sleep and a supportive and loving environment seem to be good treatment for postnatal depression. It is noteworthy that during pregnancy and whilst breast-feeding, the demands for calcium, magnesium and the B vitamins are very high, and a loss of most of these can cause changes in mood. It often is that simple.

## Complementary Therapies

There is no harm in trying a herbal or homoeopathic remedy alongside the recommendations made here. A session with the cranial osteopath after the birth will help to realign the body, and massage, especially with relaxing aromatherapy oils, would be soothing. But remember that correcting nutrient levels and environmental stresses and strains has to take first place.

## Lorna's Story

Lorna battled with postnatal depression for two years following a very traumatic delivery.

*I only had one child—I could never face having another one, as it was such an awful experience for me. My husband particularly wanted children and so I agreed to have a baby more to fulfil his needs than mine. The pregnancy was relatively uneventful, although I don't remember enjoying it much and must admit I tried to disguise my shape for several months. I did all the right things during pregnancy though, such as giving up alcohol, eating well, exercising and resting, but the effect Caroline's birth had on me was overwhelming.*

*I found delivering the baby hard work, and just after she had been born the cord ruptured whilst I was attempting to deliver the afterbirth. I remember blood pumping out everywhere and being given an emergency general anaesthetic to enable the doctor to manually remove the placenta. My husband was literally left 'holding the baby' while all this was happening before his eyes. I was given 4 units of blood and prayed that it was not contaminated—something that troubled me* for years and years afterwards. When I came round I remember seeing tubes everywhere and felt so utterly sorry for myself. I was not interested in the baby at all. When the nurse asked if I wanted to feed the baby I felt like telling her to get lost.

I was in hospital for ten days and home for a week before we moved house. The move had been planned before Caroline was born. Although I did want to settle in the new house, with hindsight, moving so soon was probably a very bad idea. My husband, sensing I needed help, offered to take extra time off work but being very independent I assured him I could manage. Consequently I was left at home attempting to go through the motions of looking after Caroline in our new house but spent most of the day crying while she cried. I can remember rocking the pram so hard to try and quieten her down that she almost fell out.

I did not go to see my GP as I was ashamed of my feelings and felt that I should have been able to pull myself together. I know I wasn't in my right mind at the time. All I could feel was the baby encroaching on my space, preventing me from leading my life. I remember one night when my husband was away, she was screaming with earache and I could not get her to take any medicine or calm her down. In the end I closed the door to her room and went off and left her. I felt so bad about it afterwards that I started drinking alcohol. I suppose I was trying to numb my senses.

My husband has since told me that he was convinced he would come home from work one day and I would have gone, leaving Caroline behind. I was awful and felt ill. I had diarrhoea at least six or seven times a day which was totally out of control and my wrist bones became so painful that I couldn't even lift the baby out of the bath.

My health visitor suggested I take evening primrose oil, which did help a bit. I made an appointment to see a psychotherapist privately and had three sessions of talking my problems through. This seemed to help too.

I eventually settled in to a routine of having horrendous premenstrual syndrome, and this is what eventually drew me to the WNAS. With my new knowledge from the WNAS and a lot of hindsight I realise that a combination of being unprepared for the baby, lack of sleep once she was born and inadequate levels of important nutrients affected my brain chemistry, and as a result, badly affected my sanity. I had no training to be a mother and, it seems, no instinct. I feel looking back I could have looked after my cat better than I looked after Caroline. I feel so guilty about the way I treated her.

Thankfully I have really sorted myself out completely now. I don't have any more PMS, I don't drink alcohol and I absolutely adore Caroline. The WNAS was my refuge I honestly feel it saved my sanity and since going on my *programme I have been able to find my emotions and develop a very wholesome relationship with my daughter. There is nothing I wouldn't do for her and I would certainly like to make up for my lack of mothering in the past.*

# DERMATITIS (ALLERGIC)

Dermatitis literally means irritation of the skin, and the term is sometimes used to mean the same as eczema. However 'dermatitis' is now used to describe an irritating red, sometimes scaly, rash that has followed contact or exposure to a number of possible agents.

Common irritants include:
◆ washing-up liquid
◆ acids
◆ alkalis
◆ many cleaning agents
◆ glass fibre as used in insulation

Usually it is the area of skin that is most exposed to the irritant that develops the rash.

Sometimes an allergy develops to something that is in contact with the skin. In this situation even very small amounts of the allergen will cause a rash in some, unlike common irritants. The culprit agent may have been used without difficulty for years as sensitivity may take a long time to develop. Common agents causing allergic dermatitis include:

◆ Cosmetics, perfumes, hair bleaches and dyes, chemicals used in 'perms', lanolin or wool fat
◆ Metal, mainly nickel, found in cheaper jewellery, studs in jeans, wrist-watch bands
◆ Rubber, from rubber gloves, scuba diving suits and elastic bands to condoms!
◆ Foods, when handled—garlic and citrus fruit are particularly troublesome

- Medicines, local anaesthetics, antibiotic creams and even steroid creams
- Other compounds, wood, plants, rosin from pine trees which is found in paper and glossy magazines, plastics, dyes used in leather, pesticides and other garden chemicals

## What Your Doctor Can Do

- Skin patch testing will help to identify the cause of the dermatitis. This is particularly important when employment is affected.
- Avoidance is always important and can not only resolve the problem but may after several years lead to a clearing of the sensitivity.
- Steroid creams are useful for severe acute episodes.

## What You Can Do

- Make sure that your skin is as healthy as possible, as dry, cracked or broken skin makes it easier for contact allergies to develop.
- Use cotton-lined rubber gloves when doing the dishes, or when your hands are in water.
- Use hypo-allergenic soaps and cosmetics, and wash your clothes in non-biological washing powder or liquid.
- A healthy diet and supplements of multi-vitamins and zinc might be useful if the skin is particularly poor quality, and you do not eat as well as you might. Supplements of evening primrose oil are worth considering if your skin is very dry.

## Complementary Therapies

These may not be very successful as the cause really needs to be addressed, and this is usually physical. Herbal treatments may be worth considering.

❖

# DERMATITIS (SEBORRHOEIC)

This is a red, greasy, scaly dermatitis which develops usually on the face, especially around the sides of the nose and the ears, on the front of the chest or at the back between the shoulder blades. Dandruff, eyebrow and even eyelid scaling can also develop. Mild forms of this are often referred to as 'combination skin', with some parts of the face being greasy and others dry and scaly. In some cases the rash is worsened possibly caused by the presence of a superficial yeast infection with *Pityrosporum ovale*. Anti-fungal treatments can be very effective.

## *What Your Doctor Can Do*
- Ointments based either on mild steroids or salicylic acid can be used on the face and trunk.
- An ointment of lithium and zinc (Efalith) can be quite effective.
- Scalp scaling can respond to tar-based shampoos, and anti-fungal shampoos (ketoconazole, Nizoral).
- Anti-fungal creams are sometimes helpful.

## *What You Can Do*
In certain deficiency states, very similar skin problems develop. This applies to deficiencies of vitamin B (especially pyridoxine, B6, riboflavin, B2, and biotin) as well as zinc.

So try the following:

- Eat The Very Nutritious Diet.
- Take a vitamin B supplement providing 50 mg of B6 and B2, a supplement of biotin, at least 300 µg per day, and 30 mg of zinc.
- Sunbathe. This sometimes helps.
- Try using some plant oil extracts, some of which come as shampoos, as these may have anti-scaling and anti-fungal properties. Tea tree oil and juniper berry are two suggestions.
- Possibly try dietary exclusion, but this is probably only worth considering as a last resort or if there is an element of eczema present as well. True sensitivity to yeast does seem particularly likely if there is facial eczema.

## Complementary Therapies

Try homoeopathy and herbalism. Some plants and plant oil preparations could have anti-fungal activity and be quite effective.

## Raylene's Story

Raylene looked every year of her forty-eight. Her red puffy face was covered by a fine, dry, scaly rash. This was bad enough, but it was her severe scalp scaling that really troubled her. Scalp irritation had been unrelieved by many types of shampoo, and even a steroid scalp application. The cause of the rash was unclear. It had possibly been triggered by a reaction to a hair-dye applied six months earlier, but this did not explain why it was persisting so severely.

She had been under considerable stress over the past year and as a consequence had been smoking 20 to 25 cigarettes daily, and drinking perhaps up to 20 units of alcohol per week.

The failure of her scalp and skin conditions to respond to more standard treatment suggested that there may have been an untackled nutritional cause. Investigations revealed evidence of moderate deficiency of the vitamin biotin, and there were reduced levels of some of the essential fatty acids derived from vegetable and fish oils.

She was asked to halve her cigarette and alcohol consumption, eat a healthier diet and to take supplements of high strength vitamin B with biotin, together with evening primrose oil and fish oil.

The response was gratifying. Over six weeks her scalp irritation diminished considerably, and the rash on her face and scalp scaling improved markedly. Over the next three months the transformation was nearly complete.

On reflection it was felt that her increased alcohol intake had placed a strain on vitamin B metabolism that had cost her her previously good complexion. It is interesting how, in the development of a deficiency, the body will probably, quite correctly, 'sacrifice' the nutrient levels in the skin before other parts of the body are affected. This has good survival potential for vital organs such as the liver, kidneys and brain, but does mean we become less beautiful. At least this gives us some outward sign that all is not well internally.

# DIABETES MELLITUS

The term diabetes, used without qualification, is taken to mean diabetes mellitus. In this condition there is a chronic rise in the level of glucose in the blood which routinely spills out into the urine. This gives the condition its name: diabetes meaning 'a flowing through' and mellitus 'sweet'. Thus the urine is passed in excessive amounts because the high level of sugar in the urine pulls water along with it. Thus the typical presenting symptoms are:

◆ increased passage of urine
◆ increased thirst
◆ a craving for sweet foods
◆ fatigue due to the effects of this upon the body's metabolism

Other features include changes in visual acuity, recurrent thrush, muscle cramps, tingling in the feet and hands and constipation.

Blood glucose levels are controlled by what we eat, a variety of hormones and the function of the liver and muscles. In medicine there is in fact a wide variety of situations, many of which are rare, where blood glucose control is disturbed. Understandably this happens with liver and muscle disorders and a number of exotic hormonal conditions, as well as in some pregnancies. The most important hormone in blood glucose control is insulin, which is produced by the pancreas, a gland situated in the abdomen. The role of insulin is to help glucose pass from the bloodstream into cells, especially the nervous system, muscles and the liver. To all these organs glucose is a source of energy, and uniquely for the nervous system it is the only source of energy that it can use.

Diabetes used to be simply divided into two main types—insulin-dependent or IDDM, and non-insulin dependent, NIDDM. In the insulin-dependent variety there is a lack of the hormone which must then be given by injection. In the non-insulin dependent form there is plenty of insulin or related forms of the hormone, but the tissues of the body are relatively insensitive to it. This type does not need insulin but a diet and drugs that improve the body's response to insulin.

There is now a more complicated classification based upon not only the need for insulin but the probable cause(s) of that type of diabetes.

## What Causes It?

This is one of the great questions of twentieth-century medicine, and it is being answered in a curiously piecemeal way. The pieces of the jigsaw include the following.

◆ Genetic factors are particularly important for the insulin-dependent diabetic. It is predominantly a disease of Caucasians, but not exclusively from the northern parts of Europe. There are many environmental factors too: if members of a low-risk population, such as the Japanese, emigrate to a high-risk country like the USA, their risk pattern follows that of USA residents.

◆ Genetic factors also appear for the non-insulin dependent diabetic. This, usually adult onset form of diabetes, seems to run in the female line of the family, may be linked with other conditions affecting muscles, and also with a tendency to high blood pressure and raised blood fats.

◆ Immune changes causing the body to produce antibodies that attack the insulin-producing cells of the pancreas. This may be genetically determined and triggered by some viral infections.

◆ Food allergy! This is a possibility, as some researchers report that the antibodies involved in cows' milk allergy can also react against the pancreas. This seems particularly relevant to children.

◆ Being overweight is an extremely important risk factor especially for the elderly with NIDDM.

◆ Being small at birth has also been shown to be a risk factor, perhaps reflecting a reduced ability to produce insulin in a form that is functional. This risk does not appear until later life, and can become marked if the individual is obese, has high blood pressure and elevated blood fats.

◆ Diseases where the pancreas is damaged or destroyed.

◆ In association with various types of malnutrition in Third World countries.

◆ In association with a number of other hormonal problems affecting the adrenal glands, the ovaries.

◆ Rare genetic disorders.

- Following drug therapy, especially thiazide diuretics if deficient in potassium.
- In pregnancy resulting in the birth of a large baby.

This is a fantastically diverse list. In practice, for the majority of those with, or at risk of developing, diabetes, dietary factors are the most important area that we can do something about on an individual level.

## *What Your Doctor Can Do*

- Make the diagnosis using blood and urine tests. Sometimes this is easy if there are large amounts of sugar in the urine or blood. The presence of ketones in the urine detected by a simple dip test means that insulin will need to be given.
- Treat with insulin. This is necessary with the majority of young patients where the diabetes is due to a lack of insulin from the pancreas. There is a variety of different types of insulin and varying treatment regimes which may need to be adjusted to suit a person's lifestyle. Injections several times per day are usually required. Minute pumps that provide insulin on a continuous basis rather like the human pancreas are being developed.
- Treat with drugs. There are two types which are most suited to older patients where there is a supply of insulin but the tissues are relatively insensitive to it. One type, the sulphonylureas, acts by increasing the amount of insulin released and is the main type used. The second, biguanides, is usually used in conjunction with the sulphonylureas and they act by altering the metabolism of glucose in the liver and other organs. Both are always used when diet alone has not worked.
- Advice on diet. This has assumed increased importance over the years. It is clear that the control of blood glucose, the risk of serious and less serious complications are to a large degree influenced by the diet. The standard recommendations are as follows:
  - ◇ Eat an appropriate amount of kilojoules to achieve a reasonable weight. For most NIDDM patients this will mean losing weight. This may well be all that is required to normalise blood glucose levels.
  - ◇ Eat regularly; consume three meals a day and, where necessary, snacks between meals. These are likely to be

needed by children, those who are physically active, and pregnant women, provided they are not overweight.

◇ The diet should contain a large amount of foods that are slowly digested and therefore cause only a small rise in blood sugar. This means excluding or severely limiting the consumption of sugar, cakes, biscuits, white and, to a lesser extent, wholemeal bread. Desirable foods are beans, peas, lentils, pasta, oats and oat products, whole-wheat cereals, sweetcorn and most fruits.

◇ High-fat foods are to be limited. Intake of saturated fats in particular should be curbed. This means consuming low-fat dairy products, including low-fat cheeses, trimming all visible fat from meat before cooking (by grilling or baking), not eating the skin of poultry and fish and not eating fried foods.

◇ Suitable oils for cooking are those high in polyunsaturates, e.g. sunflower, safflower, corn and soya. Olive oil can be used in small amounts as can walnut oil. Butter should not normally be used and margarines high in polyunsaturates used.

◇ High-cholesterol foods should also be limited, especially if the blood fats are high. Up to eight eggs per week can be consumed.

◇ Further dietary advice may well be needed for those with heart or kidney disease, or who are pregnant, or for those whose diabetes is particularly difficult to control.

◆ Monitor your progress. Regular attendance at a clinic, either at your general practitioner's or at the local hospital, will allow the early identification of problems and their treatment. These checks involve measurement of:

◇ weight

◇ blood pressure

◇ measurement of glycated haemoglobin which gives a good long-term measure of blood glucose control

◇ examination of the urine for sugar, protein and blood

◇ examination of the eyes for blood vessel changes

◇ examination of the heart, occasional checks on blood cholesterol and triglycerides

◇ examination of the feet to check circulation and nerve function

These measures need to be looked at alongside your measures of progress (see below) in order to get the full picture.

◆ Treat complications as they occur. Hopefully at an early stage. Changes in the eyes, kidneys, nerves, blood vessels affecting circulation to the heart, feet and brain are all possible and may respond to treatment with drugs, surgery or better diabetic control.

◆ Tackle special situations. Infection, surgery, pregnancy and coma. These often require the services and expertise of several specialists in a hospital setting.

## What You Can Do

◆ Learn all about your diabetes. Telephone Diabetes Australia for information. Be a professional patient.

◆ Monitor your diabetes. This means regular, usually daily, tests of blood sugar for all those with IDDM, urine tests of sugar and sometimes protein. The intention is to keep the blood sugar level between 4 and 9 mmol/l, though this may vary from person to person. There should be no glucose in the urine if kidney·function is normal.

◆ Be strict with your diet. A high intake of beans, for instance, may cause an increase in abdominal wind and bloating. Be patient, this should settle after two or three months. Ask your partner to be considerate too.

◆ Exercise regularly. This helps keep weight down, reduces blood cholesterol, lowers blood pressure and may improve blood glucose control. The minimum is to walk for 30 minutes four times per week.

◆ Don't smoke.

◆ Limit alcohol intake. This should be kept to an average of no more than 2 units per day, with up to 4 units on special occasions.

◆ Be aware of hypoglycaemia. This is low blood sugar and could be dangerous! Symptoms include light-headedness, confusion, anxiety feelings, palpitations, hunger, shortness of breath and sweating. Unfortunately some diabetics have little warning of these episodes and loss of consciousness develops quickly. This is very important if they are driving or in charge of machinery.

◆ Take some nutritional supplements. This is a very difficult but potentially important area. Many small reports associate diabetes with a lack of essential nutrients; this is most common if diabetes has been present for many years, if there is a poor response to insulin, and in older diabetics or those with complications. This lack of nutrients may not be corrected by a standard diabetic diet.

Potentially important nutrients are:

- Vitamin B1. Thiamine is needed to metabolise glucose. Those first beginning on oral medication, alcohol consumers and the elderly are at risk. Fatigue, muscle pains in the legs and loss of feeling in the hands and feet are early symptoms.
- Magnesium. Lack may develop with vitamin B1 deficiency, especially if the diet is poor. Lack of response to insulin and increased risk of damage to the blood vessels at the back of the eye can be features of a lack of this nutrient.
- Chromium. This is a curious trace element worthy of a particular mention in diabetes. It is involved in influencing the tissues response to insulin which is clearly important in the elderly diabetic with NIDDM. So much so that marked chromium deficiency produces a state virtually indistinguishable from this type of diabetes and is also associated with an increased risk of cardiovascular disease. Potentially correcting a deficiency of this trace mineral could be beneficial to many diabetics. We will have to wait for more research to be performed to be certain about the role of chromium.
- Zinc. This is easily lost in the urine in diabetics. Poor resistance to infection, poor wound healing and possibly reduced response to insulin may be features.
- Vitamin B6. Pyridoxine has been used successfully to help control the diabetes that develops in pregnancy.
- Anti-oxidants. These include vitamins E, C, A as beta-carotene, and selenium, and they are all involved in minimising the damage to tissues that occurs as a part of ageing or with an altered metabolism. They may prove to be important in the progress of vascular disease, heart disease and cataract formation in the diabetic.
- Polyunsaturated fatty acids. These are essential nutrients, and high intakes of the Omega-6 series from vegetable oils may reduce the risk of developing problems with the blood vessels at the back of the eyes. Specialised forms of these fats, such as

evening primrose oil, have been used with a little success when the nerves are damaged by diabetes. Fish oils might be beneficial too in reducing blood stickiness, but there could be problems with this.

Expert advice and individual assessment would seem the best way forward until there are large and long-term trials to assess the benefits of using these types of supplements. It should be remembered that they are no substitute for good dietary control and, where necessary, insulin and drug treatment.

**Important note**
Do not take vitamin and mineral supplements, except perhaps for low-dose preparations, without the permission of your doctor. At times their use could alter insulin requirements and blood glucose control. Hypoglycaemia, a low blood glucose, could occur as a result.

## Complementary Therapies

There is no substitute for standard care. Some homoeopathic remedies are reputed to affect blood glucose control but you need to see a medically qualified practitioner, especially if you are taking insulin. Acupuncture could be helpful when there are problems with the nerves, especially in the legs.

## Sophie's Story

Sophie is a forty-four-year-old veterinary nurse who has been diabetic since puberty. She also had a history of repeated viral infections, including meningitis and shingles, and there was a strong suspicion that a virus infection had triggered her diabetes. Once, before attending the clinic, she had another viral infection that was just a bout of flu, which left her feeling very tired indeed, so that she had had to give up work. Her diabetic control had deteriorated and she had made several attempts to improve this by adjusting her dose of insulin.

Her fatigue every day was quite severe, with muscular aches and pains, and the diabetic specialist discovered that her sodium level in the blood was very low. Investigations also revealed low levels of many other nutrients, especially magnesium, zinc and vitamin B.

She made some changes to her diet, took supplements of all of these nutrients, except for sodium, and also took a multi-vitamin preparation. Her energy level duly improved, as did her diabetic control. Hopefully her resistance to viral infections will also improve.

Low levels of magnesium are common in diabetes and may influence the balance of other minerals, especially sodium and potassium.

*See also*: References.

# DIARRHOEA

Symptoms of diarrhoea are frequent or loose stools. 'Frequent' means having more than three motions per day, and 'loose' means that the stools are not formed, and vary from a soft putty consistency to watery. Diarrhoea mainly occurs because food has moved too quickly through the gut, and there has not been time for the water in the bowel to be absorbed.

## What Are the Symptoms?

Diarrhoea is usually associated with an urgency to go to the toilet, and is often preceded by pain or waves of muscle contractions, often influenced by diet or the environment. Most of us will have experienced examination nerves, where we have had to rush off to the toilet. Some sufferers may not experience any pain before an episode, and in these cases there seems to be relatively little bowel muscle activity. The diarrhoea can therefore be due to over-sensitive bowel muscles or to the contents of the bowel irritating the bowel in some way. The gut transit time is increased in diarrhoea sufferers from the usual 48–72 hours to a mere 24 hours. Experiencing these symptoms every day may well leave the sufferer feeling washed out and nutritionally deficient.

## Who Gets It?

There is no age limit for diarrhoea. Young children sometimes have persistent symptoms which are often linked to food allergies. Adults may suffer similarly, or notice that symptoms of diarrhoea follow a bout of gastroenteritis or food poisoning. It is not so common as constipation, but still widely experienced by women, especially around the onset of a period, when there is a brief release of inflammatory chemicals as the uterus sheds its lining. Long-term symptoms should undoubtedly be investigated by your doctor, especially if self-help measures fail.

## What Causes It?

◆ Food intolerance. This is often the underlying reason for diarrhoea, which can occur at any stage in life, particularly following stress or trauma, when the immune system is impaired.

◆ Milk. Some people, especially children and infants, may react to the protein in milk and this can cause abdominal pain (colic in an infant) and sometimes diarrhoea. Drinking reduced fat or skimmed milk won't usually make a difference, as this only reduces the fat content, not the protein or milk sugar. Other signs of allergy that may be present are eczema, asthma or rhinitis.

◆ Lactose. Milk sugar can sometimes cause problems. If there is an inability to digest lactose, then sugar passes into the small bowel and colon, where it acts as a potent laxative. The severely affected sufferer would be troubled with symptoms within an hour of consuming milk or soft cheese, although small amounts of hard cheese or milk itself may be tolerated. This type of food intolerance is quite common in those of Eastern European, Middle Eastern or Asian origin.

People who are truly lactose intolerant may be able to tolerate lactose-free milk, which is available in some supermarkets, and hard cheeses, as they contain relatively small amounts of lactose.

◆ Wheat and other grains. Sensitivity to wheat, oats, barley and rye has been recorded as a cause of diarrhoea, especially in women. It seems that very sensitive individuals do react to wheat which can cause some minor but definite damage to the lining of the gut which results in diarrhoea. This situation is similar to, but not so severe as, coeliac disease. This is by no means accepted as conventional medical wisdom, even though a group of ten such patients were described as long ago as 1980 by one leading group of gastroenterologists from Birmingham in the UK.

◆ Eating a large meal. When the stomach becomes distended a reflex contraction of the muscles of the colon occurs which is known as the gastro-colic reflex. This explains why many people need to empty their bowels within an hour of having a large meal. It is not the meal we have just eaten coming through, but probably the day before's moving on.

◆ Fatty foods, too much and too little. When fat remains undigested in the small bowel it can be broken down into irritating acids by bacteria in the large bowel, which again can result in diarrhoea a few hours after eating a large or rich meal. This is most evident in those with digestive problems, and in the elderly, especially if there is weight loss.

At the other end of the scale, fat in smaller quantities actually slows down the rate at which the stomach empties and food moves along the small bowel. As it takes time to digest fat from a meal, the gut may become sensitive to its presence. Certain foods containing oleic acid, such as olive oil, almonds, hazel nuts, Brazil nuts and avocado pears, are particular offenders. The low-fat theory may explain why toddlers and children who consume low-fat cows' milk products suffer with diarrhoea, and are more prone to acute gastroenteritis.

◆ Coffee. This, unfortunately, is an excellent bowel stimulant. Both ordinary varieties and decaffeinated coffee can have the same effect on the gut. It stimulates a wave of contractions through the bowel, and whilst it is a useful tool for constipation sufferers, it should be avoided by those suffering with diarrhoea.

◆ Hot drinks. These may also stimulate a wave of contractions through the bowel. If you enjoy hot drinks, leave them to cool a little first.

◆ Artificial sweeteners. Sorbitol, an artificial sugar that cannot be digested, can cause diarrhoea. It is used in some 'sugar-free' chewing gums, sweets and mints. As it passes through the gut it attracts water in the same way that mineral laxatives do.

◆ Spicy foods. These can have a laxative effect on some people as presumably they irritate the bowel. In others it seems that both red chilli pepper and cayenne pepper actually slow the rate at which food passes through the small bowel, allowing more time for digestion. This one is down to individual observations.

◆ Smoking cigarettes. This can increase the contraction of the gut in sensitive individuals. For many a cup of coffee and a cigarette is their way of stimulating their gut into action, and thus is good for constipation.

◆ Alcohol. Alcohol is only likely to cause diarrhoea in those who drink excessively, and if you fall into that category, you will have already discovered why you should be reducing your consumption.

## What Your Doctor Can Do

If you have not already consulted your doctor about your diarrhoea, and it has persisted for some time, then you need to make an appointment, especially if you have lost weight, are aged over fifty, or if the self-help tips that follow do not help.

◆ Examination and investigations. These will look for a cause of the diarrhoea, and assess the likelihood of nutritional deficiencies. Blood tests for anaemia and measurement of vitamin B, iron and zinc are now widely available.

◆ X-ray of the bowel. This is done using a barium meal or barium enema. Barium is a heavy mineral liquid which shows up as dense white on X-ray and allows a good impression of the bowel and its lining to be obtained.

◆ Endoscopy of the bowel. This involves passing a sophisticated flexible telescope through the upper and lower gut in order to inspect the bowel lining for inflammation. Samples or biopsies from the gut lining can also be taken for further examination.

◆ Arrange for a stool examination. This would show up parasite infections, blood in the stool or undigested fats. If the diarrhoea is due to poor digestion, and difficulty digesting fat, excesses of fat may be discovered in your stool, which if untreated might lead to nutritional deficiencies.

◆ Prescribe a drug. Loperamide (Immodium) slows the passage of material along the gut, increases the amount of water absorbed by the gut and increases the tone of the anal muscles. Codeine phosphate is an old-fashioned drug derived from opium, which if taken in small doses, is relatively free from side-effects. Sodium cromoglycate (Nalcrom capsules) is an anti-allergy preparation used in spray form in the treatment of asthma. It can also be used in the form of capsules taken by mouth for those with true food allergies. One trial in Australia found that it also benefited 10 out of 20 patients with diarrhoea due to irritable bowel syndrome, in whom food allergy had not originally been suspected. This preparation is worth considering as it has very few side-effects.

◆ Prescribe a vitamin supplement. Certain nutritional deficiencies can occur in association with diarrhoea as the gut transit time is so fast the body does not have chance to digest or absorb the nutrients. It may be appropriate for your doctor to prescribe high-potency vitamin B complex or multi-vitamins, depending on the results of your investigations.

## *What You Can Do*

◆ Consider avoiding wheat, oats, barley and rye.

◆ Consider avoiding milk, yoghurt, cream and cheese. Other foods containing these or lactose (milk sugar) should also be avoided.

◆ Eat moderate-sized meals and eat every two to three hours. This will prevent overburdening your digestive system.

◆ Eat slowly and chew your food well. This may give your stomach and digestive system a much better chance to digest food properly.

◆ Adjust your fat intake. It is a good idea for many to ensure that there is a moderate amount of fat in each main meal.

◆ Stop or reduce your intake of coffee. Both ordinary and decaffeinated can cause diarrhoea. Consider drinking ordinary tea instead, as this can slow the passage of food through the gut in about 50 per cent of people. Cut down on hot drinks generally if you think that they make symptoms worse.

◆ Avoid excessive use of the artificial sweetener Sorbitol. Watch out for 'sugar-free' chewing gum and mints that contain Sorbitol.

◆ Avoid spicy foods, if they upset you. In theory taking large amounts of chilli and other hot spices might slow the gut down and help prevent diarrhoea.

◆ Reduce or stop smoking. Try to pace yourself between cigarettes so that you gradually smoke fewer each day.

◆ Reduce or stop drinking alcohol. Try to cut down to no more than three drinks per week initially.

◆ Change drug therapy. If you suspect that a drug you are taking might be causing your diarrhoea, discuss this with your doctor or specialist. A change of drug therapy may be necessary.

◆ Take some strong yeast-free vitamin B complex. Those with a high alcohol intake or diarrhoea following antibiotic usage or following gastroenteritis are particularly likely to benefit. A dose providing 50–100 mg of most of the B vitamins, including vitamin B3 or nicotinamide, is recommended as a daily dose. This should not be taken without your doctor's approval if you are known to be anaemic, have recently lost weight or have had stomach or bowel surgery.

◆ Avoid stress. Take steps to cope with stress and avoid stressful situations if you can.

If these tips are going to help you should notice some improvement within four weeks. If this is not the case, then you should check with your doctor.

## Complementary Therapies

Doctors have used hypnotherapy to assist with bowel problems with reasonably good results. It is worth having a session of hypnotherapy if you are a severe sufferer, or alternatively master the art of self-hypnosis to see whether this works for you. Acupuncture is very good at slowing down a rapid metabolism by addressing the root cause, and a herbal medicine practitioner will mix you a potion to try. Both of these avenues are well worth exploring.

......................................................................................................................

## Julie's Story

Julie, a thirty-year-old PE teacher, suffered with severe diarrhoea. Her symptoms were so bad that her job was on the line, her social life non-existent, and her relationship with her husband in jeopardy as well.

*I suffered with PMS for years, and IBS was diagnosed two years before I met up with the WNAS. My most embarrassing symptoms were my loud tummy noises, and constant diarrhoea. It was almost like being incontinent, which made me extremely nervous. I'm a teacher and was afraid of having an accident during a lesson and having to run off and leave the children.*

*I used to pass froth rather than motions and despite medical investigations was convinced I had bowel cancer. My mother read about the WNAS in a magazine and persuaded me to contact them. At my appointment I was given a programme to follow which involved cutting out orange juice, tea, cola, and chocolate, and asked to eat more fruit and vegetable fibre and oily fish. In addition I took multi-vitamin and mineral supplements and more personal exercise and relaxation.*

*Within two months my symptoms were under control, and within six months I was feeling wonderful. No diarrhoea, no IBS at all and even the PMS had gone. I haven't looked back. My husband is delighted too and now we are expecting our first baby.*

*See also*: Irritable Bowel Syndrome, Coeliac Disease, The Simple Exclusion Diet, The Strict Exclusion Diet. Plus Recommended Reading List (*Beat IBS Through Diet*) and References.

# EATING DISORDERS

Eating disorders can be broadly divided into two groups, anorexia nervosa and bulimia nervosa. Both are conditions found predominantly in women aged between ten and forty years, and are seen particularly amongst those of middle-class origins. Both conditions can be regarded as diseases of 'society' as much as they are diseases of the individual.

## *Anorexia Nervosa*
Anorexia nervosa has three main features.

◆ Very low body weight, usually at least 15 per cent below the expected weight.
◆ Disordered attitude towards body weight. Despite their thinness, the individual considers they are overweight, or still need to lose weight, in order to achieve a better shape. This disturbed thinking underpins the methods achieved to lose weight which may include fasting, exercise, self-induced vomiting and laxative abuse.

- Absence of periods in women who would normally be expected to menstruate, and who are not taking the oral contraceptive pill.

Other common co-existing features of anorexia include:

- depression
- mood swings
- obsessive behaviour
- thoughts of suicide
- limited outside interests
- being socially withdrawn
- disturbed relationships with parents
- physical characteristics of malnutrition

Physical features of anorexia may include:

- muscle wasting
- abdominal bloating
- scalp hair loss
- a development of fine downy hair over the body (lanugo)
- dry skin
- poor circulation in the hands and feet

There are a number of secondary hormonal changes which are mild and reversible. These include changes in pituitary and thyroid hormone in particular. Mild anaemia, raised blood cholesterol and disturbances in the balance of certain minerals may also be present.

Laxative or diuretic use can lead to loss of potassium and magnesium in particular. Interestingly, delayed emptying of the stomach and delayed bowel transit times leading to constipation are present. These features may lead to the complaint of fullness after eating only small amounts of food. If untreated severe malnutrition may develop bringing irrevocable damage to organs, and in severe cases girls become so ill they die.

## What Your Doctor Can Do

Usually people with anorexia nervosa do not present themselves for treatment. Invariably they are forced to do so by concerned parents or friends. All anorexics (and bulimics) require psycholog-ical treatment as well as nutritional support. The doctor must:

◆ Establish a rapport and relationship with the sufferer and family members and friends. This is a vital first step.
◆ Weigh the sufferer and test her blood for anaemia and mineral and vitamin deficiencies.
◆ Search for predisposing factors and explore the anorexic's per-ception of stress factors that may have contributed to depres-sion and disordered eating habits. This may include being overweight in the past and needing to diet, relationships with boyfriend or partner, work or domestic stresses.
◆ Aim to educate about the dangers of low body weight. Explaining that nutritional deficiencies may influence mood and energy level, that hormonal disturbances may prejudice chances of fer-tility in the future and predispose to osteoporosis, may all be ways of promoting the patient's understanding and cooperation.
◆ Work to improve the anorexic's perception of her well-being and examine the stress factors that she perceives as playing a role in her condition.
◆ Consider in- or out-patient treatment, with the need for coun-selling and psychiatric support.
◆ Decide whether drug treatment is required. This is rarely the case. Antidepressants are used, but should never be relied upon alone.
◆ Consider specialist feeding. Feeding by tube or intravenous methods should only be required in the minority of cases who are severely malnourished.

## *What You Can Do*

◆ Be prepared to discuss your feelings honestly with the doctor, psychotherapist and family members.
◆ Acknowledge that there is a physical and mental health problem.
◆ Attend your doctor or psychotherapist regularly. This may mean daily, or at least weekly, consultations.
◆ Make a list of those foods you like most and those you dislike. Discuss this with your therapist who obviously will need to advise you which foods will be even more nutritious and appropriate for you to consume.

◆ Take some high-potency multi-vitamin and multi-mineral supplements initially. Other specialist supplements may be required when you get the results of your tests but consider the following:

◇ Vitamin B1. A severe deficiency of this causes a clinical picture indistinguishable from anorexia nervosa, with delayed gastric emptying, loss of appetite, weight loss, fatigue and depression. Supplements of 50 mg per day may be required.

◇ Zinc. A deficiency is also reported in anorexia nervosa and correction might improve appetite.

◇ Calcium. Supplements are probably prudent in all women with prolonged amenorrhoea. 500–1000 mg per day may help minimise the future development of osteoporosis.

◇ Other deficiencies. Deficiency in the other B vitamins, in magnesium or the trace elements, chromium and selenium are all possible in malnourished individuals.

◆ Reduce your level of exercise if you have been over-exercising obsessively. Aim to restrict your exercise to three or four sessions per week.

◆ Recognise the support of close family members and friends and try not to be manipulative. Be honest and open with them or you will lose their friendship and support. Treat them as you would wish to be treated yourself.

## Complementary Therapies

Though none is of proven value, if you feel that one or more of these appeal to you or have been helpful in the past, then consider them now. Aromatherapy and massage may help relieve feelings of tension. Acupuncture might help balance the body's chemistry or nervous system, and some herbal preparations might act as a tonic. In all these cases a good relationship with a complementary therapist is vital.

# Bulimia Nervosa

Bulimia nervosa is now the most common eating disorder seen by psychiatrists and psychotherapists. It is not the opposite of anorexia nervosa, rather a variant of it. There seems to have been a genuine and substantial increase in its recognition over the last twenty years. There are three characteristic features:

- Binge episodes with the consumption of a large amounts of food, most frequently refined carbohydrates, and usually accompanied by a sense of loss of control.
- Use of extreme behaviour to control body shape and weight, such as self-induced vomiting, often after a binge episode, and laxative or diuretic misuse.
- A disturbed attitude towards body shape and weight.

Again women predominate with bulimia nervosa. They tend to be slightly older than those with anorexia although there is considerable overlap.

The features that distinguish bulimia nervosa from anorexia are:

- The body weight is usually normal.
- Periods are not necessarily absent although they may be irregular.
- There are frequent bulimic 'bingeing' episodes. Considerable secrecy surrounds these episodes with parents or partners being often unaware of the problem.
- The binge episodes may lead to the consumption of massive amounts of carbohydrate, up to some 12 600 kilojoules (approximately two days' energy intake).
- Occasionally alcohol bingeing or drug abuse are present.

Other features may include weakness and lethargy, erosions to the teeth because of the effect of vomited stomach acid, and signs of malnutrition, peripheral or facial swelling, enlargement of salivary glands, or signs indicative of specific nutrient deficiencies.

Laboratory investigations may uncover low levels of potassium, especially in those who abuse laxatives or diuretics. Other possible nutrient deficiencies are magnesium, zinc and vitamin B. Prolonged repeated vomiting is a known and potent cause of vitamin B1 deficiency, as is a high intake of refined carbohydrates e.g. cakes, biscuits, chocolates, sweets.

## What Your Doctor Can Do

As with anorexia, virtually all patients should be seen by a psychiatrist or psychotherapist specialising in this area. The GP and specialist should:

- Establish a rapport with the bulimic and her family members.
- Examine for signs of nutritional deficiency.
- Assess the level of depression which, if severe, may require treatment with antidepressants or hospital admission.
- Perform tests to assess the level of electrolytes, especially potassium and vitamin B1.
- If there is prolonged vomiting, refer for psychological treatment which will usually involve several months of cognitive behavioural therapy. This is designed to encourage insight into the person's condition leading to changes in their behaviour.
- Explain techniques, such as keeping a daily diary of:
  - ◇ diet
  - ◇ behaviour and thoughts
  - ◇ setting of limits and goals on binge eating
  - ◇ advice and direction on healthy eating
  - ◇ stressful situations that lead to binge eating, and how to avoid them
  - ◇ exploration of the thoughts and attitudes that may underlie this disordered behaviour. (Such an approach normally requires weekly consultations over several months and is tackled on a step-by-step basis.)
- Antidepressants can sometimes help but are less important than cognitive behaviour therapy.
- Set treatment programmes have a potentially excellent outcome in bulimia. Key elements include:
  - ◇ regular contact with the therapist
  - ◇ use of a written contract agreeing to maintain weight
  - ◇ agreeing to follow certain dietary goals about eating regularly
  - ◇ the amounts of certain foods eaten and recommendations on healthy eating
  - ◇ agreeing to maintain a regular food intake despite bingeing and vomit episodes

## What You Can Do

- Be honest with yourself and your therapists.
- Make a list of those stress factors in your life or situations that you feel contribute to episodes of bulimia. Bulimia is often worse premenstrually, and some of the dietary and supplement advice for PMS may also be relevant.

- With your therapist, set goals as to the frequency of bingeing, types of foods you will binge on and the amounts you will consume.
- Do not worry if you do not achieve these goals initially. Work towards them; it may take a while.
- Take any supplements prescribed regularly. Supplements of multi-vitamins in particular may be required as well as foods rich in potassium. These latter are mainly fresh fruits and vegetables, especially bananas and oranges. Fruit juices are another good source.
- Socialise with others. Enjoy yourself in the company of your family and friends, and when you are ready, be prepared to discuss these problems with them.

## Complementary Therapies
As for Anorexia.

# ECZEMA

This is a predominantly inherited condition, also known as atopic eczema or atopic dermatitis, affecting 1–3 per cent of the population. It often starts in childhood and is linked to asthma and rhinitis. Itchy skin is the most noticeable feature, with the skin being red, scaly and dry. The distribution varies. It may be widespread, or confined to the bends of the elbows and knees; it may affect just the face and neck, or settle in one or two other areas of the body. People with atopic eczema are more prone to asthma, rhinitis, allergic reactions to drugs and abdominal symptoms due to food allergy.

## Who Gets It?
Eczema has become increasingly common. It seems to be more common in higher social classes with the risk rising with the level of the parents' education. Having one or both parents affected by eczema or other allergies is relevant and additionally eczema has

become more common in children from African and Asian families—a perplexing combination of genetic factors. Events in the first years of life and possibly exposure to environmental chemicals seem to be at work in determining who gets it.

## What Causes It?

Eczema comes about because of a failure to control certain aspects of the immune system. A variety of different white cells which make up much of the immune system are normally busy fighting infections. Nowadays, with many of these controlled, the immune system has less to do and has had to reduce its level of activity. In the patient with eczema this has failed to occur and the white cells themselves, or proteins called antibodies that they produce, are targeted at a variety of everyday agents with which we all have contact. In practice it is allergy to these substances, which include housedust mites, foods and bacteria, that can be considered to be the cause of eczema.

It should be noted from the outset that though patients with eczema may have many allergies, and benefit from their identification and avoidance of the relative substance, only a few will subsequently experience complete resolution of their rash and itching.

Possible allergens include:

◆ Foods. Cows' milk, cows' cheese, hens' eggs, wheat, corn, yeast (baker's and brewer's), fruits and nuts are all commonly implicated.
◆ Infective agents. Bacteria that are frequently present on the skin surface, viruses including *Herpes simplex* and fungi including *Candida albicans* can all play a part in eczema. Relief of symptoms may follow measures to treat these infections or reduce the amount of bacteria on the skin surface.
◆ Housedust mite. This is a common allergen, and seems to be important in some cases of eczema as well as asthma. (For control of housedust mite see Asthma.)
◆ Others. Pollens and animals may aggravate eczema in the susceptible individual.

## What Your Doctor Can Do

Your doctor can help in the identification of possible allergens and in the treatment of the skin condition itself.

### Allergy tests

Allergy tests come in many guises and all have their limitations.

♦ Skin prick tests, where a small amount of the suspected culprit agent is placed on the skin which is then scratched, can show a reaction in 10 minutes. This is useful at identifying allergies to housedust, pollens and sometimes foods. Many non-eczematous individuals show positive test results.

♦ Blood tests that measure the level of antibodies against foods and other agents are available. The RAST or radioallergosorbent test can detect a number of quick-acting food allergies. Other tests are being developed to look for delayed allergies to foods, but their role is still uncertain. Even if a test shows a number of allergies, there is no guarantee that other foods not tested for do not cause problems.

### Treatments

♦ Steroid creams and ointments will, if the dose is high enough, damp down the irritation and rash. Typically this is the mainstay of treatment for severe eczema and is useful in smaller doses for mild or intermittent eczema.

♦ Moisturising agents will help with the dryness, and are useful for widespread or localised eczema where dry scaly skin is a problem. Several good ones are available without prescription and may be all that is needed for dry affected hands.

♦ Treatment for any associated infection. This applies especially to bacterial infection on the skin. Creams that combine antibiotics and steroids, antibiotics by mouth, or antiseptic washes to add to the bath can all be used. Occasionally treatment of thrush, infection with *Candida albicans*, may help eczema.

♦ Other medicines include powerful drugs to alter the immune system and allergic response. One medicine is worthy of special mention for those with known food allergies. Nalcrom (oral cromoglycate capsules) is a drug that when taken by mouth is not absorbed from the gut but blocks the development of immediate allergy reactions that take place in the gut wall. It has very few side-effects because it is not absorbed, and can therefore allow those with food allergies to respond better to dietary exclusion and consequently be more relaxed with their diet. Nalcrom has to be taken just before meals to be most effective.

◆ Evening primrose oil is useful for very dry, widespread eczema. It is best combined with a high polyunsaturated fatty acid diet (see below).

## *What You Can Do*

◆ Change your diet.   You could try either The Strict Exclusion Diet (with the approval of your doctor), or try The Simple Exclusion Diet for two or three weeks. Cutting out specific foods one at a time is not very successful and is not recommended except for children where exclusion of just cows' milk, eggs, tomatoes and artificial colours is sometimes worth a try. For young children, those with severe eczema, or those with asthma or a history of severe allergic reactions such diets must only be performed with medical supervision, as the re-introduction of a food after its withdrawal can sometimes lead to a severe allergic reaction.

◆ Avoid irritants. Many agents will worsen the eczema even though they are not the cause. Wear rubber gloves, cotton lined if necessary, when in contact with water. Use non-biological washing powders and liquids. For clothes that you wear next to your skin choose those made from cotton or silk as they are often less irritating.

◆ Take some nutritional supplements. Deficiencies of vitamin B, zinc and the essential fatty acids can all affect skin quality. You may need to take supplements for two or three months to see the full effect. They are often usefully combined with supplements of evening primrose oil.

◆ Go on holiday and get some sunshine. This is known to help for a number of possible reasons: the rest and relaxation are good for the immune system; the change in diet or the sunshine helps to kill off some of the surface bacteria; or the warmth and light stimulate the skin's metabolism.

◆ Reduce your exposure to housedust mite. After years of suspicion it is now acknowledged that careful avoidance of this allergen can help those with eczema who are known to be sensitive to it. A simple skin prick test will give an indication of this. In severe cases there may be a case for medical desensitisation to housedust. This is only undertaken at specialist centres.

◆ Treat any associated premenstrual syndrome. PMS is associated with a worsening or pre-existing eczema, and some of the dietary and self-help measures for PMS can sometimes benefit any associated eczema.

## Complementary Therapies

Homoeopathy is perhaps the most established complementary therapy for eczema. There are many remedies and their selection depends upon the type of eczema, the patient's response to it and any distinguishing features. Two common remedies are Sulphur and Graphites. These are given as tablets and are usually administered several times per day for a few weeks. More than one remedy may need to be tried before benefit is experienced.

## Sheryl's Story

Sheryl's partner had been a patient some years before and when her life-long eczema flared up she decided to seek our advice. The eczema indeed stretched back to infancy and had required her to use steroids intermittently. She had observed that her eczema was better in the sun and worse after contact with water which seemed to aggravate the itching rather than the rash. A variety of allergy tests in the past had suggested multiple sensitivities to inhalant allergens which caused her some nasal stuffiness.

Some simple skin prick allergy tests for foods were performed, but there were no clear-cut reactions, and we therefore decided to proceed straight-away to a strict exclusion diet. There was a good improvement, but after a few weeks the diet became very tedious. It took nearly a year of introducing and re-introducing foods before the picture was clear. There seemed to be delayed reactions to dairy products, egg, chicken and fish, and we were still uncertain about a variety of other foods.

Blood tests had shown a potential important abnormality. There were very low levels of some of the Omega-6 series of essential fatty acids, especially gamma linolenic acid, the active component found in evening primrose oil. Her GP was willing to prescribe this for her, and it produced further improvement in her skin quality, especially a lessening of the dryness. It became increasingly clear that she had a wide number of food allergies, and as her diet was difficult to follow completely, she began a course of Nalcrom (oral cromoglycate). This allergy-blocking drug, when taken by mouth, may help minimise the adverse reactions to foods that may underlie some patients' eczema.

Sheryl was very pleased with the further progress, and her skin was better than it had been for over a decade. Furthermore she was able to deviate from her rather restricted diet without experiencing any severe reactions. Shortly after this she became pregnant. Calcium supplements were needed to ensure adequate intake of this mineral, and she already had been taking supplements of vitamin B and folic acid. She was asked to be extra vigilant during her pregnancy and whilst breast-feeding as her allergy to certain foods may in some way be 'transmitted' to her baby. Avoidance of common food allergens by mothers with eczema seems to reduce the risk of their offspring developing eczema as well.

# EYE PROBLEMS

For much of our lives our eyes are designed to take care of themselves. They are cleansed by our tears, which naturally contain chemicals that kill bacteria. Our eyes are vulnerable, and at times become the victims of infection or allergy, or may be affected by some other medical condition, like hayfever or seborrhoeic dermatitis.

As we age, our eyes change shape. When they change shape from back to front we become short-sighted, and when the change occurs from top to bottom we become long-sighted. Taking care of ourselves generally will also help to preserve the health of our eyes.

## Loss of Vision

According to iridologists our eyes are a reflection of what is happening inside the body, not something that conventional doctors would agree with. Orthodox medicine acknowledges, though, that hardening of the arteries may be detected in older folk by checking for a pale ring around the iris. Another eye problem that can occur in later life is glaucoma, in which there is an increase of tension within the eyeball as a result of blocked drainage from the eye. Although the symptoms may initially appear like conjunctivitis, with red and bloodshot whites, glaucoma may be a threat to our sight. The tension can be reduced by drugs, or the blockage will need to be cleared rapidly, and so it is important to be examined early.

Two major causes of loss of vision are cataracts and macular degeneration.

## Cataracts

A cataract is a gradual clouding of the lens of the eye, in which a jelly-like substance grows over the lens of the eye. They are a major cause of blindness all over the world. A number of risk factors for their formation have been identified, some of which are nutritional, and these include:

◆ age
◆ diabetes
◆ sunlight exposure, especially ultra-violet B radiation
◆ poor diet with poor intakes of vitamin A, in the form of carotene and its relatives, which are found in spinach and other dark green vegetables
◆ possibly consumption of dairy products with an inability to digest milk sugar or lactose
◆ use of steroid drugs and other medicines
◆ diarrhoea (both in the Third World and in the Western world). This is possibly due to loss of nutrients or as a reflection of poor general health

The treatment of cataracts usually involves the surgical removal, with sometimes replacement, of the lens. As yet there is no evidence that they can be prevented, although progress has been produced by use of nutritional supplements, but this may change with time.

Some protection may be achieved in those taking low-dose aspirin or similar analgesic (often for arthritis but also for the prevention of heart disease). And long-term usage of a vitamin C supplement has also been associated with a lower risk, but only after ten or more years.

## Macular Degeneration

The macular is the most sensitive part of the retina at the back of the eye that perceives the majority of fine vision. Healthy function of this part of the eye is necessary for reading, driving, writing and any fine work.

The degeneration of this part of the eye is mainly age-related and is a major cause of irreversible blindness among those aged sixty-five years and more. Again, studies have been performed to look at risk factors for the development of age-related macular degeneration. Attention has focused on nutrients. So far we know that the risk of this condition's increase is influenced by:

- smoking, which increases the risk
- atherosclerosis, or a narrowing of the arteries in the neck, may be an additional risk factor in the elderly
- a low intake of carotenoids in the diet. Agents like beta-caro-tene (vegetable vitamin A) do not have any vitamin function. High concentrations are found in spinach or collard greens
- low intake of vitamin C from foods, though this effect is small

In practice what this means is that eating healthily in your formative and middle years may help retard the rate of decay of tissues in later life. Smoking once again seems to accelerate this risk of tissues degenerating.

### What Your Doctor Can Do

Not much really, except refer you to a specialist.

### What You Can Do

- Follow The Very Nutritious Diet.
- Ensure that your diet is rich in fresh fruit and vegetables, especially spinach, tomatoes, carrots and any dark-green vegetables.
- Consider taking a multi-vitamin supplement with beta-carotene and zinc.

# FATIGUE AND CHRONIC FATIGUE SYNDROME

Tired when you go to bed, tired when you wake up. Tired at work, tired when you get home. It's a familiar story, and even if you are not a habitual victim of chronic fatigue you probably know someone who is. It is one of the commonest complaints for which we consult our doctors, and more women suffer than men.

There are of course, different types of fatigue. Most of us have, hopefully, experienced fatigue after a period of hard and fruitful work, and then noticed a return in our energy after a good night's sleep or a relaxing holiday. Some of us, however, suffer from fatigue day in, day out, despite the amount of sleep or rest we have. The causes of this problem vary, from the physical to the psychological, and both aspects need to be considered in the majority of those suffering from significant fatigue. This chapter deals with *severe* fatigue that is troublesome enough to cause the individual to change her lifestyle in some way.

During the last ten years there has been a great deal of research and publicity about severe fatigue, particularly ME or myalgic encephalomyelitis. This term is now replaced by Chronic Fatigue Syndrome, which also replaces other similar terms such as post-infective or post-viral fatigue. Chronic Fatigue Syndrome, CFS, often—but by no means always—follows an acute infectious illness, such as a sore throat, glandular fever or gastro-enteritis.

## What Causes It?

The interest of doctors in these chronic fatigue syndromes is a landmark in medical thinking, with research being focused on a symptom, for which there are many possible causes, and not a single disease state. There are serious and not so serious causes of fatigue, so it is important to determine which category an individual falls into. Research has shown that up to 10 per cent of those with severe fatigue have some underlying health problem.

Some sufferers may have a physical illness which may not yet be fully developed, some may have recently experienced acute infection, and others may be mainly depressed. The first step must be to eliminate the possibility of any serious underlying cause *before* progressing to self-help measures.

As a rule of thumb, fatigue which is persistent or prevents you from working and requires you to make drastic changes to your home life and social calendar, should be regarded as possibly being due to a serious cause. This also goes for fatigue that is associated with weight loss, fever, significant pain or any other troublesome symptoms. This should always prompt you to check with your doctor as your first course of action.

*Causes of fatigue (not so serious)*
◆ lack of sleep
◆ stress or overwork
◆ lack of physical fitness
◆ poor quality diet

*Causes of fatigue (serious)*
◆ physical illness, e.g. heart, liver or kidney disease
◆ after viral or other infection, e.g. glandular fever or flu
◆ depression
◆ rarely, a continuing infection, e.g. tropical

Wide-ranging surveys have revealed a pattern connecting common non-serious health problems with mild to moderate fatigue which includes muscular aches and pains, bowel problems, headaches, premenstrual syndrome and sleeping difficulties including snoring, and allergies. Addressing these problems can often result in a reduction in the associated fatigue.

When a doctor has to assess a new patient with significant fatigue it is probably best for her to consider the following four broad groups:

1. It can accompany any acute infectious illness, such as flu or a cold. Occasionally, an infection is hidden and this can be the case in some tropical illnesses or parasitic infections. If anyone with fatigue has a fever usually more than 37.5°C, then they should be carefully checked for a possible hidden infection.

2. Fatigue can also follow an infection. After the acute episode has resolved, the individual can be left with fatigue, which instead

of resolving in a week or so, drags on for months and even years. This condition is sometimes called ME or myalgic encephalomyelitis. It simply means inflammation of the muscles and nervous tissue, and there is now evidence that patients with ME can have, at times, evidence of damage or alteration to either the muscles, the nervous system or immune system. It seems in some ways that the infection, after causing an acute illness, goes into a slow or hidden phase which sometimes can reappear. This is particularly true for the glandular fever virus, but may also be true of other virus infections.

The term ME has now really been replaced with Chronic Fatigue Syndrome, or CFS. This is used to describe significant fatigue present for at least three months which typically, but not necessarily, has followed one or more infections. Several of the following features should also be present:

◆ the fatigue is worse after exercise
◆ headaches
◆ forgetfulness or poor concentration
◆ muscle aches and pains
◆ recurrent sore throats
◆ painful enlarged glands in the neck or elsewhere

Doctors still disagree about this definition. In practice, if this picture is present and continuing infection, other underlying illness, drug or alcohol abuse, or severe depression are excluded, then this allows at least a working diagnosis of CFS (or ME).

3. Fatigue can also be caused by a wide variety of physical illnesses, including heart conditions, arthritis, conditions affecting the immune system or nervous system, kidney problems and so on. These conditions should be suspected in older patients, those who experience weight loss or have other unusual symptoms. They will usually be detected by blood and urine tests, together with X-rays. In order to eliminate the possibility of any underlying sinister problem, it is important that all those suffering with severe fatigue do see their medical practitioner for a check up.

4. Fatigue of varying degree is often caused by nutritional factors. This can either be a lack of vitamins or minerals, or can sometimes be due to other dietary problems. Though we are often told that the average diet in countries like the United Kingdom, Australia

and New Zealand should provide all the vitamins and minerals we need, careful scrutiny of the evidence from both Government and other sources, doesn't always support this claim. In fact mild nutritional deficiencies are not uncommon, especially among women of child-bearing age, the elderly and the ill, and these can affect muscle and brain metabolism and result in loss of energy. This is easily underestimated by the medical profession through lack of knowledge, and may consequently be overlooked.

A 1993 CSIRO dietary survey revealed that up to 20 per cent of adults have a dietary intake below the recommended dietary intake. This applies particularly to the minerals iron, magnesium and potassium, as well as some of the B vitamins. Deficiency of any of these nutrients can cause fatigue. Most are essential to the function of muscles, nerves and the immune system. There is good evidence that deficiency is particularly common in certain groups.

For example, 70 per cent of premenopausal women and 60 per cent of adolescent girls do not get sufficient iron in their diet. This is mainly because of heavy or prolonged periods and may explain why fatigue is more common amongst women. Mild fatigue in such women has long been shown to respond to iron supplements, and is a good example of how a mild or severe nutritional deficiency can be a cause of chronic fatigue.

| WHO MAY LACK NUTRIENTS? | DEFICIENCY |
| --- | --- |
| Women with heavy or prolonged periods | Zinc and iron |
| Tea- and coffee-drinking vegetarians | Iron |
| Those eating junk and fast food | Vitamin B and magnesium |
| Those who drink too much alcohol | Vitamin B and magnesium |
| Women with premenstrual syndrome | Magnesium |
| Those suffering from depression or anxiety | Vitamins B and C |
| Those who eat little fruit and vegetables | Vitamin C, magnesium and potassium |
| Heavy smokers | Vitamin C |
| Those suffering any illness resulting in weight loss | Vitamin B and others |
| The ill and elderly | Vitamin B and others |
| Those with poor resistance to infection | Zinc, vitamins B and A |

Iron deficiency is most likely in women who are having periods, particularly if they are heavy, and in vegetarians or people who don't consume much meat.

Mild deficiency of the B group of vitamins is also quite common, particularly in those who complain of anxiety, depression or mood changes. This may often accompany fatigue. Again, a poor diet, smoking, and drinking too much alcohol, are all significant risk factors for lack of vitamin B.

The mineral magnesium has attracted considerable interest in recent years. This mineral is essential for nerve and muscle function. In our own surveys of women with PMS we have repeatedly found that over 50 per cent of women with PMS have low magnesium stores.

## Go to Your Doctor If You Suffer Serious Fatigue, and . . .

◆ you have a fever (a temperature above 37.5°C)
◆ you are losing weight
◆ you have enlarged glands in the neck, armpits and groin
◆ you have pains which disturb your sleep or daily activities
◆ your facial appearance or colour has changed
◆ you have travelled abroad, especially to Asia, the Far East, the Mediterranean, or South, Central or North America
◆ you have had contact with animals other than known pets
◆ you are troubled by any joint swellings and pains
◆ you have bowel problems such as diarrhoea, a change in the colour of your stool or severe abdominal pains

## What Your Doctor Can Do

Establish whether there is a serious underlying cause to your symptoms by:

◆ Taking a history of your symptoms and giving you a thorough physical examination, with routine blood screening, including a full blood count—to look for anaemia or evidence of infection, serum ferritin—to check your iron stores (particularly useful for menstruating women), thyroid function to assess the status of your thyroid, biochemistry tests to assess kidney and liver function, measurement of blood calcium, sodium and potassium to assess mineral imbalances.

◆ Enlightened doctors may care to measure your red cell magnesium level. This is a simple test that can be performed at district hospital level. Reduced red cell magnesium is associated with fatigue, PMS, muscle cramps or fibromyalgia (see page 89).

◆ Make some assessment of your nutritional state, and look for evidence of vitamin B deficiency in particular. Lack of vitamin B12 and vitamin B1 can be serious, and fatigue may be one of the earliest symptoms.

◆ Consider referring you to a specialist for further assessment. This is most likely if the fatigue is severe and prolonged, or has caused you to make major lifestyle changes as previously discussed.

◆ Treat depression if this is a major component of your illness, but this should not stop them from looking for underlying physical or nutritional causes.

◆ Refer you to a specialist unit, or a behavioural psychologist, as simple coping techniques have been shown to help speed up the recovery process.

## Maureen's Story

Maureen, a forty-seven-year-old nurse, lectured in further education. She suffered chronic fatigue and, as a result, her moods were wildly out of control. She was in the process of disciplinary action at work, and finding life generally difficult, when she approached the WNAS.

*I had experienced symptoms for nearly twenty-five years, but they had become markedly worse in the past three. My doctor had prescribed numerous forms of hormone treatment which seemed to make the symptoms worse. My total exhaustion, irritability, anger and aggression had almost totally alienated me from the world. I was struggling along on the contraceptive pill continuously as my doctor felt my symptoms may improve if we could suppress ovulation.*

*I had a lot of time off because of exhaustion and my wild moods. I had reached the point where I was afraid to go out of the house. I was so tired that I could not get out of bed in the morning without a friend phoning to command me through the procedure, limb by limb. My doctor had sent me for counselling and had even referred me to a psychiatrist, but I walked out halfway through the appointment as I was so angry with his suggestion that I should pull myself together. I often felt like ending my life. I had upset so many people and had lost most of my friends. At work I was regarded as unreliable, and regarded as an oddity.*

*Then one day I read about the book, Beat PMS Through Diet in Woman and Home magazine, and decided to read it. To my utter amazement my fatigue and mood changes were almost exactly the same as many of the case histories. I made some changes to my diet myself by following the instructions in the book whilst I was waiting for my appointment with the WNAS. After an in-depth consultation I was asked to make considerable changes to my diet. I cut out certain grains, caffeine, and biscuits, which I used to eat day and night. I also took supplements of Optivite and went back to exercising, which I had let slip from my routine.*

*At my follow-up appointment six weeks later, I was able to report that I had been on an even keel with no wild mood swings, and was feeling so energetic that I had taken to early-morning walks. I could hardly believe it, and nor could my friends and colleagues, especially those who had previously had to resuscitate me in the mornings. I came off the Pill too, and my headaches also disappeared.*

*Within three months I had lost 3 kg in weight, I was wonderfully stable each day and had regained my energy and enthusiasm for life. I had renewed my friendships, applied to do an MA in education which had been a goal I never dared hope for, and within six months was promoted to coordinator at work. It has now been two years since my treatment with the WNAS. I feel alive again and can't sing their praises enough.*

## What You Can Do

Many treatments or cures have been put forward, some showing some very high success rates, and there are many self-help measures that can be implemented to help overcome symptoms of fatigue.

- Follow the recommendations for The Very Nutritious Diet and the suggested menu for fatigue in this section.
- Tidy up your diet by concentrating on good sources of magnesium—green leafy vegetables and most wholesome foods—and avoid sugar, sweets, and soft drinks which contain hardly any magnesium at all. Women with PMS often have low levels of magnesium, and it seems that the same is often true of people suffering with fatigue.
- Many other nutrients, if deficient, are known to affect the function of the immune system. These include vitamins A, C, E

and the trace element, zinc. A healthy diet and a strong multi-vitamin supplement with 20 to 30 mg of zinc should be adequate. Specialised fats and oils, as found in evening primrose oil and fish oil, have been used to help those with chronic fatigue. In one placebo-controlled trial a supplement of Efamol Marine at 8 capsules daily helped a high proportion of those whose fatigue was post-infective in type. Again this should be combined with eating healthily and possibly a multi-vitamin preparation.

◆ In addition to deficiency of certain nutrients, sometimes other dietary problems can cause fatigue. There is evidence in those who have certain types of allergy, that fatigue may be one of the associated symptoms. Intolerance to certain foods seems to be a factor, and this can be suspected if there are symptoms of allergy, including eczema, asthma, nettle rash, migraine headaches and bowel problems including irritable bowel syndrome. In one study, allergy to wheat protein was linked with increased complaints of fatigue, headaches and bowel problems. It is not known how commonly this is a cause of chronic fatigue, but it does seem to be worth considering.

◆ Symptoms such as anxiety and depression, often accompany fatigue. In fact many physical problems can also cause mental symptoms. Stress, in any form, may also aggravate mental symptoms, and even reduce the ability of the immune system to fight infection. So if you are feeling stressed it is important to find a workable way of overcoming the stressful factors and to spend a little time every day relaxing.

◆ Exercising regularly to the point of breathlessness and losing weight, if you are overweight, can also help mood and stimulate the immune system. You should only exercise regularly if your fatigue is mild and you have no underlying illness.

Of course, frantic modern living is likely to contribute to us feeling tired all the time. Many of us devote insufficient time to preparing food or taking adequate exercise or relaxation. Not enough sleep, stress at home or work, lack of exercise and a poor quality diet can all reduce our energy level. Addressing the problem directly by taking a much-needed holiday, embarking on a regular exercise programme or taking steps to improve your nutritional intake may well be all that is needed to restore your vitality.

Working long hours and not eating wholesome food regularly is likely to make your blood glucose levels fall, which results in symptoms of tiredness. The solution is not merely to suddenly eat more glucose, as the body finds it hard to adjust to the rapid rise and fall that this causes. Rather eat wholesome food little and often. So aim for three good meals, with nutritious between-meal snacks, such as fruit, nuts and raisins, a sandwich with cheese, meat or fish, or rye crackers and peanut butter, which give a more sustained rise in blood sugar.

Some people seem excessively tired and dopey just after a meal. Men seem particularly prone to this phenomenon, which is likely to be worse at lunch time or after a large meal, and is aggravated by drinking alcohol. A smaller, lighter lunch, especially one of salad with meat, fish or vegetarian protein, avoiding alcohol and taking a twenty-minute walk afterwards will usually prevent this form of transitory tiredness. The alternative is to have a siesta after your midday meal. This is what the Mediterraneans and the lions do, and is simply their response to the physiological need to rest while digesting a large meal.

So in less serious cases, excellent results can be gained by making sure you get a little more sleep, cutting your workload a little to combat the associated stress, taking more exercise, improving your diet, and having a holiday if possible.

*Fight fatigue*
- eat three meals a day, with wholesome snacks in between
- cut down on sugary foods, refined carbohydrates and chocolate
- eat three servings of fresh fruit per day
- eat three portions of fresh vegetables, including a green leafy one, per day
- eat protein-rich foods at least once a day
- avoid bran and bran-based cereals and use corn and oat alternatives
- limit bread to 2–4 slices per day
- keep alcohol consumption down
- consume 300–600 ml of milk per day and 112–225 g of cheese per week
- cut down on tea and coffee and try herbal teas and alternative coffees
- enjoy your food

## Complementary Therapies

Although most of us prefer not to be given a serious diagnosis for our symptoms, when the verdict is 'no apparent underlying cause' it can be immensely frustrating. As well as implementing the advice given in this chapter is would be worth enlisting the help of one or more complementary practitioners.

Acupuncture would regard symptoms of fatigue as a deficiency syndrome. The practitioner would be looking for deficiency of Qi or the life-force in the blood, and will treat the deficiency.

There are numerous homoeopathic remedies that are available for the different sorts of fatigue including Apis melifica, useful for aches and pains, Lycopodium clavatum for symptoms of fatigue and inertia, Natrum muriaticum, a remedy for the pale and weak, and Pulsatilla, for the frail, pale female with changeable symptoms, and useful for those who do not tolerate stress well. You could try these yourself, or consult a qualified homoeopath.

The herbal practitioner also has a lot to offer, and would be worth consulting if symptoms persist. There are many different herbal remedies for fatigue including St John's Wort, Vervain, Yarrow, Echinacea and Stinging nettle.

Cranial osteopaths consider that the membranes around the brain and spinal cord can become 'tight' and cause ill health. Relaxation, massage and a consultation with a cranial osteopath may be very helpful.

*See also*: Recommended Reading List (*Tired All the Time*) and References.

# FLUID RETENTION

This is also known as idiopathic oedema: 'oedema' is the medical term for swelling; 'idiopathic' means that the cause is unknown and is just a clever way of doctors disguising their ignorance. Though there is a variety of causes, the commonest is simply the retention of salt and water in the subcutaneous tissues. This shows up particularly in the feet, in the fingers and sometimes in the abdomen. In severe cases the face may be affected.

It is well known that fluid retention is much more common in women and is very often worse in the premenstrual phase. Some studies have shown that it can be associated with fatigue and a tendency to depression, but before deciding that the swelling is simply 'idiopathic', care should be taken to exclude other causes.

## What Your Doctor Can Do

◆ Consider the possible causes of swelling including heart failure, underactive thyroid, kidney failure, swelling due to blocked lymphatic drainage following infection, or possibly due to a familial disorder.

◆ If simple idiopathic oedema is diagnosed, a low-salt diet is recommended, and this should always be the first line of treatment. Careful studies conducted by doctors at Charing Cross Hospital in London clearly demonstrated that a restriction of sodium (salt) leads almost always to clearance of idiopathic oedema. Our bodies are composed of 70 per cent water, and the reason we retain fluid is because each cell in the body has a mechanism to balance sodium and other minerals. It is primarily sodium that governs the retention of water and it seems that some women are particularly unable to tolerate large amounts of salt in the diet. Our Western diet has become laden with salt, with intakes some ten to fifty times our actual requirements.

◆ Prescribe diuretics if all else fails. This is very much a poor option and a last resort, although it is indeed a common treatment. Low-dose mild diuretics often do not produce lasting benefit as the body adjusts to the effects on their chemistry.

## What You Can Do

◆ Be vigilant with The Low-salt Diet; if you recall, we consume far more salt than we need and most of the sodium salt in our diet comes from hidden sources rather than added salt in cooking or at the table. This means doing without crisps, other salted savoury snacks, bacon, sausages and greatly limiting the intake of bread.

◆ Fluid restriction is not required although it is inadvisable to drink very large amounts. Watch out for some mineral waters which actually contain significant amounts of sodium, and choose those rich in calcium and magnesium if possible.

- Lose weight if you need to.
- Restrict your alcohol intake to no more than two units per day.
- Follow The Very Nutritious Diet. High intakes of magnesium and potassium will help the body get the balance of sodium right.
- Take supplements of magnesium and multi-vitamins (see Pre-menstrual Syndrome, for further advice).
- Put your feet up. Lying down aids clearance of fluid from the legs and also the body's ability to pass it out in the urine.
- Have a cup of coffee? This has modest diuretic effects. Perhaps a cup of coffee first thing in the morning, whilst putting your feet up for a couple of hours to read the newspaper, may help you offload some of the fluid that has accumulated overnight.

## Complementary Therapies

Most herbal remedies have diuretic properties, so see a qualified herbalist for advice. A homoeopathic remedy, Agis mel, is traditionally used to treat this sort of problem. These avenues are worth exploring but will not replace the need for a low-salt diet.

## Alison's Story

Alison, a thirty-eight-year-old welfare worker with two children, suffered severe water retention which made her life a misery. She felt swollen and tired for two weeks each month which was severely disrupting her life.

*For two weeks before my period each month, with unrelenting regularity, my body would begin to swell. Within days, my middle swelled so much that I looked at least five months pregnant. My waist would increase by inches and my face would puff up. My eyelids felt tight and my breasts sore because of the swelling. I could hardly fit into my bra, and even walking felt uncomfortable.*

*Every month I'd be so bloated, I felt like a pudding, and everything was an effort. I was lethargic and lacking in energy. My doctor prescribed progesterone suppositories which made me feel even more bloated. When I returned to ask for further help he told me I needed to see a psychiatrist. I felt insulted as I knew that my symptoms were not psychological. I went off and tried to help myself with vitamin B6 and evening primrose oil. They did help a bit, but not significantly. My doctor's reaction had put me off trying to get help, so I struggled on for another couple of years.*

*My husband read an article in the newspaper relating to the work of the WNAS*

*in which one of the patients reported symptoms similar to mine. I wrote off imme-
diately to ask for help. The detailed questionnaire and diet diary arrived shortly
after, and I set about completing it. The WNAS worked out a programme for me
that involved cutting out chocolate bars, which I used to crave, and bread, tea and
coffee had to go too. Instead I was asked to concentrate on fresh foods. Every day
I had to eat lots of vegetables, salad and fruit. I drank herbal tea and fruit juice,
and small amounts of decaffeinated coffee. As well as the fresh foods, I had to
take vitamins and minerals to help speed up my recovery, and to exercise regularly.*

*I had a constant headache for the first week and felt sluggish. Once the first
two weeks were over I felt smashing. Within two months I was really feeling slim
and positive. The bloating disappeared and my breasts were no longer tender.*

*Six years on, I'm still full of energy, my skin looks smooth, my nails no longer
split and break, and I no longer have cravings for food. I am 12.6 kg slimmer now
without dieting, I'm more confident and can honestly say that I feel like a different
person. I'm really amazed.*

*See also*: Standard References.

# FOOD CRAVING

Just as cars need regular petrol and oil, so our bodies have specific
nutritional requirements in order to keep them running efficiently.
Too little 'nutritional fuel' results in us running out of steam and
having difficulty maintaining our body weight. Equally, too much
food and drink can leave us feeling wiped out, both physically and
mentally. Craving food, particularly chocolate, is very common. It
is not uncommon for women to get into a routine of eating in
excess of six bars of chocolate each day, sometimes whole packets
of fun-size bars, followed by biscuits, cakes and sweets. A little of
what you fancy does you good, but excessive consumption does
little for our self-esteem, or our waistlines.

## What Causes It?

The brain and nervous system require a constant supply of good
nutrients in order to function normally. Eating nutritious food little

and often would probably provide all that was needed, and indeed is the way we were designed to sustain ourselves. In the mid-1930s, for example, we were eating on average four proper meals per day with one in-between-meal snack, whereas now in the late 1990s, our habits have changed, and we are consuming one or two proper meals per day, with four or five in-between-meal snacks. To make matters even worse, many of us are not shopping regularly for fresh food or spending time in the kitchen preparing proper meals. We often rely on pre-prepared meals and fast food in order to satisfy our hunger, without realising that these do not fulfil our need for nutrients. Then, little by little, we reach for these sweet foods in order to give us a boost, which they undoubtedly do, but it is short lived. A biochemical merry-go-round develops, which becomes less and less under our control as time progresses. The progress and results of this are listed below.

- When we haven't eaten for a while or consumed much nutritious food our blood sugar levels drop.
- The brain, which requires glucose in order to function normally, sends out a red alert asking for more glucose, ideally in the form of nutritious food. Unfortunately as we are not educated about nutrition, we often supply the body in the form of a sweet processed snack, or chocolate, which are largely composed of refined sugar, which doesn't contain any vitamins or minerals whatsoever, but does demand good nutrients in order to be metabolised.
- The result of eating the refined sugar snack is that the blood sugar levels shoot up rapidly, flooding the blood with sugar.
- The brain then sends another message to say that there is too much sugar in the blood, which triggers the release of the hormone insulin, whose function it is to drive the sugar back into the cells. It does this so efficiently that the blood sugar levels then go back to low again, and the whole cycle begins again as a result.

The trick is knowing how to break this cycle, which often develops into a real addiction, and just like alcohol, drugs or smoking, involves a period of withdrawal.

*Low blood sugar*

Low blood sugar levels usually follow some traumatic event in a woman's life, or alternatively can occur gradually due to poor nutritional intake. Very often women feel low after pregnancy and periods of breast-feeding, when the nutrient demands placed on our bodies are greater than at other times in our lives. Following a broken relationship, we often become vulnerable, so we shun normal meals in favour of comfort eating. Equally, when life becomes stressful, whether with financial pressures, dissatisfaction at work or loneliness, we often find our way to the chocolate counter. It is not simply lack of will that stops us taking control, but real biochemical needs that develop as a result of poor dietary management over a period of time. There is nothing wrong with enjoying food and eating modest amounts of chocolate after a proper meal, but when the cravings take control of you it is time to do something about it.

The WNAS has undertaken several surveys on low blood sugar and food cravings, and some fascinating factors were revealed:

- Women, it seems, suffer more commonly than men, probably because of their hormone cycle, and because the nutritional demands that are placed on their bodies vary throughout the stages of their lives.
- From a sample of 1000 patients, we initially discovered that just under 80 per cent suffered with cravings for sweet food in their premenstrual phase, in the days before their period was due.
- A further survey of women of 500 women of all ages showed that 78 per cent admitted wanting to eat less chocolate, and 60 per cent claimed it was a problem for them.
- Weight gain, poor skin quality, fatigue and flagging self-esteem were the commonest resulting problems experienced.

The most recent survey we undertook on 295 women also revealed that 74 per cent crave sweet food, and the following:

- Sweet food consumption was related to age and occupation.
- Most felt worse after eating sweet food, with fatigue being the worst complaint.
- Women who consume lots of sweet food tend to drink more

coffee, smoke more cigarettes and eat a less healthy diet.

◆ Retired people, housewives and unskilled workers consume far more sweet food than managers and directors.

◆ Chocolate and cakes were the most popularly craved foods.

◆ Severe sufferers burned their way through at least $30.00 per week in order to satisfy their cravings.

*Hypoglycaemia*

There are three main types of hypoglycaemia. The most common type is that caused when an insulin-dependent diabetic either injects too much insulin or fails to eat soon enough, or to eat an adequate amount of food after an insulin injection. The effect of an excess of insulin is to lower the blood glucose to levels that can cause a marked reaction.

Hypoglycaemia can also occur as a result of certain diseases. Very rarely, a tumour of the pancreas may cause secretions of insulin and profound hypoglycaemia, particularly if the person goes without food for several hours. Additionally it can accompany disorders such as liver disease, especially alcoholic liver disease, over- or under-activity of the thyroid gland, as a side-effect of some drugs, after operations that change the emptying pattern of the stomach and after alcoholic binges.

More severe forms of low blood sugar, often referred to as reactive hypoglycaemia, can be measured and dealt with medically, and indeed persistent symptoms should be medically investigated. Reactive hypoglycaemia is the term used to describe a fall in blood sugar following a rise brought about by eating a meal with a high content of starch or refined carbohydrates, sucrose or glucose. There has been much debate over the significance of reactive hypoglycaemia. It is probably much less common than was at first thought. The exact nature of the chemical signals involved has not yet been worked out, but it probably involves changes in carbohydrate and protein metabolism in the brain.

Low blood sugar can cause profound changes in mental function as well as physical ability and our mood.

| SOME SYMPTOMS OF LOW BLOOD SUGAR | | |
|---|---|---|
| Irritability | Hunger | Palpitations |
| Faintness | Nausea | Sweating |
| Dizziness | Headache | Apprehension |
| Weakness | Fatigue | Anxiety |

## What Your Doctor Can Do

It is fair to say that food craving (as opposed to low blood sugar) is not really recognised as a syndrome, and because of lack of education about nutrition, it is not something that most doctors would be equipped to deal with. Your doctor can:

◆ measure your fasting blood sugar levels
◆ investigate for any other underlying medical problem like diabetes
◆ assess your dietary habits to see whether you have an eating disorder

## Gail's Story

Gail, a thirty-six-year-old working mother with two young children, had been suffering with uncontrollable premenstrual bingeing since she finished breast-feeding her youngest child.

*I've always been a vegetarian—very health conscious and sporty. Not the type you'd think would suffer PMS. But all that changed after I had my second baby. When my periods returned, they returned with a vengeance. I suddenly found myself craving bars of chocolate and junk food. At first it was just one or two bars of chocolate a week but, within months, my craving for chocolate was insatiable and I was eating only junk food.*

*I'd raid the house for anything chocolatey and if I couldn't find anything, my poor husband would have to go and get me my 'fix'. I'd eat five or six bars in one sitting and still fancy more, even though I didn't really like the taste of it. I'd even raid the children's chocolate box. This went on for twenty-one days out of my twenty-eight-day cycle. I put on so much weight, and experienced feelings of violence and aggression which were vented on my family for no reason.*

*I visited my GP and was told that my symptoms were psychosomatic. I felt guilty and sure I should be able to control my cravings. During my one clear week each month I'd tell myself that next time it would be different. But, of course, a week later I was that madwoman all over again—cramming my face with chocolate and hating myself for it.*

*Thank heavens I read about the work that the WNAS were doing. Their programme helped me to withdraw from chocolate and caffeine. The first couple of weeks were awful. I had headaches and suffered terrible withdrawal symptoms. But I had been warned to expect this and so persisted with the programme. Within a few months I was completely back to normal. I had no cravings and began losing weight. All my premenstrual symptoms were gone.*

*It's been five years now and I've never looked back. Personally and professionally, thanks to a resurgence of self-belief and awareness brought about by the WNAS programme, life is wonderful. For the past three years I have studied incessantly to increase my knowledge of financial services, and practise as a financial advisor. I have since been adopted as a partner—all thanks to the WNAS.*

## What You Can Do

The most recent report produced by the UK Committee on Dietary Reference Values recommends that we cut down our non-milk extrinsic sugars by 50 per cent—this includes any foods or drinks containing sugar. It is not necessarily an ideal recommendation, as it really depends on how much you were eating in the first place. However, it does present an achievable goal that should bring about substantial improvements in both dental and general health.

◆ Avoid obesity. Obesity is associated with poorer blood sugar control, and at its worst can sometimes precede a diabetic state. The message is to keep your body weight in the normal range for your height and bone structure.

◆ Reduce intake of alcohol. Alcohol can cause liver damage, which can lead to significant hypoglycaemia. Replacing a meal with two or three gin and tonics, for example, can cause a profound rise and subsequent fall in blood glucose levels, producing all the symptoms of hypoglycaemia.

◆ Stop smoking. Smoking can increase the release of insulin and glucagon, another hormone which causes a rise in blood glucose, which is also released by the pancreas. Smoking is a powerful appetite suppressant in the short term. If a balanced meal is not consumed, blood glucose levels will inevitably fall.

◆ Cut down on tea and coffee. If these are consumed in large amounts, they can also cause an increase in the release of insulin. Large amounts of sugar consumed in tea or coffee can contribute to an unstable blood glucose level.

◆ Eat regularly. Irregular eating can lead to swings in blood glucose levels. This is particularly significant for insulin-dependent diabetics. Missing a meal or fasting will cause blood glucose levels to fall to the lower end of the normal range in susceptible individuals.

◆ Take exercise. This is the one factor that can improve the control of blood sugar, as well as having many other health benefits. Exercise increases the sensitivity of the body's response to insulin, leading to smoother control of blood sugar levels. Ideally you should be doing at least four sessions of exercise per week to the point of breathlessness.

## Useful Tips

◆ Consume nutritious food little and often. Eat breakfast, lunch and dinner each day, with a wholesome mid-morning and mid-afternoon snack to keep the blood sugar levels constant.

◆ Eat fresh, home-cooked foods wherever possible.

◆ Eat foods that are intrinsically sweet like dried fruit, fresh fruit, nuts and seeds.

◆ Relax whilst you are eating and enjoy your food.

◆ Plan your meals and snacks in advance.

◆ Take wholesome snacks out with you so that you don't get caught short.

◆ Always shop for food *after* you have eaten.

◆ Concentrate on a diet rich in chromium, magnesium and vitamins B and C. Although we need a constant supply of all the important nutrients, these three specific groups of nutrients have been shown to be needed to maintain normal blood sugar control. B vitamins are also necessary for optimum function of the brain and the nervous system, as is magnesium, which also is necessary for normal hormone function, and incidentally, is the most common nutritional deficiency amongst women of child-bearing age. Chromium is a curious mineral of which we have only tiny amounts at birth, and these gradually lessen as the years go by. Chromium, like magnesium and B vitamins, can be sourced in food, but we have to know where to look for it, so this calls for a little study of The Nutritional Content of Food lists (Appendix I).

◆ At the WNAS we recommend nutritional supplements of vitamin B, magnesium and chromium in the form of a preparation called Normoglycaemia, which acts as a short-term nutritional prop to regulate blood sugar levels.

◆ Take regular physical exercise, five sessions per week to the point of breathlessness.

◆ Use the Menu for Sugar Craving as a guide.

*See also*: Obesity, Alcoholism, What's Wrong with Present-day Diet and Lifestyle?, Nutrition Is the Key to Health, The Very Nutritious Diet, Menu for Sugar Craving. Plus Recommended Reading List (*Beat Sugar Craving*) and References.

# GALLSTONES

Gallstones are formed in the gall bladder, whose function it is to collect and concentrate a dark green fluid produced by the liver called bile. This fluid aids the digestive process, especially that of fats, and contains cholesterol, other fats, calcium and pigments derived from the breakdown of blood cells.

Gallstones form slowly, usually over many years, when the concentration of cholesterol, calcium and other chemicals normally found in the bile is so great that they can no longer remain in solution. Often the presence of a small amount of bacteria acts as the focus for the onset of gallstone formation. There may be just one stone or many small stones. Often the stones are 'silent'— being present, but without any symptoms. Their presence, however, may cause pain or other symptoms relating to digestion and the liver.

## What Are the Symptoms?
The pain caused by gallstones is often severe, episodic and can last up to 2 hours. The sufferer is likely to be doubled up by pain,

which is usually, though not always, located in the upper right-hand side part of the abdomen. Typically the episode passes off after a few hours. Minor episodes may occur, and can be associated with a feeling of sickness, or alternatively an aversion to large or fatty meals which may indeed trigger the attacks. Sometimes infection also develops in the gall bladder in which case there may be a fever, the pain is more prolonged and the sufferer is visibly unwell. If the gallstone moves and blocks the passage of bile from the liver to the bowel then the person becomes jaundiced and the stools become pale.

So much for the full-blown picture. We now know that gallstones are in fact very common and may cause milder intermittent symptoms of abdominal discomfort, nausea and aversion to fats. In this situation the picture is similar to that of irritable bowel syndrome or of a peptic ulcer. The treatments for these three common conditions are very different, so doctors as well as the sufferer need some understanding of what is going on.

## Who Gets Them?

They are rare in children, but do develop if there is a blood condition that leads to an increase in the breakdown pigments from haemoglobin. This can run in some families. Recent surveys reveal that the prevalence of gallstones, detected by ultrasound examination (like that used to look at unborn babies) rises steeply with age, especially after the age of forty and especially in women. Figures of between 10 and 20 per cent in the middle-aged and the elderly are not uncommon.

## What Causes Them?

◆ Being female, as women carry approximately twice the risk of men.
◆ Getting older.
◆ Being overweight, especially if the fat is distributed around the abdomen rather than the hips. Obese teenagers are especially at risk, as are those who gain weight in later life.
◆ Fluctuating weight. Feasting then dieting may cause changes to the chemistry of the bile that promotes gallstone formation.
◆ A diet high in sugar and low-fibre carbohydrates, e.g. potatoes, and low in fresh fruit and vegetables.

- Lack of alcohol! Just one drink per day seems to offer reasonable protection.
- The oral contraceptive pill and some drugs cause a slight increase.
- Severe constipation in women is associated.
- Some diseases of the liver and bowel are associated.
- A high level of fats called triglycerides in the blood. This is associated with being overweight, being diabetic, or consuming a lot of alcohol or sugar.

## What Your Doctor Can Do

- Ignore them. Gallstones that are found coincidentally, and cause no or very few symptoms, require no treatment. Gallstones are a phenomenon that many us will acquire if we live long enough. However we may not all live long enough for them to be a problem.
- Remove them with an operation. This is necessary for most of us if they start to cause problems like severe pain, infection or cause jaundice. The operation may be needed as an emergency, or more usually is tackled when any acute episode is over. During the operation the gall bladder and the stone or stones are removed, and special attention has to be paid to make sure that all the stones present are found.
- Dissolve them using chemical treatments. Preparations of acids with cholesterol-dissolving properties are a possible treatment for some with stones made mainly from cholesterol. This technique is useful when the stones do not contain a lot of calcium and are contained within a relatively healthy gall bladder.
- Destroy them using high-energy sound waves. This is technically known as extracorporeal shock-wave lithotripsy. With the abdomen immersed in water, high-energy sound waves can be focused upon the gallstones when they shatter. Combining this with chemical means leads to a 90 per cent success rate in selected patients.

## What You Can Do

If you need an operation, have it. Then select those pieces of the following advice that may be relevant to you. If your gallstones are not really a problem, and there is no need for definitive treatment, the following advice may reduce the risk of their becoming worse. Increasing numbers of people will fall into this category. These measures may also be helpful if your gallstones are being dissolved by chemical means.

- Lose weight if you need to (see, The Simple Weight-loss Diet).
- Alternatively follow The Very Nutritious Diet or The Vegetarian Diet.
- Allow yourself one alcoholic drink per day.
- Don't let yourself be constipated.
- Don't miss meals. Eat regularly and always have breakfast.
- Supplements of vitamin C, 1 g per day, might help by encouraging the breakdown of cholesterol.

## *Complementary Therapies*
Traditional naturopathic texts refer to the treatment of gallstones using the juice of 6 lemons and 300 ml of olive oil. A small number of our patients have apparently used this treatment after an overnight fast. According to their testimony they have subsequently passed a number of small stones and been relieved of their gallbladder pain. This is a potentially dangerous treatment for most patients with gallstones, especially those with large or multiple stones. If any reader of this book has successfully passed stones in this way we would be grateful if they would contact us. Photographic evidence or a suitable affidavit would be required! This truly is a kill or cure treatment.

# GENITAL HERPES

The term 'herpes' is derived from the Greek word *herpein*, meaning 'to creep', and it was first described by Hippocrates. Genital herpes is a disease that is spread through sexual contact, and may be passed to new partners without either party being aware of the risk. It cannot be cured, it may cause cancer, and it may be passed on to new-born babies who either die or become severely brain damaged. When compared to genital herpes, syphilis and gonorrhoea appear to be relatively mild diseases.

The virus that causes genital herpes is the *Herpes simplex* virus type 2 (HSV-2). This is one of a family of five herpes viruses that cause a wide range of human ills, including chickenpox, shingles, infectious mononucleosis (glandular fever), and birth defects such as mental retardation. Research suggests that HSV-2 is a complicated virus, with over 100 000 different strains or varieties of its basic structure. HSV-1, the virus that causes cold sores can also cause genital herpes as well. As people 'swap' mucous membranes during sexual intercourse, it is likely that either of these types of virus may be present in genital herpes.

## What Are the Symptoms?

Genital herpes affects the vulva, perineum, buttocks, cervix, the vagina, thigh or anus, and sores can erupt in any of these areas.

| SYMPTOMS OF GENITAL HERPES | | | |
|---|---|---|---|
| Itching | Burning | Blisters | Open sores |
| Fever | Painful urination | Immobility | Headaches |
| General malaise | Swollen lymph glands | Painful bowel movements | |

When genital herpes repeats itself, as it does, particularly in the first year following the primary attack, some of these symptoms may recur. The attack usually begins when a person experiences an itchy tingling sensation over a reddened area of the skin, which is followed hours or days later by a single blister, or cluster of highly infectious fluid-filled sores that will erupt in one to two days, and then crust over after three or four days. These sores usually appear on the cervix, in the vagina and in the urethra, and in men the sores are generally on the penile shaft.

The primary outbreak may involve intense pain for as long as three weeks, but subsequent outbreaks tend to be less and less severe as time passes, and in some cases they are almost unnoticeable.

## What Causes It?

The virus can be passed to a woman in any of the following ways:

◆ sexual intercourse with an infected partner with active sores
◆ sexual caresses from a partner with herpetic whitlows, sores on the fingers
◆ oral sex with a partner who has a herpes sore on the mouth

It can also be triggered by internal stimulation of the latent virus which has been hiding in the body by any of the following:

◆ emotional stress
◆ over-exertion
◆ sunburn
◆ fever
◆ ultraviolet light
◆ onset of a period
◆ anxiety or depression over the illness
◆ persistent vaginal discharge
◆ chafing
◆ impaired immune system which may be caused by some of the above and by a lack of essential nutrients

## What Your Doctor Can Do

◆ Prescribe Acyclovir (Zovirax), the only effective anti-viral agent. It can be given as a cream for those suffering their first attack, but this does not help recurrent episodes. In tablet form it is not always well absorbed. A dose of 200 mg five times per day for five days can be used to treat repeated attacks, but to be of any use it needs to be taken as soon as symptoms begin, often before there is definitive evidence of the infection. This means your doctor giving you a prescription to carry around with you in the event of a further attack.

Long-term use of Acyclovir to prevent attacks is sometimes used. The dose is 200 mg per day. This is only rarely required.

◆ Assess you for the presence of other genital infection especially candida.
◆ Assess and treat your partner.

## *What You Can Do*

◆ Report early when you have symptoms.

◆ Use symptomatic treatment to control the discomfort, which includes painkillers, e.g. aspirin or paracetamol, especially if there are generalised 'flu'-like symptoms, and local applications of iodine ointment (messy but effective), ice packs, or used tea bags (an old folk remedy).

◆ Refrain from sexual intercourse—just in case you wondered.

◆ Wear underpants in bed at night to minimise the risk of spread to other parts of the body, e.g. the hands and eyes.

◆ Wash your hands thoroughly every time you go to the toilet.

◆ Try supplements of lysine. Lysine is an amino acid found in foods and can replace the chemically related amino acid arginine which is needed by the virus to replicate itself. Supplements of lysine have been used in the treatment of oral herpes with some benefit. Not all studies have been positive. The dose is 50 mg three times per day. Some advise taking it with vitamin C, 1 g three times per day.

◆ Follow a diet rich in lysine and low in an opposing amino acid, arginine. This means avoiding nuts, chocolate, carob, oats, wholewheat and soya beans. You can eat more of fish, chicken, meats, milk, cheese, mung beans and other beans but not soya.

◆ Try supplements of multi-vitamins and zinc in the longer term as a means of improving resistance to infection. Also follow The Very Nutritious Diet.

◆ Avoid those factors that seem to precipitate an attack.

◆ Do not get pregnant until this problem is sorted out. You should probably see a venereologist if your genital herpes is recurrent, and you and your partner are planning a pregnancy. It is possible for a woman with genital herpes to bear a normal healthy child, if medical screening procedures are methodically followed prior to delivery. If the screening shows that the infection has become active near or during labour, the baby can be protected by being delivered by caesarean section.

## *Complementary Therapies*

Anything that helps to strengthen the immune system may help to increase your rate of healing. The main four therapies—cranial osteopathy, acupuncture, herbal medicine and homoeopathy—are all geared to do this in their own way. It is a matter of preference which combination of therapies you try.

.....................................................................................................

## Jennifer's Story

Jennifer, a thirty-six-year-old mother of three, works as a receptionist at a family planning clinic. She had suffered with herpes for thirteen years, and although she and her doctor tried all sorts of medication nothing really kept the herpes at bay.

*I had been suffering with herpes for so long and they have been much worse for the last couple of years. I remember when we went on a family holiday in the sun, and my whole top lip swelled up. It really ruined the holiday. I also had boils on my chin to accompany the herpes which made me feel like nothing on earth. Last year we went on holiday again, and there wasn't even any sunshine, but I still had an attack. In fact, when I think about it I have had herpes every couple of weeks for years and it seems to last for about ten days each time so I have been rarely free of an ugly cold sore on my lips.*

*My doctor had prescribed all sorts of products. We have tried antiseptic, and I have even tried antibiotics, but nothing seemed to help. In fact, some of the products for herpes seemed to make the sores spread.*

*I approached the WNAS for some help with my premenstrual syndrome, after reading their book on PMS. Not only is my PMS relatively non-existent now but I haven't had an outbreak of herpes or boils since I began. I can't really believe it and I am thrilled to bits. We are off to Cornwall this year and I am looking forward to a normal family holiday.*

*See also*: References.

# HAEMORRHOIDS

Women are particularly prone to haemorrhoids, or 'piles' as they are commonly known, which are varicose veins that form inside the rectum. Sometimes after childbirth or following an episode of constipation, because of the straining and pressure in the area, they become external, and resemble a small bunch of grapes. They can vary from being mildly uncomfortable to extremely painful, and they often bleed, as their thin walls may be ruptured by a passing motion.

Our veins contain valves, which prevent blood flowing backwards. When the vessels are healthy and strong, this system works well. However, when the valves themselves become weak and inefficient, blood flows backwards and pools at certain points making the vessel wall swell out into a varicose vein.

## What Are the Symptoms?

- pressure and a feeling that 'everything is falling out' of your rectum
- soreness, irritation and sometimes sharp pains in the rectum
- itchiness around the anus
- small amounts of fresh red blood in the stools

## What Causes Them?

- The constant pressure of carrying a baby during pregnancy can precipitate haemorrhoids in a woman who has not previously been a sufferer.
- Straining on the toilet when constipated can weaken the vessel walls in the area.
- Lack of adequate nutrition—for example we know that vitamin C and bioflavonoids are necessary for the health of the walls of our blood vessels.
- Lifting heavy goods on a regular basis.
- Bouts of coughing.

## What Your Doctor Can Do

- Examine your back passage to determine whether haemorrhoids are present, or whether there is likely to be any other physical problem, like a tear or a growth.
- Prescribe some soothing cream, suppositories or topical anaesthetic to help relieve the pain, if it is severe.
- Supply you with an anal dilator to manually replace external haemorrhoids after a motion.
- An enlightened doctor will tell you to increase your consumption of fruit and vegetable fibre, but not necessarily cereal fibre, which can sometimes make constipation worse.
- Give you, or refer you for, a course of injections, which over a period of three months cause the haemorrhoids to shrink.

◆ In severe cases, refer you for surgical removal of the haemorrhoids. This is a particularly painful operation, and there is no guarantee that the haemorrhoids won't re-form, unless you tackle the underlying cause.

## What You Can Do

◆ Keep your motions very soft by eating a good diet. Follow the recommendations for The Very Nutritious Diet or, if you think you may have food sensitivities, follow the recommendations for The Simple Exclusion Diet.

◆ Take supplements of magnesium at night to keep the motions soft, and 2 tablespoons of organic linseeds with your morning cereal to make the motions smooth, rather than dry and lumpy. The magnesium needs to be taken to gut tolerance level (see Constipation). This will prevent you from straining, which stresses the haemorrhoids further.

◆ Drink plenty of fruit juice, water and herbal tea.

◆ After each motion, gently bathe your tail end, and use some soothing herbal cream, either from the health-food shop or ask your herbal practitioner to make up a prescription for you.

◆ If you have external haemorrhoids, take care to manually replace them with an anal dilator greased with herbal cream.

◆ During an acute episode, keep your feet up when you can, until the pain and soreness has diminished.

◆ Make up a small bag of frozen peas and sit on it for 10 minutes. This should be repeated throughout the day when symptoms flare up, and will help to reduce the swelling and inflammation in the area.

◆ Take warm baths or showers rather than hot baths, as the intense heat may encourage even more blood into the area.

◆ Take regular exercise, including exercises for your pelvic floor and your tail end. Draw your muscles in as if you are trying to stop the flow of urine mid-cycle. Hold it for the count of ten, and then slowly release. You can repeat this exercise at convenient moments during the day.

## Complementary Therapies

Acupuncture, homeopathy, herbal medicine and cranial osteopathy all have something to offer in their own way. Improving the flow of fluid around the body will help to unblock the areas of stagnation. Addditionally acupuncture may also be able to help strengthen the walls of the vessels.

*See also*: Standard References.

# HAIR LOSS

There are different patterns of hair loss in women and men. In men there is often a receding hair line which is due to action of the male hormone testosterone. Women may occasionally experience this pattern, but more usually have either generalised diffuse hair loss or alopecia areata.

Alopecia areata involves discrete patches of hair loss. It is common in young adults, and often recovers spontaneously. Treatment sometimes involves injection of steroids and always patience. There seems to be little that the patient can do to speed up the natural turn of events.

Diffuse hair loss is exactly what it says it is, with generalised thinning and loss of hair from the top of the head. Generalised, often mild, scalp hair loss can also accompany any disease of the scalp such as psoriasis and eczema.

## What Your Doctor Can Do

Your doctor can investigate the cause by checking for:

- an underactive thyroid gland or other hormonal disturbance
- a pregnancy
- a fever or any severe illness
- a side-effect of drugs
- iron deficiency, even a mild lack, for example following blood donation

## What You Can Do

- Eat The Very Nutritious Diet.
- Take a supplement of iron if you are anaemic or if the haemoglobin level is normal but at the lower end (11.0 to 12.5 g/dl). A small supplement such as 1 tablet of Ferrous Sulphate taken

daily with fruit juice for six months is safe, and should correct any mild deficiency. You will need to take it for six months, though, as recovery is slow.

◆ Supplements of zinc and multi-vitamins might be helpful. Again they will need to be taken for several months.

## Complementary Therapies

Watch out for some unusual shampoos. Local applications are unlikely to make much difference and sensitisation can occur. For advice see a qualified trichologist (see *Yellow Pages*).

# HALITOSIS

Bad breath, or halitosis as it is medically known, in most cases is detected by someone other than the sufferer themselves. It is not a very social topic of conversation, and even dentists, who are responsible for keeping us orally fit, are sometimes embarrassed about mentioning it to a patient. Dental health problems were among the health conditions reported most frequently in the Australian Bureau of Statistics 1989/90 National Health Survey.

The mere thought that our breath may be unsavoury does little for our self-confidence, and is likely to make us feel introverted and nervous. If you think you may be a sufferer check it out with your partner or a close friend, and ask them to be absolutely honest. A bad taste in your mouth doesn't always translate to a bad smell, and it is difficult to smell your own breath. If you do suffer, you need to know so that you can deal with it without delay.

## What Causes It?

◆ The most serious cause is an infection of the gums, where the bone supporting the teeth is eaten away after plaque (bacteria in the mouth) has been allowed to stagnate in the pockets of gum surrounding the teeth. Plaque becomes rotten and smelly as it ages, which is what causes the odour.

◆ The milder form of gum disease is known as gingivitis, which means inflammation of the gums, and a more advanced form, which involves bone resorption, is called periodontitis or periodontosis. Not all gum infections cause bad breath though. It usually has to be an acute flare up or advanced gum disease before it affects the nostrils of others. Acute ulcerative gingivitis, or trench mouth as it more commonly known, will make the breath smell foul, and should be treated quickly.

◆ Stomach disorders such as hiatus hernia can create an oral odour.

◆ Infections of the tonsils and respiratory tract may also make the mouth smell.

◆ Hormonal changes, particularly a rise in the level of the hormone progesterone, can cause gums to be swollen, resulting in a bad taste and sometimes a bad smell. This is why symptoms are sometimes worse before a period or during pregnancy.

◆ A dry mouth, which can arise from stress or other illnesses, or simply as a result of too much exertion and not enough fluid, often causes bad breath.

◆ Food allergies often cause a reflux, food returning to the mouth after it has been digested, which is smelly.

◆ Crash diets affect the flow of saliva, and this is the body's natural mouth wash, flushing away odour-producing bacteria. Some drugs like sleeping pills can also dry the mouth.

◆ Constipation can be associated with halitosis.

## What Your Doctor Can Do

◆ Check to see whether you have a hiatus hernia, upper respiratory tract infection, like infected tonsils, or constipation. If so, these should be treated and the problem will resolve by itself.

◆ If you are on medication, check to see whether you are suffering a dry mouth as a side-effect.

## What Your Dentist Can Do

Check for the presence of any form of gum disease, and if so treat it, see pages 328–9. Gingivitis can be eliminated by careful toothbrushing and flossing between the teeth, over a period of weeks or months. More severe forms of gum disease, where pockets of calculus (old, hard stagnated plaque) have developed between the gum and the tooth, may involve dental intervention. The pockets can be cleaned out by the dentist or the hygienist, and in severe cases where bone loss has occurred, but substantial bone still exists, the bones can be remodelled. Once the mouth has been cleaned up, your breath will undoubtedly feel fresher.

◆ Diagnose AUG (acute ulcerative gingivitis) or trench mouth (see page 329) which needs urgent treatment with metronidazole—a special form of antibiotic.

......................................................................................................................................

## Julia's Story

Julia, a thirty-six-year-old part-time sales assistant with two children, had developed halitosis—bad breath—which made her feel extremely self-conscious.

*With hindsight I think my problem started years ago when my two children were small. Our eldest child had open-heart surgery as a toddler and I knew that he would need a further operation when he reached his teens. We also had concerns about the little one at school. My mouth and throat became dry, which I presumed was directly related to the anxiety. My husband eventually confirmed my worst fears, that my breath was very smelly, particularly in the two weeks before my period. I had a foul sour taste in my mouth, and when I ran my tongue across my teeth I was aware of an equally unpleasant smell.*

*My first thought was that I must have a dental problem. I was extremely dismayed when my dentist could find nothing wrong with my teeth, and only minor inflammation on the gums which I corrected with improved brushing. I read that halitosis can be caused by a number of illnesses, like lung disease and gastric ailments like hiatus hernia. But my doctor confirmed that there was nothing wrong with me in these departments.*

*I began to wonder if my problem had something to do with the food I was eating, so I made a point of avoiding all the acknowledged obnoxious smelling foods like onions, garlic and blue cheese. I brushed my teeth several times each day, flossed between them, gargled with mouthwash and chewed and sucked fresh-breath sweets and gum. Nothing worked and I became so embarrassed about the problem that I made sure I stood well away from people when I spoke to them. I even got into the habit of covering my mouth with my hand when having a conversation.*

*I felt very humiliated and self-conscious. I was used to being such a lively and outgoing person, it's hard not to be inhibited when you are trying to keep your mouth firmly shut. Most people are too polite to comment, but I knew they could smell my bad breath, which was so distressing. What didn't make sense was that* the smell was worse for two weeks before my period, and seemed to improve after my period had begun. I had been having other premenstrual problems for many years which eventually led me to the solution.

I read an article in a magazine about premenstrual syndrome, and not dreaming that my breath problem could be connected, I wrote for information. When I received the questionnaire from the WNAS I was stunned to see that bad breath was one of the premenstrual symptoms they asked about. I came to discover that life events and stress can upset the brain chemistry which influences our hormones. It turned out that I had an allergy to wheat, which seemed to cause a chemical reaction in my body, particularly before my period. Once I tidied up my diet and avoided wheat the bad breath cleared up completely. The only problem was that I had cravings for pasties in the two weeks before my period, and each time I indulged I'd feel the bad breath taste welling in my mouth. Once I tuned in to my body I realised that the pasties and other foods containing wheat affected my gut too. This explained why my breath was worse premenstrually.

It's ten years since I kissed my bad breath goodbye. Occasionally I get the cravings for a pasty, and if I do indulge I feel that old familiar taste return. I managed to overcome the other premenstrual symptoms too and feel totally in control. It's wonderful to be able to smile and chat without having to be self-conscious.

## What You Can Do

- ◆ Follow The Good Oral Hygiene Plan on page 335.
- ◆ Omit from your diet any foods that you are aware upset your tummy, and of course avoid the known smelly foods like garlic and onions.
- ◆ Use an anti-bacterial mouth wash before brushing your teeth which helps to decrease the plaque levels, and thus reduce the smell.
- ◆ Coffee and cigarettes can dry your mouth, so it's best to cut these down, or better still, cut them out altogether.

*See also*: Allergies, Constipation, Asthma, The Simple Exclusion Diet. Plus Recommended Reading List and References.

# HAYFEVER AND ALLERGIC RHINITIS

Nasal irritation, discharge, sneezing and blockage are the hallmarks of rhinitis which literally means 'inflammation of the nose'. This can occur at fixed times of the year, being related most frequently to pollens and is known as hayfever. Non-seasonal rhinitis may occur separately, or as well, and is often related to housedust mite allergy, but there are other possible causes. The symptoms of nasal irritation may be accompanied by throat itching, irritation in the ears, conjunctivitis with red watery eyes and, in more severe cases, asthma.

The basic mechanism involved is that cells called mast cells present in the nose and lungs are stimulated by an allergen (a substance to which the individual is allergic), and subsequently release a variety of powerful irritating chemicals, including histamine. These chemicals produce the symptoms of rhinitis, and in particular stimulate the production of mucus, possibly in an attempt to 'wash away' the triggering allergen as though it were a serious threat to health. The mast cell contains, on its surface, specific antibodies of a type called IgE that interacts with specific antigens. Other chemicals and cells found in the lining of the nose determine the degree to which the body produces this sensitising IgE antibody.

## Who Gets It?

Something like 20 per cent of Australians and New Zealanders suffer. The most common causes of hayfever are the housedust mite, grass pollens and cats. However, almost anything can cause hayfever, from air pollution and cigarette smoking to aspirin and some foods.

There is some association with other allergic conditions such as eczema and asthma, and there is therefore probably a genetic component in determining who is likely to suffer.

## What Causes It?

It will be useful to separate seasonal and non-seasonal allergies.

*Seasonal allergies*

Spring and summer can be months of sheer misery for the two million sufferers of seasonal hayfever in Australia and New Zealand. A recent book, *The Low Allergy Garden* by Dr Mark Ragg, looks at the role of plants in causing allergies and lists which ones to plant and which ones to avoid. The book also includes month-by-month pollen calendars for Australia and New Zealand.

♦ Tree pollens are present in the spring and continue throughout the summer months.
♦ Grass pollen is abundant again throughout the spring and summer months.
♦ Weed pollens.
♦ Sensitivity to mould is again not uncommon. There are many varieties present from June until the autumn. Moulds are Mother Nature's dustbin men, breaking down vegetable matter, and releasing millions of invisible spores. Depending upon the variety, this can occur in either warm summer weather following rain, or after a heavy dew. In the house, damp dark places, especially cellars, attract moulds. In the garden, compost heaps, piles of grass cuttings and the soil are all places where some moulds proliferate.

*Non-seasonal allergies*

♦ Housedust mites are the commonest perennial allergen. They are abundant in most homes and live on shed human skin scales, thriving in the warm, moderately moist conditions that are the norm in most centrally-heated modern homes. Carpets, bedding materials and furnishings are the major preferred residences for these common allergens. Housedust mite counts tend to peak in the spring and autumn, and their level is greatly influenced by the type of materials found in the home, and cleaning habits.
♦ Animals, especially domestic pets, are again another common source of allergic material. This is often from the saliva of cats which is passed on to their hair but can also be present in the air and mixed in with housedust. Dog, rabbit and horse hair as well as feathers are other possibilities. Sensitivity to an animal's urine can also develop in farm and laboratory workers.
♦ Cockroaches in semi-tropical climes and now some inner city

buildings are again a potential source of allergic rhinitis.

◆ Occupational exposure to animal products, chemicals, flour, yeast, enzymes in biological washing powders and in flour improvers, and rubber are all possibilities.

◆ Foods are a possibility, though this is an uncertain area. From adult and child experience it would seem that sensitivity to artificial colours, dairy products and oranges are especially likely. Only repeated withdrawal and challenge will determine the issue.

◆ Sulphur dioxide is worth a special mention. This is a chemical pollutant found in the air, especially in relation to inner cities and industrial areas. Some are particularly sensitive to it as it readily irritates the lining of the nose and lungs. Small amounts of this and related chemicals called sulphites are used as a preservative in foods and beverages (E 220–227). It is a surprisingly common additive in wine, especially cheap acidic white wine and in some this tipple will aggravate symptoms of rhinitis and asthma. Concentrated squashes are another possible source.

## What Your Doctor Can Do

◆ Help identify the allergen from your history, from skin prick tests or, occasionally, blood allergy tests.

◆ Advise about allergen avoidance.

◆ Offer drug treatment with steroid nasal sprays, antihistamine tablets and nasal sprays, and a nasal spray of sodium cromoglycate which blocks the allergen's interaction with IgE and the activation of the mast cell.

◆ Rarely desensitisation is used for isolated grass-pollen sensitivity.

## What You Can Do

Avoiding the allergen is a central part of treatment for most sufferers.

◆ For seasonal allergens it may be difficult to completely avoid them. Staying indoors with windows and doors closed, during times of high grass pollen count is for many a thing of the past because of effective drug treatments. For some, going to the seaside and sitting on the beach with an on-shore wind blowing is a way to reduce one's exposure to pollen.

- If mould sensitivity is a problem, make sure that you are not being exposed to mould in the house. Watch out for damp patches with dark discoloration of wallpaper, and treat such patches with an antifungal paint. If there is a lot of damp, then a builder may need to be consulted. Treat any dry, as well as wet, rot that affects wooden structures. It may be advisable to remove houseplants which encourage mould growth.

- Measures to reduce exposure to housedust mite can be highly effective though this can take two or more months before the full benefit is experienced. The following measures are recommended in approximate order of importance and cost:

  - Use a modern powerful vacuum cleaner with an efficient filtration system once or twice weekly in the bedroom and main living areas.

  - Vacuum the carpets, furniture and the mattress and pillows.

  - Clean sheets and duvet covers weekly on a hot wash.

  - Renew pillows, opting for a synthetic and not feather filling.

  - Use a synthetic-filled duvet rather than wool blankets and sheets.

  - Put the pillow and duvet out into bright sunshine on a dry day for several hours each week or month when possible. This helps to kill off dust mites.

  - You can also wash pillows and duvets from time to time.

  - Putting pillows into the freezer for 24 hours and then into a tumble drier for 30 minutes will help curtail the mite's activities.

  - Keep the temperature and humidity in the bedroom low.

  - Minimise use of soft furnishings, cuddly toys and carpets in the bedroom.

  - Buy a new mattress.

  - Use specialised occlusive covers for the mattress and pillows. This is worth considering if symptoms persist despite simple measures, or if mite sensitivity is a factor in asthma which is severe enough to require regular treatment with substantial amounts of steroids.

  - In the case of animal sensitivity, remove the animal from bedrooms and main living areas. Many children with asthma, without obvious animal sensitivity, are well advised not to have cats or dogs as pets in case they develop a sensitivity.

◇ In the case of exposure at work to a possible allergen, expert advice may be needed, particularly in the case of asthma that is severe enough to affect the quality of life.

◆ If food sensitivity really is suspected then try The Simple Exclusion Diet (but only with medical supervision if you have asthma).

◆ Try limiting exposure to sulphites in foods and beverages (this latter will include some beers and many cheaper acidic tasting wines).

◆ Exercise might help! A run or 40 minutes' aerobics is a pretty good way of clearing your nasal passages. Regular exercise over several weeks might reduce the overall degree of sensitivity of the lining of the nose.

◆ Avoid drugs that might worsen nasal congestion. Sensitivity to aspirin is a not infrequent problem. Be suspicious of this if there are also nasal polyps, a personal history of asthma, or a family history of aspirin intolerance. Paracetamol is usually a safe alternative. Those who are very sensitive may need expert advice, and may benefit from a specialised diet low in fruits, vegetables and other foods containing salicylates.

◆ Vitamin C, 1 g twice daily, has a moderate antihistamine effect. It's simple, cheap and free from side-effects.

◆ Supplements of vitamin B or multi-vitamins might help. Vitamin B6, pyridoxine, is needed by the body for the breakdown of histamine.

# HEADACHES

Headaches are familiar to practically everyone, being the most common human complaint. At least 80 per cent of the population suffer with tension headaches at some point, and they are essentially due to contractions of the muscles of the scalp, neck and face. It is primarily an adult problem, with women affected three times as often as men. About half of those afflicted will have headaches that are severe and disabling, and it is thought that between 10 and 20 per cent will consult a doctor about their headaches, as a primary symptom. Unlike migraine, which occurs periodically, the tension headache is often a daily occurrence. It usually gets worse as the day goes by, and it is not associated with visual disturbance.

## What Are the Symptoms?

The symptoms of a tension headache usually consist of an aching or squeezing discomfort on both sides of the crown, temples and forehead. The description most often used to illustrate the headaches is 'It feels like a tight band around my head, like a skull cap' or 'as if a clamp or vice was squeezing my head'. Others feel as if their head is about to 'burst or explode', and they stress that there is a feeling of pressure as well as pain.

The neck is often involved, and so too, sometimes are the nose and jaw. The headaches may only last for a few hours, but can last for days, weeks and even months.

## What Causes Them?

Tension headaches are frequently associated with spasm of the muscles of the scalp, neck or shoulders. Anxiety and depression are other emotional associates. A somewhat different view is that of cranial osteopathy, which believes that tension headaches often come about because of stress to the fascia, the connective tissue structure under the skin. This can apparently be the result of physical, mental or emotional trauma.

The cause is usually a combination of overwork, stress, lack of exercise or an emotional crisis of some sort which causes the muscles to go into spasm.

Whilst headaches may stand alone as a problem, they may also be a manifestation of various general medical diseases, or problems affecting the nervous system or the head. The risk of headaches being due to a serious condition increases after the age of sixty-five years of age. Other possibilities include bleeding or leakage from blood vessels at the base of the brain, and only very rarely a brain tumour.

## What Your Doctor Can Do

◆ Examine you physically, and take a history of the problem, which is important for three reasons: firstly, to eliminate the possibility of the symptoms being anything other than a tension headache; secondly, to locate the source of the headache, such as the neck, which may have been forgotten; and thirdly, to put your mind at rest. Anxiety about an underlying brain haemorrhage or something will only serve to make the headaches worse.

◆ Once the cause is located, it may be that drugs are unnecessary. However, analgesics, and even sedatives, tranquillisers and other tension-relieving drugs are sometimes used. If drugs are used they should only be limited to short courses.

◆ Refer you to a neurologist if there is any cause for concern.

## What You Can Do

◆ Eat a good diet. Follow the recommendations for The Very Nutritious Diet.

◆ Avoid excessive amounts of tea, coffee and alcohol.

◆ Never miss a meal, as low blood sugar can often precipitate a headache.

◆ Talk through any problems you face, and aim to get a workable solution underway.

◆ Learn to manage your time, so that you have time for regular relaxation.

◆ Try to reorganise yourself so that you can avoid further stressful situations recurring.

◆ Take regular exercise, preferably in the fresh air and sunlight when available.

◆ Massage your own scalp, forehead, temples and ears regularly, or treat yourself to a regular massage. Use some of the gentler and more relaxing aromatherapy oils like lavender, ylang ylang or geranium.

◆ Take daily supplements of strong multi-vitamins and minerals, with a high-potency B complex. Add an extra supplement of magnesium, in the region of 300 mg per day, as magnesium acts as a muscle relaxant. It may take two or three months before it is fully effective.

◆ When you feel the stress is getting the better of you, try going for a walk or doing some deep breathing.

◆ Try chewing some ginger, either root or crystallised, as this old remedy can often reverse the process of a headache if caught in time.

## Complementary Therapies

Cranial osteopathy is the first choice of treatment, and may sort out the underlying physical cause of your headaches. Other therapies like herbal medicine, homoeopathy and acupuncture all have something to offer.

*See also*: References.

# HEART FAILURE

At its simplest, this is a failure of the pumping action of the heart. For a variety of reasons the heart may not be able to pump enough blood forwards around through the lungs and around the body. The heart has two sides: the right side pumps blood to the lungs where oxygen is collected and carbon dioxide released; the refreshed blood returns from the lungs to the left side of the heart from whence it is pumped around the body. This requires a greater degree of force and consequently the left side of the heart is bigger than the right side. Blood is prevented from flowing back in the wrong direction by a series of valves and chambers in both sides of the heart.

## What Are the Symptoms?

◆ shortness of breath, especially with any activity, or at night when lying down
◆ fatigue
◆ ankle swelling
◆ cough
◆ irregular breathing pattern when asleep
◆ poor appetite
◆ sometimes, loss of weight

## Who Gets It?

The elderly are the largest group at risk, and heart failure is now one of the commonest reasons for admission to hospital throughout the developed world.

## What Causes It?

Often there is more than one cause. The main ones are:

- high blood pressure
- ischaemic heart disease
- disorders of the heart muscle or the heart valves
- alcoholism
- nutritional deficiencies
- rarely, infections

## What Your Doctor Can Do

- Assess the cause and severity. This often requires specialist referral for blood tests, X-rays, ECG—electro-cardiogram, an electrical heart tracing—and ultrasound examination of the heart.
- Treat the failure with diuretics or water pills, digitalis (a very old-fashioned but effective drug derived from foxglove), and drugs that help to open up blood vessels and reduce the pressure under which the heart works. These latter drugs, called ACE Inhibitors, have greatly improved the outlook for many with heart failure.
- Advise about the need for supplements of potassium which may be deficient or in excess as a result of drug treatment.

## What You Can Do

- Rest in bed with your feet up. This helps in the removal of excess fluid in acute episodes of heart failure.
- Follow The Low-salt Diet, as salt in the diet contributes to a build-up of water in the body and creates more work for the heart to do.
- Make sure the diet is adequate in essential nutrients, especially protein, vitamin B, potassium and magnesium.
- Spread the meals out in the day, as eating little and often is a good rule for you to follow.
- Avoid all alcohol. It is actually a poison and damages the heart muscle.
- Take supplements of multi-vitamins and magnesium, with your doctors approval, as these may well make a difference if you are not eating very well.
- Weigh yourself regularly, as rapid weight loss or weight gain may signify deterioration in heart function.

◆ Exercise. Amazingly, very careful graded exercise is appropriate for those with mild to moderate heart failure once any acute episode is over. In fact this can lead to considerable improvement and actually helps correct the underlying weakness of the heart muscle in a way not achieved by drug therapy. Again specialist advice from your doctor is needed.

# HIGH BLOOD PRESSURE

The blood in our body circulates around due to the pumping action of the heart which causes the blood leaving the heart in the arteries to be at a higher pressure than that which is returning to the heart in the veins. When the heart contracts, the pressure rises to reach a peak called the systolic pressure, and between contractions the pressure falls to what is termed the diastolic pressure.

When you have your blood pressure measured, both these levels are recorded and are expressed as the systolic value over the diastolic value. They are measured as millimetres of mercury which are written as 'mm Hg'. Elevation of either can be associated with an increased risk of a stroke and other disorders of the circulation. The clear association of a raised blood pressure with stroke risk, and the now-established benefit of reducing blood pressure, means that doctors commonly measure blood pressure during routine examinations and patient visits.

Blood pressure values vary considerably from one person to another and from country to country. Furthermore our own blood pressure shows a substantial variation during the course of the day rising with stress, physical pain, exercise and sexual intercourse. There is usually a modest rise with age in most urban populations and much of this age-related rise has been attributed to the relatively high intakes of sodium salt found in the diet of developed communities.

Definitions of high blood pressure vary. In the United States and now in most other developed countries, many experts accept that if the blood pressure is consistently greater than 140/90 mm Hg, then this is worthy of a diagnosis of hypertension, and more importantly a signal to do something about it. For most adults a rise in either the diastolic or systolic readings above these values is associated with an increased risk of premature death. Values up to 160/95 are considered to be mild hypertension and may be improved by non-drug approaches. Severe hypertension with blood pressure values above 160/110 almost always needs drug treatment and, if not tackled vigorously, is associated with greatly increased risk of early death usually from a stroke, kidney damage or a heart attack.

The risk of all three rises as blood pressure rises, and there is also an increase in the furring up of arteries in the legs which leads to peripheral vascular disease. These conditions are dealt with elsewhere in this book.

The mechanisms behind these diseases are damage to the walls of the arteries that are subjected to this increase in pressure. The artery wall becomes thickened, the lining damaged and more prone to the deposition of cholesterol, particularly if the blood level is elevated. The risk of blood pressure to health is thus greatly magnified if the person is overweight, smokes cigarettes, drinks excessively, has an elevated blood cholesterol or eats a diet low in fresh fruit and vegetables.

The symptoms of a high blood pressure are few and far between. Usually with a mildly elevated pressure there are none, and the diagnosis is made by chance at routine examination. Headaches, giddiness, a sensation of fullness in the head are all possible symptoms, but equally have many other causes. Dangerously high blood pressure can cause these as well as visual disturbance, symptoms relating to nerve damage, and even epilepsy or loss of consciousness. Symptoms relating to another condition causing the high blood pressure may also be present.

## Who Gets It?

The prevalence of high blood pressure obviously depends on the criteria set for its diagnosis. In the United States 33 per cent of white men and 38 per cent of black men in the age range eighteen to seventy-four years have a blood pressure above 140/90. The rise in systolic blood pressure with age means that the risk of high blood pressure is greater in the older population. Generally high blood pressure is more common in women compared with men, mainly from the age of fifty onward. In the UK the rates of high blood pressure in whites, Asians and blacks are similar. Urban populations tend to have higher pressures than those from rural communities. If Australian Aborigines return from an urban to a rural existence there can be a substantial fall in blood pressure as well as reduction in other heart disease risk factors such as obesity and altered blood-fat levels. Reductions in salt and alcohol intake are top of the list of necessary changes.

## What Causes It?

The causes of high blood pressure have been one of the most hotly contested topics for the last thirty years. There are usually many minor contributing factors which produce a noticeable effect. This has important implications for treatment. Causes can be divided into three main categories:

- genetic
- environmental (e.g. diet)
- disease (e.g. hormonal disorders)

### Genetic factors

These would seem to account for about 30 per cent of the variation in blood pressure, and are less important than environmental factors. The genetic mechanism may involve other factors such as weight, hormonal changes and a propensity to retain sodium. The effect of these is in turn capable of being reversed by appropriate dietary changes.

### Environmental factors

There are many environmental factors considered below under the section 'What You Can Do', which interact with each other, and there is potentially substantial benefit in addressing most of them in every person with high blood pressure.

Two environmental factors that should be mentioned at this point are the effect of oestrogen and environmental poisons.

- The oral contraceptive pill and hormone replacement therapy, HRT, can cause a rise in blood pressure in a small percentage of users. This is in the region of 1–2 per cent of users only, but necessitates the doctor to monitor blood pressure levels when prescribing these or similar hormonal treatments.

◆ Steroid drugs and occasionally other medicines cause an elevation of blood pressure and require an alteration of the dose or change of treatment.

◆ Rarely a raised blood pressure is due to past exposure to lead or possibly cadmium. These are two toxic minerals that can damage the kidneys and as a consequence cause high blood pressure as well as other health problems. A history of working with these minerals, no matter how long before, should make one suspicious.

*Disease factors*

These are relevant to probably less than 10 per cent of newly diagnosed patients, and are for the most part outside the scope of this book. Brief details only will be given about these possible causes. Blood pressure can be raised in a wide variety of conditions, including:

◆ kidney disease
◆ an underactive or overactive thyroid gland
◆ excessive production of adrenaline, cortisone and related substances
◆ structural abnormalities of the main artery leaving the heart
◆ occasionally metabolic disorders

Many of these conditions are rare but their importance is that their management may be very different from 'ordinary' high blood pressure and in some instances a cure can be genuinely achieved. Such conditions should be suspected if:

◆ there is a very high blood pressure, especially if it is not easily controlled by standard means
◆ there is a family history of these rare causes or hormonal disorders
◆ there is a personal history of kidney or urinary problems
◆ there are persistent or severe headaches, palpitations or sweating and in all young people with a very high blood pressure

Careful physical examination, blood tests, urine tests and a chest X-ray will detect the majority of them, and consequently all patients with high blood pressure should be carefully assessed by their doctor before beginning treatment.

## What Your Doctor Can Do

◆ Assess your blood pressure by measuring it on three separate occasions. You should be sitting or lying down, relaxed and with no restrictive clothing on the upper part of the arm.

◆ Assess any possible damage that may have developed as a result of an elevated blood pressure. Enlargement and weakening of the heart, damage to the kidneys and changes to the blood vessels at the back of the eye are all possible, though now much less common due to the benefits of good treatment.

◆ Assess the possible causes, especially the presence of underlying medical conditions even if they are rare. The nature of any associated symptoms, examination, and results of simple blood and urine tests usually serve as a guide to these possibilities.

◆ Assess associated risk factors. An elevated blood pressure by itself may have relatively little health implication for the individual. Add one or more of the following and that can change dramatically: high alcohol intake, cigarette smoking, obesity, an elevated blood cholesterol, a poor diet and lack of exercise. These should all be discussed as appropriate by your doctor and the necessary advice given.

◆ Treat your blood pressure with drugs. There are many different types of drugs, and within each type of drug a variety to choose from. Commonly used drug types are:

◇ Diuretics. These are now usually given as a very low dose, and are very useful in the elderly.

◇ Beta-blockers. These act by blocking the action of adrenaline. They are more suited to young and middle-aged patients, especially if they suffer from coronary artery disease.

◇ Calcium antagonists. This family of drugs is useful for those with coronary artery disease. Some may cause ankle swelling as a side effect.

◇ Angiotensin converting enzyme inhibitors. These act by counteracting one of the hormonal mechanisms that underlie high blood pressure. They are particularly suited to those who have a weakened heart, and diabetics. Chronic dry cough is a common side-effect.

◇ Alpha-blockers. Another type of drug that also acts against adrenaline. It may be particularly suited to blacks and diabetics.

◆ Monitor your progress, which is vital. Regular frequent checks at the start of therapy are needed, and when control is achieved these can reduce to once- or twice-yearly checks. Those with a very high blood pressure, heart disease or diabetes will need more careful monitoring with regular urine and occasional blood tests and X-rays.

## What You Can Do

Once upon a time there was nothing for the patient to do except to have faith in their doctor and the treatment. That has changed. In fact it is probably fair to say that today the patient's efforts are as important as the doctor's. You can choose whether or not to address the environmental factors that so often play a part in high blood pressure, and the doctor should direct you to the most important areas to address, and work out how to combine them with appropriate drug therapy.

To explain it all a little further, there is a collection of factors relating to our day-to-day existence that determine our blood pressure. These probably interact with any genetic predisposition for the blood pressure to rise.

For example, blood pressure levels, both systolic and diastolic, rise with age in virtually all communities around the world. The rise is quite substantial in some, but does not develop in those communities where there is a very low intake of salt. It seems likely that this environmental factor, salt intake over many years, will influence blood pressure, especially in those who are predisposed to respond this way. As you will see, salt intake is one dietary factor in the development of a raised blood pressure.

Another important factor is the age of the person, and how long these environmental factors have been at play. Initially blood pressure readings may fluctuate considerably with high levels being recorded intermittently. This is termed 'labile hypertension'. Eventually this usually leads to an established raised blood pressure, though it may take many years. If you set about tackling some of the environmental factors in the early stages it is likely that you will achieve substantial results, whereas in an older person with persistently elevated blood pressure, drug treatment is more likely to be needed in order to achieve satisfactory control.

The most important areas that may need to be tackled, and can be tackled by you, are:

◆ Weight. Obesity is a major determinant of blood pressure, which also influences blood cholesterol, heart disease and stroke risk. Weight reduction is often all that is needed to control mildly elevated blood pressure that is newly found in an overweight person. Follow The Simple Weight-loss Diet.

◆ Alcohol. Consuming anything other than very modest amounts can raise blood pressure. This can happen temporarily the day after an evening's socialising, but again in regular heavy drinkers the elevation in blood pressure can be very substantial. In one study of young heavy-drinking Australian men, the drop in blood pressure after several weeks' abstinence was better than the improvement achieved by use of standard drug therapy. Modest consumption of alcohol may protect against heart disease, so a reasonably conservative guide for those with a raised blood pressure would be 7 units per week for women and 10 for men which is half the maximum safe amount.

◆ Salt. As we have already mentioned, this seems to be an important determinant of a community's blood pressure. For individuals, modest salt restriction, reducing sodium intake from the current average of around 150 mmols per day to half this value, can produce a small fall in blood pressure of usually no more than 5 to 10 points in either systolic or diastolic. Very severe salt restriction can be more effective, but such diets are very difficult to follow in the long term. It is rare that this measure alone is enough to control a raised blood pressure. However it would seem unwise not to advise those with an elevated blood pressure to not make some restriction of their salt intake. See The Low-salt Diet.

These three factors are the most important and should really be considered by all those with established or labile hypertension. The remaining factors are worth considering, particularly as they may be relatively easily corrected by making simple dietary changes and because these same changes may bring other important health benefits.

◆ Potassium. Increasing the balance of this mineral, which broadly speaking is the antagonist of sodium, also helps to lower blood pressure. The effect is small and it is no longer considered advisable to use supplements of potassium too freely as they can easily cause stomach irritation. A high dietary intake of fresh fruit and vegetables, which are the main sources of this mineral, will normally suffice. This is sound advice for almost all of us, as high fruit intakes are associated with a reduced risk of having a stroke.

◆ Magnesium. The sister of potassium. Poor or barely adequate intakes are common in adults, and losses can also occur as a side-effect of some diuretics (water pills) used in the treatment of high blood pressure. One Scandinavian study showed that supplements can help lower blood pressure levels slightly in women, but not all similar studies have shown this small effect. Magnesium supplements can help improve the balance of potassium. Consider trying a daily supplement of 200–300 mg. It should not be taken by those with kidney problems without medical advice.

◆ Calcium. The big brother of magnesium, at least so far as the bones are concerned. It too may have a mild blood pressure lowering effect. This is small and of uncertain value until the results of further current trials are published. To its advantage it is simple, cheap and safe, and of course mostly worth considering for older people who may also need to minimise their risk of developing osteoporosis. An effective dose is not clear, but probably between 500 and 1000 mg per day.

◆ Fats and oils. Cutting down on saturated fats, which come mainly from animal sources, and increasing the intake of polyunsaturates, can also help lower blood pressure slightly. There does seem to be some particular effect of fish oils, particularly the Omega-3 essential fatty acids, in this respect.

◆ Avoiding liquorice. The black chewy sweetmeat of our childhood, prepared from the root of a Mediterranean and Asian plant, has one interesting side effect: it encourages the retention of salt by the body which can lead to a rise in blood pressure, so avoid it.

◆ Exercise. There are many reasons for doing it, and yes, you can add controlling high blood pressure to the list. Experts recommend a daily jog or brisk walk or any other pleasurable and easy-to-do regular exercise of your choice. Some 40 minutes three times per week is a good goal. It lowers blood cholesterol and is also associated with lowered risk of heart disease, stroke and osteoporosis. So what are you waiting for!

◆ Stress avoidance. This is now broadly accepted as being effective. Relaxation exercises and even meditation have been successful in controlling blood pressure. Do it the simple cheap way and fit it in with your lifestyle and daily schedule. Try relaxing very fully at home.

Everyone with high blood pressure should be careful about their weight, should not drink excessively, should limit salt intake and follow the general recommendations for The Very Nutritious Diet with an emphasis on a good daily intake of fresh fruit and vegetables and exercise. There is a great deal you can do to influence your blood pressure.

## Complementary Therapies

Relaxation therapies, acupuncture and herbalism are all possibilities to be considered. Whichever of these you choose, make sure that your blood pressure is monitored by your general practitioner. Alternatively you can, with his approval, buy a blood pressure machine called a sphygmomanometer and record it yourself at home. If you want to do this then you should keep a careful record of the readings you obtain and check these results with your GP who should oversee the whole activity. A very high blood pressure is a danger and the consequences of it remaining untreated or under-treated are substantial.

## Kathy's Story

The reason Kathy wanted to see us was because of her long-standing rheumatoid arthritis which had begun thirty years before and had required her to take low dose steroids for the last ten years. Weight gain had become inevitable and had probably contributed to the recent deterioration in her arthritis. However, this did not prove to be her main problem.

Indeed she was overweight at 83 kg, and many joints, especially those of her hands and knees, had been severely damaged by the arthritis. Her blood pressure was very high, recorded at 250/140, and her weight was increased to 84.5 kg. There were changes in the blood vessels at the back of her eye indicating that this elevation in blood pressure was not just a one-off. Routine blood and urine tests were fortunately satisfactory.

She was immediately begun on a weight-reducing, low-salt diet, together with a beta-blocking drug. Within two weeks her weight was down to 81.75 kg and her blood pressure had fallen to 185/104. The headaches that she had barely mentioned at her first appointment had cleared up and she felt a lot better in herself.

Over the next three months her weight finally came down to 80 kg and blood pressure to 160/100. She was eventually changed to a lower dose beta-blocker with a small amount of diuretic, followed her reduced-kilojoule, low-salt diet, and took supplements of calcium and magnesium together with multi-vitamins.

If left untreated, this very high blood pressure would almost certainly have brought substantial consequences.

# HYSTERECTOMY

The term 'hysterectomy' originates from the Greek words *hystera*, meaning uterus, and *ektome*, meaning to cut out. The earliest hysterectomies on record were performed 1600 years ago in Greece, and despite the high death rate, this method of treatment continued. The procedure involves the removal of all or part of the female reproductive organs. When the ovaries are removed (oopherectomy) as well as the uterus, the procedure is referred to as a full or radical hysterectomy, and when the uterus alone is removed, it is known as a partial hysterectomy.

It is one of the most common operations performed on women these days, surpassed only by caesarian section. It is offered, mainly for the control of heavy bleeding, to 50 per cent of women in the USA, 22–34 per cent of Australian women, and 20–25 per cent of women in Britain. Despite these large percentages, there are many unanswered questions about the appropriateness of performing a full or radical hysterectomy on many of the chosen women, and the effects that this operation then has on long-term health and life expectancy.

Although there are times when a hysterectomy may be a life-saver, as in the case of uterine or ovarian cancer, in our experience there is substantial evidence that it is often performed unnecessarily, without giving the patient sufficient information to make an informed decision. In the case of heavy bleeding, where the ovaries are healthy and there is no history of ovarian cancer in the family, it may not be necessary to remove the ovaries as well as the uterus. A full or radical hysterectomy will prematurely rob you of your supply of oestrogen, which plays a key role in keeping your body youthful. And yet, many 'uneducated women' are told that 'it is better to have the ovaries removed at the time of surgery in order to avoid further trouble later'. Let us now test this premise.

Apart from obvious fertility, some women associate their uterus with femininity, and feel that its presence makes them more sexually appealing to their partner. This may be particularly relevant in societies where the ability to reproduce is a highly respected function. At the WNAS we have encountered numerous patients who went into hospital believing that they were having relatively minor surgery, and woke up to find that they had lost both their uterus and their ovaries. Surely we are all entitled to fully informed consent, no matter what the operation. In the case of a radical hysterectomy, the consequences may be great, and it is impossible to turn back the clock. All too often we hear of gynaecologists who suggest a radical hysterectomy after childbirth, assuming that as no further children are desired there is little point in retaining the reproductive organs. This is still occasionally recommended for the treatment of PMS, which is totally unacceptable.

## *The Advantages of Hysterectomy*

◆ no more periods
◆ an end to heavy bleeding and period pain
◆ no further risk of pregnancy
◆ no need to use contraception
◆ elimination of the threat of cancer of any of the reproductive organs
◆ no further need for cervical smears
◆ no more gynaecological operations needed

## The Disadvantages of Hysterectomy

◆ an earlier menopause, with increased risks of the bone thinning disease, osteoporosis, and heart disease. The risks of this latter are reduced by taking HRT, but not all women will tolerate this

◆ little further protection by oestrogen from ageing

◆ surgery and an anaesthetic required

◆ possible complications, either at the time of the operation or afterwards

◆ time needed to convalesce after the operation

◆ help needed at home during the recovery period

◆ the prospect of needing to take HRT in the long term, without first demonstrating that it suits you

◆ lack of fertility

◆ possible reduced sexual satisfaction for you or your partner, and less comfortable sex (the vaginal tissues dry as a result of the falling levels of oestrogen)

## The Reasons for Hysterectomy

The most common reasons for performing an hysterectomy are heavy periods or fibroids (lumps of fibrous tissue that grow inside the uterus).

◆ Heavy bleeding. When periods become heavy, especially if there is flooding or associated anaemia, your doctor may suggest hormone therapy treatment with tranexamic acid, which affects blood clotting, or a hysterectomy.

◆ Fibroids. Usually, with careful surgery, these can be removed, and the uterus left intact.

◆ Prolapse. Where the uterus has dropped down in the pelvic cavity, but this can usually be repaired.

◆ Endometriosis. Where the lining of the uterus grows outside the uterus, around other organs. This can often be improved by non-surgical means.

◆ Pelvic inflammatory disease. This includes all manner of infections and pelvic pain, which should be treated with drugs, antibiotics and natural means, with an hysterectomy being the last resort.

◆ Cancer. It goes without saying that a hysterectomy should be performed quickly in any life-threatening situation. Cancer of the uterus, ovaries and cervix are major killers, which means there is no room for hesitation.

A study by the Australian Institute of Health and Welfare of the estimated 30 000 hysterectomies performed in Australia each year demonstrated that:

- fibroids accounted for 22 per cent
- heavy menstrual bleeding for 18 per cent
- prolapse 7–21 per cent, depending on the type of hospital and the State
- endometriosis and adenomyosis (endometriosis growing within the thick wall of the uterus) 6–23 per cent
- cancer 1–12 per cent
- pelvic inflammatory disease 2–8 per cent

A number of other reasons were given for the remaining hysterectomies.

## Types of Hysterectomy

- Total hysterectomy. The removal of the uterus, the cervix and the supporting ligaments, leaving the fallopian tubes and ovaries intact.
- Partial hysterectomy. The removal of the upper two-thirds of the uterus only, leaving everything else intact.
- Total hysterectomy with salpingo-oophorectomy. The removal of the uterus with the cervix and supporting ligaments, together with one or both sets of ovaries and fallopian tubes.
- Radical hysterectomy. The removal of the uterus, cervix, supporting ligaments, both ovaries and fallopian tubes, as well as lymph nodes in the area, and the upper portion of the vagina. In women with cancer that may have infiltrated other areas, there may be little choice but to choose this option. For others there may be some flexibility.

## Surgical Alternatives to Hysterectomy

Various techniques have been developed in the last few years to destroy the endometrium, the lining of the uterus, rather than removing the uterus itself. These methods, in principle, are usually performed through the vagina, possibly under local anaesthetic.

They are far less invasive and traumatic, and the recovery time is a fraction of that for a hysterectomy. They are useful tools for women who suffer heavy bleeding that is resistant to drug therapy, or where there are side-effects to the drugs, and for women who are intolerant to general anaesthetic, or for whom anaesthetic may be life threatening (the obese, for example). However, they are not thought to be so suitable for women with large fibroids, endometriosis or a retroverted uterus (tilted backwards).

The methods use lasers, an electrically heated rollerball, and more recently a thermal technique, which involves passing hot water through the uterus, and are collectively known as 'endometrial ablation and resection'. As they are relatively new procedures, there is still much research to be done. We already know that they are not risk-free procedures, but the risks seem to be lower than for hysterectomy. They can cause infection, bleeding, damage to other organs, vessels or fluid overload. The worst scenario is that two women in every 10 000 die as a result of these procedures, compared with between two to six women out of every 10 000 that have a hysterectomy.

It is acknowledged that doctors performing these techniques need to be experienced, previously performing between ten and eighty operations, so as not to cause damage or perforate the uterus itself. Having said that, there are many satisfied customers. Periods may continue after surgery, but they are usually light. The stay in hospital is likely to be only one night, and women are often back at work within two weeks. Those with fibroids may need the procedure repeated in the future, and some even resort to a hysterectomy eventually.

## What Your Doctor and Consultant Can Do

♦ Give you an honest appraisal of what is physically wrong with you. So if you have fibroids, for example, you want to know how large they are and whether they could be removed without taking the uterus with them. It is possible to remove very large fibroids with skilled surgery, leaving the uterus intact.
♦ Give you a rundown of the treatment options available, before considering an hysterectomy.
♦ Assure you that, if the removal of your uterus seems necessary, the ovaries will remain, unless they are diseased. Even leaving part of an ovary puts you at an advantage.

◆ Have a respectful attitude towards your reproductive organs.

## What You Can Do
◆ Read widely on the subject (see Appendix III).
◆ Take your time making a decision, and discuss the pros and cons with your partner.
◆ Follow the recommendations relating to your problem in this book for three or four months to see whether there is any improvement before agreeing to surgery.
◆ If you do have surgery, and cancer has not been diagnosed, explore the alternatives to hysterectomy with your surgeon, and put your views and requests relating to your ovaries in writing to the consultant before the operation.

## Complementary Therapies
Many of the complementary therapies have a great deal to offer in helping with period problems. Herbal therapy is top of our list. Vitex agnus castus was shown in one early study to reduce heavy bleeding in 60 per cent of the patients included. There are other herbs and homoeopathic remedies that may be useful, and acupuncture is worth a try. Follow the recommendations for your specific problem by referring to the appropriate chapter.

# INDIGESTION

One of the main functions of the stomach is to produce acid of a strength great enough to dissolve metal! Dangerous stuff, but only if not confined to a healthy stomach. Leading into the stomach is the oesophagus which carries swallowed food from the mouth down through the chest, pierces the diaphragm and, via a muscular valve-like mechanism, joins the top of the stomach. This muscular valve is intended to keep the contents of the stomach in the stomach and prevent them from washing back up into the oesophagus. But if this happens, this acid reflux (as it is known) will irritate the delicate lining of the oesophagus, causing pain and spasm. It can even trigger chest problems and asthma.

A common factor with indigestion in middle-aged and older people is a hiatus hernia. This is when a small portion of the stomach passes up through the diaphragm. The protective valve-like mechanism is lost, and indigestion results.

## What Are the Symptoms?

Typical symptoms include burning discomfort at the top of the abdomen and the lower part of the chest, which is often worse shortly after eating if bending or lying down. There may also be a desire to belch wind and a loss of appetite when it becomes difficult to swallow. It raises the possibility of scarring of the lower end of the oesophagus as a result of long-standing acid reflux, or even of a cancerous growth causing a partial blockage.

## What Causes It?

There are a number of factors that can lead to acid reflux with or without a hiatus hernia. They all have the potential to relax the muscular valve mechanism, stimulate an excessive amount of acid from the stomach or damage the protective covering of mucus that lines the lower end of the oesophagus. They include:

- smoking
- alcohol
- being overweight
- tea and coffee
- fatty foods
- possibly other foods to which there is an intolerance
- stress

## What Your Doctor Can Do

- Assess the severity of your symptoms.
- Investigate those with swallowing difficulties or who fail to respond to drug treatment.
- Prescribe one of three types of medicines:
  - Alkaline medicines based on magnesium or aluminium to neutralise the acid. These are suitable for mild symptoms.
  - Drugs that stop acid production. These can be very effective, especially Omeprazole (Losec).
  - Drugs to help the muscles of the stomach to pass its contents out of the stomach.

- Rarely, refer patients for surgical correction of a hiatus hernia. This once common operation is now rarely needed as drug therapy has become so effective.

## What You Can Do

- Stop smoking. Tobacco increases stomach acidity and releases the muscular valve at the lower end of the oesophagus.
- Lose weight.
- Eat slowly. Chew your food well too.
- Avoid very fatty foods. Follow the recommendations for The Very Nutritious Diet.
- Don't eat late at night. If you do, when you go to bed your stomach will still contain a significant amount of food and acid when you are lying down in bed.
- Prop the head of your bed up. Place books under the top legs. A pair of telephone directories will do the job nicely. This reduces the flow of acids upwards from the stomach.
- Avoid spicy food. This may be best, although, despite its reputation it only rarely causes problems.
- Reduce tea and coffee consumption. Use alternatives.
- Avoid foods that commonly cause digestive problems. These include wheat, especially wholemeal bread, bran, and wholegrain breakfast cereals, eggs, dairy products, citrus fruit and foods containing yeast. You could try The Simple Exclusion Diet if all else fails.

## Complementary Therapies

Acupuncture, homoeopathy and herbalism may all have something to offer.

## Ingrid's Story

Ingrid was a fifty-three-year-old licensee with two grown-up children. When she began taking HRT to address her menopausal symptoms, she developed a mystery gum disease and rather severe gastric reflux.

*I hadn't had any problems with my gums or my digestion before I started taking HRT, and for the first two and a half years didn't link the two. My gum problems came on gradually and eventually became extremely painful. They felt very irritated, almost as if the gums were too big for the spaces between my teeth and no matter how much I cleaned them or rinsed them with mouthwash, the symptoms persisted. The gastric reflex also began about the time I started taking HRT, but my doctor insisted that neither of these conditions were related to the medication.*

*I eventually went off to see my dentist who said there was nothing wrong with my teeth. I simply had gingivitis, inflammation of the gums. He gave me a series of mouthwashes and dental paste to use which masked the problem for a while, but did not seem to get to the root cause. I saw the dental hygienist every two months. She agreed there was a problem but also could not put her finger on what was causing it. I felt so miserable, in constant pain, it really wore me down.*

*I read about the natural approach to the menopause in the Daily Express and did not waste any time contacting the WNAS for some help and advice. I felt certain inside that the HRT was not really helping my gums, plus I was still experiencing menopausal symptoms despite taking it.*

*The WNAS programme involved making dietary changes and taking supplements aimed at helping my menopausal symptoms plus also extra vitamin C to help with my gums. During the first month I noticed that the gum problem was easing and that the reflux was calming down. Before I could not eat a meal without feeling bloated, nauseous and experiencing heartburn. The worst side-effect of the reflux was breathlessness where I felt I could not fill my lungs easily, which made me panic. My doctor's explanation was that the acid from the gastric reflux was tipping into my lungs. However, it got to the point where I was vomiting after eating and drinking which made me feel awful and obviously restricted my social life.*

*Now, six months later, I am happy to report that my gums are healthy, the gastric reflux has gone and I don't experience any sickness or even feel sick after eating or drinking. I can eat almost everything. Occasionally I get an acid feeling after overdoing it, but that really is rare now. I feel so much happier and the quality of my life has improved beyond belief. I'm grateful for every symptom-free day.*

# INFERTILITY

Although many women manage to conceive without any difficulty, approximately one in six couples experience problems. There are many underlying causes, which include the woman's age, the man's sperm count, and an assortment of other factors. About one in ten couples take more than a year to conceive, and one in twenty take more than two years.

There is no need to rush to be investigated if you are under thirty-five, unless you have been trying to conceive for over two years. If you are over thirty-five, having had regular sexual intercourse for a year, and are experiencing a disturbed menstrual cycle, it would be acceptable to be investigated without further delay.

Infertility is best regarded as a problem of the couple, rather than the individual, and nutritional causes will often overlap, resulting in self-help measures being much the same for both. To fully understand the causes, it is best to separate them into female and male.

## Causes of Female Infertility

By the time a woman is born, all the eggs that her ovaries will hold have already been produced! Several million eggs are in place initially, but only about 400 of them will reach maturity. The supply is influenced by smoking, even before birth, and daughters of women who smoked during pregnancy have fewer eggs, have more difficulty conceiving, and may reach the menopause earlier that the offspring of non-smokers.

The monthly release of an egg from the ovary is known as ovulation, and occurs at approximately mid-cycle with menstruation, the monthly period, coming fourteen days later. Ovulation does not always occur with every cycle, but when an egg is released from the ovary it is picked up by the finger-shaped projections at the end of the fallopian tubes and then passes along towards the womb.

### Failure of ovulation

A guide to whether or not an egg is being produced each month is whether the periods are regular, between twenty-five and thirty-five days. Ovulation can be checked for by measuring the blood level of the female sex hormone progesterone seven days before the next period is due. Usually this is day twenty-one of a twenty-eight-day cycle, but can be day twenty-eight in a thirty-five-day cycle.

A rise in early morning body temperature of 0.5°C should also be observed in the few days after ovulation, but this is less reliable than measuring the progesterone level. Often the day twenty-one progesterone level is checked in two or three cycles in couples with fertility problems, especially if there is some uncertainty about ovulation.

Failing to ovulate can be due to:

- Hormonal problems, including an early menopause.
- An underactive or overactive thyroid gland.
- Disturbance of the pituitary gland, especially an excess of the hormone prolactin in the blood, can inhibit ovulation. Often the first clues are the presence of a milky white discharge from the nipples, known as galactorrhoea, and infrequent periods. However, only one-quarter of those with galactorrhoea will have a high prolactin level, and this then requires further investigation.
- Nutritional deficiencies, even changing your diet, can affect ovulation. Following a 4200 kilojoule weight-loss diet for six weeks may suppress normal ovulation. The World Health Organisation survey of infertility found that recent weight loss or gain was a mild risk factor for infertility.
- Any chronic illness, especially if there is weight loss.
- Stress, which can be a powerful factor.
- Excessive physical activity and an inadequate kilojoule intake, resulting in loss of weight, can prevent ovulation taking place each month. When the body is not well nourished perhaps this is Mother Nature's way of preventing a pregnancy.

### Blockage of the fallopian tubes

This is very often due to past infection, most commonly by an organism called *Chlamydia*. It is usually acquired following sexual intercourse, particularly in those who have had multiple partners, and causes lower abdominal or pelvic pain, a vaginal discharge, painful periods and sometimes a fever.

The reporting of infection with chlamydia has escalated, and damage to fallopian tubes is now the commonest cause of infertility in many developing countries because of the high prevalence of pelvic inflammatory disease (PID), an acute illness which requires treatment with antibiotics.

To confirm the diagnosis a more detailed assessment by laparoscopy, examination of the pelvic organs with a telescopic instrument passed into the abdominal cavity, and X-rays of the fallopian tubes may be performed. Blocked or damaged tubes can be corrected by surgery, but assisted fertilisation is often the simplest way to achieving pregnancy.

## *Endometriosis*

This condition, in which the cells from the lining of the womb grow outside the uterus, such as around the ovaries or adjacent to the outer walls of the womb, can cause infertility. Difficulty conceiving, very painful periods and abdominal distension are common problems of endometriosis. Diagnosis is often made after investigative surgery, a laparoscopy, to examine the pelvic organs. Unfortunately treatment is not very successful.

## *Polycystic ovarian disease*

Up to 20 per cent of the normal female population suffer with cysts on the ovaries which cause a shift in the balance of sex hormones resulting in:

◆ irregular and infrequent periods
◆ excessive hair growth
◆ reduced fertility
◆ often, but not always, obesity

## *Contraception*

Users of the oral contraceptive pill may experience delayed fertility, as it sometimes takes several months to re-establish a normal menstrual cycle after being on the Pill. Users of intra-uterine devices have a slight increased risk of PID resulting in reduced fertility.

## *Abortion*

A history of abortion does not seem to reduce the future chance of conceiving, according to recent research.

## *Medical drugs*

Many drugs can interfere with a woman's fertility. This is almost always reversible and can follow use of:

- anti-cancer agents
- hormone preparations, as may be used to treat period pains or premenstrual problems
- drugs used in the treatment of schizophrenia and depression
- drugs such as metoclopramide and domperidone used in the treatment of nausea
- drugs such as reserpine and methyldopa used in the treatment of high blood pressure, all of which can increase the level of the pituitary hormone prolactin

*Medical conditions*
Diabetes and thyroid disease can cause infertility in women, but only if the conditions are not well controlled.

*Social poisons*
Many, though not all, studies show slightly reduced fertility rates in those women who drink or smoke. Coffee consumption has also been studied, and there is a possible slight adverse effect on fertility. The same may be true of the consumption of soft drinks that have a high sugar content and contain colourings and additives. There are many other possible explanations as those consuming these social substances often have a poorer nutrient intake.

Recreational drugs, including marijuana, may reduce the chances of fertility, and are likely to have a substantial effect on pregnancy outcome.

*Exposure to environmental chemicals*
This has been shown in studies, especially in the work-place, to reduce fertility. Those who work with textile and leather dyes, lead, mercury, benzene, petroleum and related chemicals, and possibly other chemicals used in the plastics industry, are most likely to be at risk. Additionally, female dentists, anaesthetists and assistants, have been reported as having delayed conception, possibly due to their exposure to the anaesthetic gas, nitrous oxide.

*Nutritional deficiencies*
Whilst it is widely accepted in developing countries that a significant degree of malnutrition which results in severe weight loss is likely to stop women menstruating and could result in them being infertile, surprisingly little work has been done to determine if *mild*

nutritional deficiencies contribute to infertility in women from developed countries. Several small reports have documented the association of deficiencies of iron (without anaemia), vitamin B12 and vitamin B3 being associated with reduced fertility.

*Other causes*
In rare cases, fertility may be associated with:

◆ structural deformities of the uterus or vagina which may be a barrier to fertility, or prevent successful implantation of the fertilised ovum
◆ genetic problems which cause some women to fail to menstruate at all
◆ antibodies to sperm or allergic reactions to it! Some women suffer from these, but treatment with assisted conception can get round this problem

Despite careful assessment of both partners, no cause for infertility is found in some 20 per cent of couples. If spontaneous pregnancy has not occurred within three years, then some form of treatment is deemed appropriate.

## *What Your Doctor Can Do*
This depends on the discovered cause of infertility.

◆ Your doctor could treat failure of ovulation either by correcting any underlying hormonal abnormality, or by inducing ovulation through short courses of agents that encourage the ovary to release an egg. These measures might be aided by attention to diet and lifestyle which we will come to shortly.
◆ Your doctor could arrange for tubal disease—blockages in, or damage to, the fallopian tubes—to be treated by surgery to repair the damaged tube(s), or by assisted conception. Tubal repair surgery is actually not very effective as it is difficult to repair damage to the delicate tube lining, but it is useful for reversal of sterilisation procedures. Newer specialised techniques—trying to remove scar tissue from inside the fallopian tube by passing an ultrafine tube via the uterus—may be more successful.
◆ Your doctor could also advise you on assisted reproduction

techniques (ART). Women with unexplained infertility of more than three years' duration, and those with ovulation problems that have not responded to more simple measures, may be advised to choose this method. It can also help where the male partner has very few sperm or when the woman has no eggs and is willing to use donated eggs.

These techniques involve collection of a women's eggs, often after treatment with hormonal agents, collection of sperm and their careful preparation. This is followed by either in-vitro fertilisation (IVF) or test-tube fertilisation with placement of the embryo in the womb, or placement of both the prepared eggs and sperm in the fallopian tubes (gamete intrafallopian transfer or GIFT), or some of the newer techniques being piloted. In some circumstances it may be appropriate to use donor eggs from (usually) younger women together with the partner's sperm.

## Causes of Male Infertility

Sperm are produced in the testes by specialised cells, and slowly mature over four months. During orgasm they are ejected from the part of the testis called the seminiferous tubules, mix with fluid from the prostate gland and other tissues, and are released into the outside world. Millions are produced, even though only one is required to fertilise an egg. The number and quality of sperm as well as the health of the prostate gland are all important in deciding how fertile any one male is.

Sperm production takes place most efficiently at a temperature of 33°C, and thus the testicles are *outside* the body, which has a temperature of 37°C. A normal ejaculate should:

- be greater than 2 ml
- contain at least 20 million sperm per ml
- have 30 per cent or more with a normal shape
- have 50 per cent actively mobile (it is quite normal for some 50 per cent of sperm to be 'duds')

Assessment of male infertility requires asking many questions about diet and lifestyle, a physical examination and examination of a sample of sperm. Quite often a sperm sample can be collected by using a post-coital test, which will also determine whether it responds to the cervical mucus.

### Absent or deformed testicles
Sometimes testes may have failed to descend from their original position high up in the scrotum or lower part of the abdomen. New-born and infant boys are routinely checked to make sure the testes are descended. Small testes may be due to past injury, illness or sometimes developmental problems. Enlargement is most commonly due to a varicocele—enlargement of the veins around the testis—and this is present in 10 per cent of the normal population. This can raise the temperature of the testes, and contribute to a poor sperm count. Surgical treatment is often necessary.

### Blockage of the vas deferens
A blockage of the duct leading from the testicles to the base of the bladder will result in a very low sperm count or no sperm in the ejaculate. Previous vasectomy is an obvious cause, and can be reversed by surgery. Sometimes the sperm-carrying ducts are distorted as they reach the area of the prostate gland. Consequently some or all of the ejaculate does not reach the outside world directly, but passes into the bladder. Sperm are detected in the urine that is passed after intercourse. This commonly happens after surgery on the prostate gland.

### Excessive heat
The sort of heat which may be encountered by steel workers and bakers can be associated with a reduced sperm count. Severe obesity and tight underwear and trousers may play a part too.

### Damage to the testicles
The chromosomal material in the sperm itself, or the motility of the sperm, can be damaged by:

- infection, especially sexually transmitted disease like chlamydia or non-specific urethritis (NSU)
- infection with mumps during adolescence or early adult life
- drugs as used for cancer and colitis or Crohn's disease
- radiation treatment

- exposure to environmental pollutants—lead, cadmium, mercury, pesticides, herbicides and other chemicals that have effects similar to the female sex hormone, oestrogen
- cancer of the testicle

### Chronic illnesses
Diabetes, cystic fibrosis, chronic disease of the nervous system, any chronic infection or unexplained fever, an underactive thyroid gland, disease of the pituitary gland and kidney disease can all affect sperm count. Sperm counts also fall in men who are paralysed by a spinal injury.

### Social poisons
Alcohol and cigarette smoking are the most important, but marijuana and other recreational drugs can also affect the quality and quantity of sperm.

### Lack of essential nutrients
Some nutrients seem to be particularly important to sperm production, and these include zinc, and vitamins B and C. One experiment in healthy volunteers of mild zinc deficiency showed a dramatic reduction in sperm quantity and quality, and testosterone (male sex hormone) production, which took nearly a year to fully correct.

### Stress
This might also be a factor in reducing a man's sperm count.

### The modern world
A group of Danish doctors published an important review in 1992 of the fall in sperm count that seems to have taken place over the last fifty years. Looking at sixty-one papers detailing the results in nearly 15 000 men, there appears to have been a 40 per cent decline in sperm concentration and a 20 per cent decline in seminal volume over this time. Combined with the known increase in testicular cancer and developmental abnormalities of the genitals in new-born boys, this strongly suggests an environmental cause, probably due to pollution.

Smoking, alcohol and lack of some essential nutrients may also be factors.

The escalating use of the oral contraceptive pill and hormone replacement therapy, traces of which can find their way into the general environment, should also give us all something to be concerned about. Increased use of plastics and related chemicals, the pesticide DDT and the chemical PCBs used as insulators for electrical cables prior to 1970, have also been suggested as factors, because of their mild oestrogen-like effects. Decline in reproductive capacity could also be interpreted as an indication that the planet is becoming too crowded, and is Mother Nature's answer to the problem.

## What Your Doctor Can Do

This does of course depend upon the cause, but unfortunately most of the treatments tried are not very successful. Self-help measures may be more effective at improving sperm count and function than are drug therapies.

◆ A wide variety of drugs and hormonal treatments, including steroids, have all been tried with either no benefit or uncertain benefit being recorded. Steroids can be useful in those men whose infertility is due to antibodies that attack their own sperm. Hormonal treatments are only helpful for the small percentage of men with true hormone deficiency.

◆ Surgery is useful if blockage of the ducts from the testicles is causing a low sperm count. Enlargement of the veins of the testicles, a varicocele, can be treated by surgery if there is a low sperm count, when infertility has been present for two or more years, and if there is no associated hormonal disturbance.

◆ Antibiotics are necessary to treat any infection of the testicles or prostate gland. Treatment for several months may be required.

◆ Your doctor could advise on assisted reproduction techniques (ART). Test-tube fertilisation or in-vitro fertilisation, IVF, are often the best hope for many couples where a low sperm count is the main barrier to conception. Such techniques involve the collection of the partner's sperm, treatment with an agent that improve its function, bringing together the sperm and egg— sometimes by actually injecting healthy sperm into the egg— and return of the fertilised egg into the womb. In this way pregnancy can be achieved when there is a very low sperm count.

If there is no sperm, then donor sperm will have to be used, and the donor can be chosen to have similar physical characteristics to those of the male partner.

## What You Can Do

Whilst none of what follows may be as important as the hormonal and surgical techniques that have revolutionised female infertility treatment in particular, they all have their importance. It seems foolish not to take simple common-sense measures to improve health before embarking upon costly assisted reproduction techniques. Remember that most of the advice that follows will take three to six months before it has a detectable effect upon body chemistry and therefore a subsequent influence upon your reproductive ability.

Certain nutrients seem to play a crucial part in the way ovaries respond to pituitary hormones (magnesium and possibly the essential fatty acids), and in influencing female sex hormone metabolism in general (vitamin B, essential fatty acids and possibly magnesium and zinc). Severe deficiencies of these nutrients are rare except in women with very poor diets, or who are seriously ill or alcoholic. However there is now substantial evidence that mild undetected deficiencies are quite common, and they may have a modest effect upon the regularity of your menstrual cycle and ovulation.

## What You Both Can Do

◆ Cut down on alcohol and cigarettes—ideally, you should both stop. Cigarette smoking in women is associated with reduced fertility and means a lower success rate in those undergoing assisted reproduction techniques.
◆ Eat a healthy diet with plenty of fresh fruit and vegetables. Their high content of vitamins A, C and E act as anti-oxidants that help limit the adverse effects of many environmental pollutants. Ensure a good intake of protein-rich foods of either animal or vegetable origin: these are particularly important for men as they are good sources of zinc, which seems to play such a crucial role in sperm production and function.

- If you are very overweight then lose weight, and if underweight try to gain weight, but always by eating healthy nutritious foods. Rapid weight change, gain or loss, is usually undesirable, in women especially.
- If you are on long-term drug therapy ask your doctor or specialist to review your need for medication. The goal is the minimum effective dose for a drug or drugs, with the least risk of side-effects. In men, drug therapy for mental problems or Crohn's disease could be reducing sperm count.
- If you have any chronic illness that is not being adequately treated at present, then check with your doctor.
- Limit exposure to environmental chemicals. Take especial care if your work involves handling heavy metals, pesticides or industrial chemicals.

*For women*
- Follow the preconception programme (see Preconception).
- Limit consumption of tea and coffee to a total of four cups per day. More might have a small adverse effect on the chance of conceiving.
- Do not consume more than three cans of soft drink, either low kilojoule or normal type, per week. This is about 1 litre in volume.
- Consider taking nutritional supplements, depending upon your health circumstances. Expert advice is often desirable and if you are receiving infertility treatment, then you should always check with your specialist about these before commencing.
- Iron may be needed by those who:
  ◇ have heavy periods
  ◇ are poorly fed, such as vegetarians who are also tea drinkers
  ◇ have symptoms of iron deficiency, e.g. recurrent mouth ulcers or a sore tongue
  ◇ have flattened or up-turned nails
  ◇ have poor hair growth
- Folic acid should be taken by all women who are trying to or who might conceive. The dose is 400 µg per day. Those women who have had a previous pregnancy complicated by a neural tube defect will need to take 4 mg per day.
- Vitamin B complex could be needed by those who:
  ◇ eat poorly

◇ consume more than an average of two units of alcohol daily
◇ suffer from significant anxiety or depression
◇ have any illness that has caused recent weight loss
◇ have recurrent mouth ulcers or a sore tongue

◆ Vitamin B12 may be needed by vegans. All women wishing to become pregnant should be taking folic acid, and it is a wise precaution that all vegans should also take a vitamin B12 supplement.

A mild deficiency of vitamin B12 could be made worse by taking folic acid, resulting in damage to the nervous system and numbness in the hands or feet. An appropriate dose of vitamin B12 is 5 μg per day.

◆ Magnesium might be useful for those who are deficient, and have trouble ovulating regularly. Early symptoms that could indicate a lack of this essential mineral are:
◇ premenstrual syndrome—physical or mental symptoms
◇ muscle pains or cramps
◇ fatigue

An appropriate dose is 300 mg per day. Once pregnant, your need for these supplements may well change. Again check with your GP or specialist.

*For men*

◆ Avoid use of jockey-style underwear and underwear made from synthetic materials. Cotton boxer shorts will help keep the testicles at the right temperature.

◆ If your sperm is low, then rather than 'saving it all up for one good go' it would seem better to have more frequent intercourse, especially around mid-cycle. The optimum frequency of intercourse to maintain a good sperm count is two or three times a week!

◆ Do not have excessively hot baths or showers. Limit the time you spend in a sauna. Avoid exposure to excessively hot environments.

◆ Take nutritional supplements of vitamin C (about 500 mg), multi-vitamins and zinc (up to 30 mg) per day. These can all help improve sperm count, especially if you have low levels of vitamin C. These moderate doses can be safely taken in the long term, but the positive effects are likely to take three or six months at least to be felt. Supplements of other nutrients may be needed if you have deficiencies or other health problems.

Remember that all of these factors are likely to take some time to show results. Whilst getting yourselves into better condition, you will both need a little patience. If you haven't managed to conceive after two years of regular sexual intercourse you will need to see your doctor with a view to organising some specialist investigations. Most doctors do not initiate any treatment until after three years, though this can be less in older couples.

## Complementary Therapies

Whilst complementary therapies cannot be relied upon to solve the problem of infertility, it may be worthwhile having some acupuncture from an experienced practitioner or consulting a cranial osteopath in order to free any blocked energy.

## Carole's Story

Carole was a thirty-three-year-old who was experiencing problems with infertility at the time when she approached us.

*I had been investigated for infertility in the mid-1980s as we were trying for a baby for three years without any success. The doctors did not think I was ovulating although there was no concrete evidence, and eventually I managed to fall pregnant. We were hoping to have several children in quick succession but after a further two years without any success, we began investigations again. Our GP referred us to a consultant who confirmed that I was not ovulating. My periods were very irregular at the time and I was put on Clomiphene for three months and then a double dose for a further six months. However the tests didn't change: even after the treatment I was still not ovulating.*

*By this time I had developed very severe premenstrual syndrome. I think the strain of trying to conceive had got to me. My behaviour was utterly uncharacteristic and I experienced all manner of symptoms ranging from migraine to mood swings bloating and irritability, from which I seemed to have no respite. When I was not knocked out by migraines or an upset stomach I was prone to violent mood swings and at one point tried to attack my husband. I regularly wept for no apparent reasons. I felt so ill I was never in the mood for sex, which affected both our marriage and our plans to conceive. My husband actually phoned the Samaritans* at one point because I was so emotionally out of control. He had asked me why I was unhappy and I replied, 'I'm not unhappy, I am just ill'. Of course it was difficult for him to understand.

My doctor said I was causing the symptoms because I wanted to have a baby so much, so eventually I decided I ought to see a psychiatrist. At about that time a close friend of mine had read an article about the work of the WNAS and suggested I bought a book called Beat PMS Through Diet. I put myself on the diet straightaway, and contacted the WNAS.

As a fifteen-coffees-a-day woman, and a Diet Coke addict, I was advised to cut these out and also to initially stop eating wheat and other grains except rice and corn. I also gave up cheese. I was told to exercise and take nutritional supplements. For the first time for as long as I can remember I had two normal regular cycles with no PMS. A week later the migraines stopped. Inside two months my erratic moods had abated. A regular cycle had re-established which I hadn't had for years, and my libido was restored. I felt so well that I decided to relax the diet, and then had a dreadful month with a fifty-day cycle.

When I went back to the clinic and went over my charts, it seemed that wheat that I had recently been eating had aggravated the situation. I was asked to cut it out again, and after having some tests I was given some extra zinc and magnesium as well as my other supplements. I am delighted to say that I fell pregnant the next month and had a very smooth pregnancy and a lovely baby daughter.

I have had to stick to the diet which I sometimes find difficult as wheat, chocolate and dairy products all seem to affect me in different ways. I have since added a herbal preparation to my supplements as it seems to help to normalise my cycle. My husband was both relieved and delighted that not only was I able to overcome my symptoms but also I was able to conceive without difficulty for the first time in years.

*See also*: Recommended Reading List (*Healthy Parents, Healthy Baby*) and Standard References.

# INFLUENZA, RECURRENT COUGHS, COLDS AND SORE THROATS

Hardly anybody needs telling, but for those few who might never have suffered, the common cold is a short-lived infective illness due to one of several easily transmitted viruses. Symptoms include nasal stuffiness with the production of profuse watery catarrh. A fever, which is not usually great, may be present too. Severity varies from person to person and depends also upon changes in the virus that allow it to bypass the immune system's defence mechanisms. In most people the illness lasts a few days and rarely more than a week.

Influenza is a viral infection that typically occurs as a wide-spread outbreak. Its name was derived from the old erroneous belief that the illness was due to divine influence. It is of course caused by several strains of the influenza virus known as A, B or C. Typical features are headache, muscle aches which can be severe, a fever, sore throat, cough and nasal catarrh. The illness lasts from two to seven days unless secondary infection with bacteria develops, causing bronchitis, pneumonia or sinus infections.

Sore throats are most often due to viral infections which may cause inflammation of the conjunctiva (red eyes), or a cough due to chest infection. Occasionally, though, they are due to bacterial infection that may need antibiotic treatment. Many of us will experience around four to six such infections each year, though half of these may be so mild as to pass virtually unnoticed.

With simple viral infections, provided they are uncomplicated, there should be little constitutional disturbance, unlike influenza. Some people seem prone to these viral infections, especially the elderly or those with poor resistance to infection.

## Who Gets Them?

We all do, especially young children. Influenza is more common in the winter months. As the virus can spontaneously make subtle changes to itself, thus evading the immune defences caused by previous infections, we are all prone to infection every few years, especially with new strains. Immunisation is effective, though not completely so, and is offered yearly to those with heart, lung or kidney disease, the elderly, diabetics, those with poor resistance to infection, and some health-care workers.

Colds and sore throats are common throughout the year, though slightly more so in the winter months. Incubation following initial contact with these viruses is one to six days.

## What Your Doctor Can Do

- For all viral illnesses affecting the upper airways there is little treatment. Prevention by immunisation is only effective for influenza, and it is only appropriate for those groups already detailed.
- Aspirin may help with the fever and pain of these infections but probably increases your chances of infecting other people. A drug called Amantidine is effective for reducing the severity of influenza caused by type A infections, but only if given before the illness starts so it can be used early on in some outbreaks.
- Antibiotics are needed if an infection with a bacterium follows causing a cough or nasal discharge with yellow or green mucus.

## What You Can Do

- Ignore it if symptoms are mild.
- Take supplements of vitamin C, 1 g three times per day, although the evidence in favour is small.
- Suck zinc lozenges three times a day: these have been shown to reduce the duration of a sore throat. The high concentration of zinc in the throat may be harmful to the virus, and the zinc that is absorbed can act as an immune stimulant.
- Have a steam inhalation. These are old-fashioned but effective at reducing the duration of symptoms, especially if there is nasal stuffiness. The steam needs to be as hot as possible. Pour freshly boiled water into a large bowl which is securely placed on a table. Sit at the table and place a large towel over your head and breathe in deeply through the nose. Do this for 10 minutes three times a day. Such inhalations are particularly useful if there is a lot of sticky phlegm on the chest or nasal catarrh that is difficult to clear. You can add some eucalyptus or menthol preparations to it if you like.
- It may be worth going on a mild fast for two or three days. Drinking plenty of clear liquids and eating mainly fruit could

help, as strict fasting can stimulate immune activity. Furthermore, if there is a degree of nasal sensitivity to a food (most commonly, dairy products) then avoiding this could benefit some. For those who have more than two upper respiratory tract infections each year, especially if this has led to taking antibiotics, then the following may be helpful:

◇ Eat The Very Nutritious Diet.

◇ Don't smoke, and drink very little.

◇ Take supplements of a moderately strong multi-vitamin, zinc 15–20 mg, and vitamin A, 4000 IU per day. A lack of the latter can make it easier for bacteria to adhere to the lining of the airways. The first two were taken in a trial of healthy elderly regularly over one whole year and were shown to approximately halve their rate of these infections and subsequent use of antibiotics.

## Pamela's Story

Pamela had had a full and busy life and now, at the age of seventy-five, she was troubled by a persistent fatigue. In fact she had felt fatigue for about thirty years, and then, when she was still bringing up three children, she had a severe viral pneumonia and felt that her energy levels had never been the same since. She had coped through her middle years, but now as an elderly lady her reduced energy level meant that she spent most of her time at home indoors and rarely enjoyed the walks and gardening that she had managed in the past. She seemed predisposed to recurrent minor infections, coughs, colds and sore throats, which never missed their opportunity to punctuate her winter months. Fortunately, she rarely required antibiotics. She had lost a few kilos in weight but there were no other features to assume that there was any more sinister cause. Indeed, she had been very thoroughly assessed by a local physician a few years earlier and all routine tests were satisfactory. She had occasionally been found to have a low white cell count in the past, and perhaps this indicated her reduced resistance to infection. However, she herself had tried taking a variety of nutritional supplements with no clear-cut benefits.

She found it difficult to keep her weight much above 51 kg. She also found it difficult to eat large or rich meals, which caused her to experience abdominal bloating and discomfort.

Nutritional investigations had shown a surprisingly low level of retinol—

vitamin A, 136 mg per litre (200–650). The level for zinc was also very reduced at 7.6 mmols per litre (11.5–20) and a number of other essential nutrients were also reduced. Low levels of zinc and vitamin A are quite strongly linked with poor resistance to infection and repeated upper respiratory tract infections, which was clearly part of Pamela's problem. Perhaps her poor digestion lay behind it. She began supplements of strong multivitamins and zinc and was advised to take some digestive enzymes with her main meal.

It actually took about six months before her nutrient levels increased and, as they did, she gained a few pounds in weight, her energy level improved and she began to experience fewer coughs and colds. There was significant improvement in her levels for zinc and vitamin A.

All the patients are predisposed to mild to moderate nutritional deficiencies, which may significantly impair their resistance to infection. For many in this situation it would seem of good policy for them to take moderately strong multi-vitamin and zinc preparations.

In Pamela's case it is not known how long she really had the deficiencies.

# INSOMNIA

Anyone who has ever suffered from disturbed sleep will be able to tell you how vital sleep is, although it is probably taken for granted by those who have never experienced problems. Whatever the reason for the insomnia, be it anxiety, bereavement or simply jetlag, it leaves you feeling washed out, with your vitality crushed. You feel unrefreshed, irritable and listless, and as you are not alert, you are prone to make mistakes.

The main features of insomnia are difficulty falling asleep, an inability to stay asleep, or waking in the early hours and not being able to get back to sleep. Sufferers usually feel frustrated because they feel they should be asleep, and they invariably feel tired and washed out the next day.

Insufficient sleep may have serious repercussions in people of all ages. In children it may cause growth retardation, it can affect the academic performance of adolescents, cause under-achievement in the workplace and contribute significantly to the cause of accidents.

- Nearly four out of ten individuals do not get a regular night's sleep, which affects their alertness.
- One-third of adults experience difficulty falling asleep or remaining asleep.·
- Approximately 60 per cent of the elderly suffer from disorders that disrupt sleep, like snoring, sleep apnoea, where breathing ceases temporarily.
- Sufferers are often more tired during the day, not sufficiently alert to even drive a car. Road traffic accidents, for example, have been associated with sleepiness in 27 per cent of cases, and in one study this accounts for 83 per cent of the deaths on the road, even more than deaths from alcohol-related accidents.

## *What Causes It?*

There is a variety of underlying factors that disrupt our sleep pattern:

- It is thought that in 50 per cent of complaints of insomnia there is underlying anxiety or depression. Stress, tension, grief or fear can all keep you awake.
- Caffeine, found in tea, coffee, chocolate and cola-based drinks, can stimulate you to the point of insomnia.
- Some drugs may produce side-effects which include insomnia, or may induce disturbing dreams which cause you to wake during the night.
- Withdrawal symptoms when coming off certain drugs.
- Alcohol in excess will also produce insomnia.
- Any painful condition, e.g. arthritis.
- Any condition that causes you to break your sleep, e.g. cystitis or diarrhoea when you need to go to the toilet.
- Day-time napping can prevent you having a sound night's sleep.
- A cold bedroom, especially for the elderly, could be enough to keep them awake at night.
- Shift work, which involves working some nights and not others is likely to severely disrupt your sleep pattern. We regularly

see nurses and air hostesses with problems that relate to their poor sleeping routine, as the menstrual cycle is disturbed by the lack of routine.

## What Your Doctor Can Do

◆ The first step is to exclude the possibility of any underlying cause, especially if there is pain. Your doctor should do a physical examination and routine blood screening to check for thyroid problems, diabetes, low iron stores, infection or other serious problems.

◆ Check to see whether anxiety or depression is keeping you awake.

◆ Give you instructions about 'sleep hygiene'—going to bed at a regular time, not napping during the day, making sure your room is warm enough, that your bedcovers are comfortable, and that there is no external noise to disturb you.

◆ Reassure you that your problem is likely to be short-lived.

◆ Prescribe sleeping pills in the very short term to break the pattern of insomnia and re-train you to sleep through the night.

◆ If you are depressed, he may prescribe antidepressants, and in severe cases refer you to a psychiatrist for further investigation and treatment.

## What You Can Do

◆ Pinpoint the reason for your insomnia, either by visiting your doctor if you feel it may be a symptom of a medical condition, or by discussing your problems with your partner or close friend.

◆ Take concerted steps to sort out the problem to alleviate your worry or anxiety. The problem may take some time to resolve, so you will need some intermediate measures to get you through.

◆ Eat well. Follow the instructions for The Very Nutritious Diet. Never miss a meal, and eat wholesome snacks between meals, especially in your premenstrual week if you are menstruating, as your kilojoule requirements are increased by up to 2100 kilojoules per day.

◆ Never go to bed on a full stomach: eat earlier on in the evening allowing sufficient time for your food to be digested. This is more important for older patients or those with digestive troubles.

◆ Take plenty of exercise during the week, at least four or five sessions, out in the fresh air when possible.

◆ Learn how to relax your body and mind by practising daily one of the relaxation techniques (see The Benefits of Relaxation, page 27). You can use these techniques before going to bed (or in the night to help you get back to sleep).

◆ Eliminate the stimulant caffeine from your diet completely, and use alternatives. Cut down gradually or you will get a withdrawal headache.

◆ Cut down on cigarettes if you smoke, or give up completely, as nicotine can act as a stimulant.

◆ Keep your alcohol consumption to a minimum, especially at night. Many people are under the misconception that alcohol is a hypnotic; it does induce sleep, but as it metabolises it acts as a stimulant.

◆ Make sure that you have a quiet, warm and comfortable environment in which to sleep. Having a good mattress with clean bedding might well help.

◆ Train yourself to go to bed at a regular time each night, before midnight, but not too early.

◆ Don't watch any scary films or upsetting television programmes before going to bed.

◆ When in bed, don't think about the day's activities, try to concentrate on something pleasant, and consciously relax your muscles.

◆ Cuddle up to your partner if you have one. The warmth of another person can help you get to sleep.

◆ An orgasm will often induce sleep—so this may be one problem that your partner will be only too keen to help you solve!

◆ Try taking some herbal tranquillisers in the short-term, like Blackmores Valerian Forte.

◆ Set your alarm for a regular time, unless you are a shift worker, as this will help you re-establish a routine.

*When you wake in the night*
◆ Instead of worrying, get up, make yourself a warm drink and read, watch a video or practice some relaxation technique,

before returning to bed. This often does the trick and takes the frustration out of the situation.

◆ Go back to bed when you feel sleepy. Practise relaxing your muscles again and getting your mind to wander to a favourite location.

◆ If you are still awake 10 minutes later, get up again, go to another room, do some more reading or relaxing.

Try not to worry or get too frustrated about not being able to sleep, as it is much more tiring than just being awake!

## Complementary Therapies

They are tremendously valuable in the treatment of insomnia that does not have an underlying physical cause. Acupuncture is very effective, but it requires a course of treatment to gradually ease you back into a proper sleep pattern. Herbal preparations and homoeopathic remedies are useful tools, but you would be advised to seek professional help, as there will more than likely be other related problems that need addressing too. It would be worth visiting a cranial osteopath to see whether there are any lesions that need attention, and having a massage before bed, with some relaxing aromatherapy oils like lavender, geranium or ylang ylang, which will help to induce sleep. A useful homoeopathic remedy is Coffea 6X, taking two before you go to bed.

## Angela's Story

Angela, fifty-six, with two children, was unable to sleep, despite being desperately tired. Her health had been so badly affected that she had retired from her job.

*For eleven years, prior to the menopause, I had heavy periods, headaches and mood swings. My last period was in November 1993. Since then I had suffered with hot flushes, my libido had disappeared and my vagina was dry. My doctor prescribed HRT which I took for five months, but the side-effects were so severe I had to stop taking it. I was unable to sleep at all and experienced terrible panic attacks, plus my curly hair went straight and unmanageable.*

*Not being able to sleep seemed to be affecting my brain. I couldn't retain anything in my mind, and was anxious about everything. I usually play bowls, but did not have the energy or the confidence to go to games. I have a super husband*

*and lovely grandchildren, but I couldn't be bothered with them either. I felt really cheated as I knew I was missing out on life, but I just wanted to be left alone to doze in the afternoon.*

*A friend recommended that I go to the WNAS clinic, which in desperation I did. I was asked to get my doctor to measure my serum ferritin levels, which is a test to detect low iron stores. I was also given a programme which consisted of making dietary changes, relaxation, supplements and exercise.*

*My doctor did find that my serum ferritin was very low, and as a result I was put on a course of iron pills. I followed the programme closely and within a month felt that my symptoms were calming down. I began to sleep for parts of the night, my flushes were calming down and I didn't feel quite so tired. The next couple of months were hampered a little because I developed diarrhoea. We eventually discovered that I was reacting to the vitamin E and ginseng which were designed to help with the flushes, and when I stopped taking them my bowel settled down.*

*I continued to make gradual progress through the year. I avoid wheat and coffee completely, even decaffeinated which seems to upset me. I feel that I am now back to my old self and have been able to cope well with two family crises that have occurred. I am able to sleep through whole blissful nights again, my social life is restored and so is my sense of humour, and as an added bonus my libido is back. My husband is relieved and we are both very grateful to our friend who suggested we visit the WNAS.*

*See Also*: Alcoholism, Cystitis, Diarrhoea, and Arthritis, if applicable, What's Wrong with Present-Day Diet and Lifestyle?, The Very Nutritious Diet. Plus Recommended Reading List and References.

# IRRITABLE BOWEL SYNDROME

Irritable bowel syndrome is the modern name for a condition that was formerly known as spastic colon. It is such a common condition that surveys reveal that about half of those who attend hospital out-patient departments with digestive problems are suffering with IBS. Some doctors feel that this is the tip of the iceberg, and that many others suffer in silence.

For a diagnosis of irritable bowel syndrome to be made, a patient must have no underlying sinister symptoms, but be suffering with either constipation or diarrhoea or both, and abdominal pain and/or bloating and wind.

A 'normal' bowel habit was considered to be anything from passing motions three times per day to three times per week, according to a large UK study published in 1965. At the time 99 per cent of the population survey fell within these limits. It was also discovered that despite this many people still complained of diarrhoea or urgency, or constipation with stools difficult to pass. A further American survey some twenty years later revealed that 94 per cent had a stool frequency of between three times a day and three times per week. However, further questioning about a variety of bowel symptoms revealed that a total of 17 per cent had symptoms indicative of bowel dysfunction.

Surveys on precisely how common IBS is vary from between 10 to 25 per cent. Many people who are troubled by it do not consult their general practitioner but muddle on alone. One wonders how the medical services would cope if everyone with IBS turned up for help!

## What Are the Symptoms?

- constipation—opening the bowels infrequently, or hard stools
- diarrhoea—loose rather than just frequent stools
- alternating diarrhoea and constipation
- abdominal discomfort or pain
- abdominal bloating
- excessive wind
- mucus or slime in the stool
- nausea and loss of appetite
- indigestion

It is usual with IBS that patients will suffer with either diarrhoea or constipation, or a combination of the two, together with abdominal bloating and some discomfort or pain. These are the most common and typical symptoms.

## What Causes It?

- Age. Many people develop IBS symptoms in young to middle age, although approximately 12 per cent of those with IBS did experience symptoms during their childhood.
- Operations. It has been observed that approximately 10 per cent of women are more likely to suffer symptoms of IBS following an operation like a hysterectomy or surgery on the ovaries. These operations can leave internal scar tissue which is thought to be connected in some way to the onset of symptoms.
- Radiotherapy. When the abdomen has been targeted by radiotherapy, scarring can occur which may then once again produce symptoms of IBS.
- Gynaecological problems. The female reproductive organs have a very close relationship with the bowels. The womb, or uterus, is next to the end of the colon and a significant amount of the small bowel sits loosely coiled on top of the uterus. Many conditions relating to the uterus can release powerful chemicals which also influence the gut. A study by Dr Prior and colleagues in the United Kingdom on a sample of 200 women found that many of them noticed improvements in their bowel functions following a hysterectomy. 22 per cent of his sample had IBS before surgery, and two-thirds reported improvement in their bowel symptoms following the operation.
- Gastrointestinal infection. Most of us have experienced a severe tummy upset whilst on holiday or after eating a take-away meal. Sudden onset of diarrhoea, sometimes accompanied by pain and fever, can either be caused by bacteria or by a virus. Usually they don't last for more than a few days, but sometimes the gut never seems to feel the same again, and symptoms of IBS develop.
- Other bowel conditions. Older people sometimes develop a condition called diverticulosis of the colon, when the weak walls of the colon begin to bulge, and this can sometimes cause symptoms of IBS as well. A lack of fibre may lie behind both conditions. Patients suffering with ulcerative colitis, a severe inflammation of the gut which causes diarrhoea and bleeding, may also experience symptoms of IBS, even when the colitis is controlled by drugs.
- Drugs. Some pain-killing drugs can cause symptoms of IBS,

either shortly after they are taken, or several months later. Antibiotics, certainly if taken in the long term, can cause diarrhoea as a side-effect, which may set up IBS type symptoms in some. This seems to be due to a build up of *Candida albicans*, the organism responsible for thrush. This is often self-limiting and passes off, but for some it persists. Sometimes supplements of iron or multi-vitamins and minerals containing iron can irritate the gut also and produce symptoms of IBS.

◆ Stress. There is now plenty of evidence to show that stress can worsen symptoms of IBS. The stress factors affect the muscles in the gut and can cause them to go into spasm, rendering the bowel inefficient, and causing pain. Chronic sufferers of IBS sometimes suffer with anxiety and depression as their symptoms remain unresolved, which produces a vicious circle.

◆ A change of diet. Food intolerances sometimes develop after a period of eating substantial quantities of the same food, or when new foods which are hard to digest are introduced. Further information on this subject can be found in the information on Allergy and Intolerance.

◆ Nothing. Strangely, it seems that symptoms of IBS occur out of the blue with no single precipitating factor. Perhaps a subtle combination of circumstances may be the underlying cause or perhaps there may be genetic factors at play.

## What Your Doctor Can Do

Twenty years ago, it used to be fashionable in medical circles to investigate patients complaining with symptoms of IBS, with a view to diagnosing a stomach or duodenal ulcer, gallstones, digestive problems or problems with the colon, or large bowel, particularly diverticulosis. IBS was a diagnosis made by the doctor when nothing else could be found. This meant that patients were often subjected to numerous tests, including blood tests and X-rays, that were unnecessary. This was frustrating for patient and doctor alike.

Times have fortunately changed. It has become recognised that IBS is often the diagnosis for young to middle-aged patients, with abdominal pain or disturbance of bowel function. There are no tests to verify the diagnosis of IBS; it is often made on a balance of probabilities.

It is important to be screened by your doctor to eliminate the possibility of any sinister underlying cause to your symptoms.

## Sinister Symptoms

It is essential for you to become familiar with some of the possible sinister underlying symptoms, which may produce IBS type symptoms, but are not IBS, and their treatment is quite different. Here is a check-list of further symptoms for you to examine:

1.  Have you recently developed symptoms which are severe? In this case it is always best to have a medical examination.
2.  Do you have severe abdominal pain? For example, can it wake you from sleep? Does it cause you to stop what you are doing? Does it put you off eating?
3.  Have you lost weight because of your bowel symptoms? Losing any more than a few kilos in weight should not be regarded as IBS.
4.  Do you regularly pass more than four stools per day? Diarrhoea from any cause can contribute to a loss of essential nutrients, even if there is no weight loss.
5.  Have you passed blood in the stool or passed dark-coloured stools? Loss of blood from the bowel requires investigation because it may not always be due to IBS.
6.  Have you had a fever with your bowel symptoms? Infection in the bowel from parasites or other causes should be considered. Some parasitic infections can be found in Australia without travelling abroad.
7.  Have you had any abdominal operations including an appendicectomy? Past operations can leave behind strands of tissue called adhesions that can interfere with normal bowel function. If your bowel symptoms followed an operation you should return to your doctor.
8.  Are you aged fifty years or more? This increases the risk of symptoms being due to bowel cancer or a polyp (a small growth inside the bowel) which may become cancerous. Again you should check with your doctor if you have not already done so.
9.  Did your mother, father, sister or brother develop cancer of the bowel under the age of fifty? If so, you should also check with your doctor. Sometimes this type of problem can run in

families affecting relatively young or middle-aged members. Early detection of those at risk is now possible with a marked improvement in outlook for them.

10. Do you have any vaginal discharge, pain on intercourse or pain very low down in the abdomen? Infection of the fallopian tubes is particularly common in young women with these symptoms, which can sometimes aggravate, or be confused with IBS.

11. Are your periods painful, heavy or irregular? A number of gynaecological problems may cloud the picture at times. Fibroid growths of the womb, cysts on the ovaries, and sometimes hormonal problems should all be considered if you have any of the above.

Once the diagnosis of IBS is made, what is on offer from your doctor will depend on whether you are suffering with diarrhoea, constipation or a combination of both. For further details of what your doctor can do, and what measures you can implement yourself, you will now need to refer to the sections on Constipation, Diarrhoea and Abdominal Wind and Bloating.

The good news is that symptoms of IBS are both treatable and curable. We have written a book called *Beat IBS Through Diet*, which is based on our success treating this condition at the WNAS.

......................................................................................

## Belinda's Story

Belinda, a single thirty-two-year-old, had been suffering with severe bowel problems for two years prior to approaching the WNAS. She was very distressed as both her work and social life were affected by her symptoms.

*Looking back I realise that my symptoms began at about the time that my relationship ended with my boyfriend. We had been together for two years, and I found it very difficult to cope with the break-up. I began to have severe episodes of bloating and constipation every day, with extreme abdominal pain. I even found it difficult to sit down at work. By the evening of each day I was in so much pain I could only go to bed and wait for the pain to subside. I felt awfully drained and lost quite a bit of weight, which I could ill afford to do.*

*I was referred to the hospital for tests, including a small bowel enema, ultrasound and X-rays, and in November 1992 I was diagnosed as having IBS, and told to go on a high-fibre diet. The hospital doctor told me there was no known cure, and when I asked in desperation what I could do as I was still in constant pain, and with a redundant wardrobe, due to the swelling, he said I would have to buy bigger clothes. I was very shocked and angry by his unsympathetic response.*

*So a vicious circle began. I took painkillers, which brought on severe constipation and distress, which could only be relieved by laxatives. My doctor prescribed Colpermin, to make eating easier, but this only brought me out in a rash, and the list of possible side-effects was quite alarming.*

*In May 1993 I went along to the WNAS clinic at the suggestion of a friend who had been treated successfully by them. I must admit feeling sceptical when I went along for my first appointment, as I couldn't imagine that diet alone would be the solution to this severe problem. I was put on to a basic diet, asked to keep daily symptom charts and was seen fortnightly for a review. While I did have some good days, I still had more bad days. After three months and very little change I was on the verge of giving up, when I was told that in addition to excluding the foods we had so far, I should also leave out rice, corn, potatoes and bananas. It was also suggested that I take linseeds with my cereals and extra magnesium at night to relieve the constipation. To my utter amazement, my symptoms calmed down. The constipation was no longer a problem and the pain and bloating subsided.*

*I am happy to live on a restricted diet as I have traded the foods that upset me for my health. I am making great progress at work and have found a wonderful new boyfriend. I am very grateful as I now look forward to each day.*

*See also*: Stress, Taking Care of Body and Soul, The Simple Exclusion Diet, The Strict Exclusion Diet. Plus Recommended Reading List (*Beat IBS Through Diet*) and References.

# ISCHAEMIC HEART DISEASE

Ischaemic heart disease is the leading cause of death in Australia, accounting for 44 per cent of total deaths.

This is a disease in which there is a narrowing and eventually blockage of the blood vessels that supply the heart muscles. These vessels, which are called the coronary arteries, carry a very substantial flow of blood and oxygen to the ever-active heart muscle.

The narrowing is due to the slow development of what is termed a plaque. This is made up of fatty deposits, and fibrous tissue which develops in response to the fat deposit. The internal diameter of the blood vessel is reduced and even a small plaque can halve the flow of blood through one of the several coronary arteries. This process of arterial narrowing and hardening is called atherosclerosis, and the same process takes place in other major arteries, leading to strokes and poor circulation to the legs.

Very often the slowed blood that is attempting to flow through the coronary arteries is sticky, and a clot easily forms and adheres to the surface of the plaque leading to a complete blockage of a major coronary artery, which in turn leads to the most important manifestation of ischaemic heart disease, a heart attack or myocardial infarction (literally heart muscle that is stuffed with old blood). Needless to say that the heart muscle previously supplied by the now occluded artery will die, and the patient will at the very least be left with a weakened heart.

The next most important consequence of ischaemic heart disease is angina. The narrowing of a coronary artery does not always lead to blockage. The artery may have an adequate blood supply for the needs of the muscle it supplies provided that the heart is not working too hard. But when walking briskly, walking uphill or running, the supply of oxygen may be inadequate. The level of certain chemicals rises in the heart muscle which leads to pain usually felt as a 'tight' pain in the centre of the chest, which may also pass into the left arm, up into the neck or through into the back. The pain is often sufficiently severe to cause the sufferer to stop whatever they are doing and rest, which in many cases is enough for the pain to ease. The whole episode may only last a few minutes but recur every time the person tries to exert themselves.

Unfortunately not all ischaemic heart disease presents in this way. Sometimes the first event is also the last. Sudden unexpected death in a young to middle-aged man is very often due to this condition. Then there is no opportunity to undertake some of the medical and preventative measures that are proving successful in this condition.

Ischaemic heart disease can also cause palpitations with changes in the rhythm of the heartbeat, and also heart failure. This latter may be as a consequence of several heart attacks, or develop slowly and silently in older patients. The diagnosis of coronary artery disease is usually made as a result of one of these clinical pictures with confirmation from an ECG, blood tests, specialist X-rays of the coronary arteries called an angiogram, or other specialist assessments. Very often the assessment of ischaemic heart disease, especially in a young person, will involve an assessment of the main risk factors as well.

## Who Gets It?

Atherosclerosis, the process of narrowing and hardening of the main arteries, and the development of ischaemic heart disease, are common. In most developed countries around the world, death from disease of the coronary arteries rose substantially in the latter half of this century and is the leading cause of death in Australia, accounting for almost half of all deaths. The situation is similar in New Zealand, the UK, USA and other affluent countries. The most important step in prevention is keeping saturated fats low in our meals and snacks. Other protective measures are important too.

The main risk factors that determine who is likely to develop ischaemic heart disease are:

- age, the risk rising from age forty to mid-seventies then falling
- being male
- race (greater risk in those from southern Asia)
- dietary factors:
    - eating too much and being very overweight
    - too much saturated (animal) fat
    - too little fruit and vegetables
    - not enough high-fibre grain products
    - possibly poor intake of vitamins B, C, E, and the minerals magnesium and chromium
    - not consuming certain 'protective' foods and beverages such as oily fish, small amounts of wine, certain nuts (walnuts, almonds and pecans)
- body shape with excess weight being deposited around the abdomen rather than on the hips (an 'apple' instead of a 'pear')
- family history (coronary heart disease in a first-degree relative under the age of fifty-five)
- cigarette smoking

- personality type: the aggressive, striving ambitious deadline-driven type A personality as it is known is more prone than the relaxed sort who could barely care if the deadline is met or not
- stressful situations at work and at home such as the death of a spouse
- soft water (soft water is low in natural calcium and magnesium)
- diabetes mellitus
- high blood cholesterol—over 5.2 mmol/L
- high blood pressure
- an early menopause and loss of the 'protective action' of oestrogen
- an excess level of blood-clotting factors
- lack of physical exercise
- poor growth in the first year of life, especially if the birth weight was low

Many of these risk factors interact. For example the level of cholesterol in the blood is in turn influenced by genetic factors, diet, smoking and exercise. Also not all these risk factors are as important as each other. A very high cholesterol, above 9.0 mmol/L, is a major risk factor, especially if combined with smoking. A slightly elevated blood pressure in a woman with no other major risk factors hardly adds to her risk of ischaemic heart disease. Once there is evidence of actual ischaemic heart disease (e.g. an actual myocardial infarction, angina when physically active or an abnormal ECG), the need for aggressive therapy with diet and drugs greatly increases. Young patients (under the age of forty) will rarely need treatment for an elevated blood cholesterol unless it is very high or they are carrying several other major risk factors. For them simple, cheap, safe, non-toxic measures will suffice (a very healthy diet, exercise and possibly supplements of vitamin E, 200+ IU per day) until they are older, when the higher risk may then justify a more vigorous diet and cholesterol-lowering drugs.

## What Causes It?
The cause of ischaemic heart disease has been the subject of intense research both of populations and in the laboratory. This has led to the identification of the above risk factors, an understanding of their interaction, and how they lead to actual narrowing of a coronary artery. A full discussion of how these risk factors

actually cause heart disease is beyond the scope of this book. What is important is to understand how some of the main risk factors work together and the potential for prevention of this major killer. Obviously there are some risk factors that cannot be changed. Age, sex and race are not under our control.

## What Causes It?—Fats and Cholesterol

There is a strong connection between the amount and type of fat in the diet, and the risk of ischaemic heart disease. Historically attention has focused upon blood cholesterol. This is influenced by two factors. About one-third of the cholesterol in the blood is derived from the cholesterol that we eat. The remainder is made in the liver, and the amount made is determined by genetic and dietary factors. We use cholesterol to make all kinds of necessary body chemicals such as vitamin D, oestrogen, testosterone and for the structure of some cells. A high cholesterol level in a form that is easily deposited to make an atheromatous plaque is dangerous. This high-risk cholesterol is called LDL, and the beneficial protective form is called HDL. These cholesterol sub-fractions can be measured from a blood sample taken usually after an overnight fast.

High intakes of saturated animal fats add to the risk of heart disease probably because such a diet will increase the production of cholesterol in the LDL form by the liver and may cause other blood changes, encouraging the depositing of that cholesterol on to the inner wall of the artery. Other fats do not have this effect, such as the oleic acid found in olive oil and canola oil and of the polyunsaturated fatty acids derived from a variety of plant and fish oils. These oils may actually shift the balance toward the good HDL cholesterol. The degree of protection that these 'healthy oils' provide is debated, and of interest not only to the general public and doctors, but also to farmers and politicians. The majority of expert recommendations recognise a need for the 'average' consumer to reduce their total fat intake by cutting down on saturated animal fats, maintaining a modest intake of the polyunsaturates and to making little change to the consumption of oleic acid. Arguments will continue to rage about the role that these different fats play in heart disease.

Many of the risk factors also influence this balance between the good HDL and the bad LDL cholesterol. Stopping smoking, correction of obesity and regular physical exercise may have a marked effect, reducing the total cholesterol and raising the proportion of the good type. In patients with furring up of their coronary arteries or of those in the legs, meticulous attention to diet and use of drugs to lower cholesterol has been shown to reverse the process of atherosclerosis. If other relevant risk factors are tackled, then the prospects for sufferers will look better still. Do not forget that the type of advice given to someone who has had a heart attack and has a high blood cholesterol level may be quite different to that given to a healthy, middle-aged woman or man with low to average risk factors.

Broadly speaking the recommendations for healthy eating take into account the main dietary risk factors for ischaemic heart disease. Their implementation will hopefully lead to the prevention of heart disease in the general population who have yet to have a heart attack. This is termed primary prevention. Our recommendations for The Very Nutritious Diet (see Part Three) are appropriate for the majority of those who wish to delay the development of ischaemic heart disease. We say 'delay' rather than 'prevent' as this problem may be inevitable for many. Remember age is a major risk factor, and for those aged eighty years and more, a heart attack could be viewed as a relatively attractive way of ending one's days.

## What Your Doctor Can Do

- Assess the severity of the condition. Those presenting with angina at a young age, those with severe symptoms uncontrolled by drug therapy, and others with certain risk factors need a detailed assessment often involving X-rays of the coronary arteries—a coronary angiogram.
- Treat the symptoms. Angina may be helped by the use of several types of drugs: nitrates help dilate the coronary arteries and can be given as a spray or tablets under the tongue; beta-blockers slow the heart rate and reduce the demand for oxygen; and calcium antagonists also open up the coronary arteries. Many of these drugs will need to be given on a regular daily basis as well as being used for acute attacks.
- Treat a myocardial infarction or a clot. Rapid response by the doctor or emergency services with use of anti-clotting treatments, aspirin, beta-blockers and nitrate drugs has resulted in

improved survival. Speed, however, is of the essence in this situation, and all middle-aged and elderly people with prolonged chest pains are suspected as having a heart attack until proven otherwise.

◆ Assess the main risk factors for atherosclerosis. This will involve measurement of blood pressure, tests for diabetes and measurement of a fasting blood cholesterol level. If the blood cholesterol is elevated then the need for advice about drugs and diet can be assessed. Even if the patient is not enthusiastic, she will often do well to use some of the newer drugs as well as diet to lower its level.

◆ Prevent further myocardial infarction by use of drugs. This often involves giving aspirin which helps prevent blood clotting, beta-blockers to slow the heart rate, or calcium antagonists. The choice of these depends upon factors such as patient tolerance, blood pressure, diabetes and any weakening of the heart.

◆ Prevent further myocardial infarction by lifestyle changes such as cessation of smoking, reduction in weight, changes to the diet, drugs to lower blood cholesterol, and a carefully supervised exercise regime to improve fitness.

◆ Consider the need for surgical correction of coronary artery narrowing. In selected patients who have had a myocardial infarction or are at risk of one, either open-heart surgery and by-passing the blockage, or the newer technique of opening up the blockage from within the artery—coronary angioplasty—can be highly successful, and be associated with an improved life expectancy. Coronary artery by-pass graft survival is very much influenced by the control of blood cholesterol and lifestyle factors.

The last twenty years has seen a substantial improvement in the outcome for those affected with ischaemic heart disease. For both the patient with just angina on exercise, and the patient who is recovering from her (first) myocardial infarction, there is much she can do to reduce the risk of more angina, another infarction and sudden death. The wise patient should regard the diagnosis of ischaemic heart disease as a signal to make some changes and regard that day as the first day of the rest of her life.

## *What You Can Do*
Plenty!

- Make sure that you get proper medical treatment as above! The provision of good care together with appropriate monitoring are not automatic. Expert assessment is very often needed for those with severe angina, those whose lifestyle is significantly altered as a result of a myocardial infarction, those who have had several infarctions, those with diabetes, those with a high blood cholesterol unresponsive to simple dietary measures and those with a weakened heart.
- Don't smoke. You're crazy and probably dead if you do.
- Don't be overweight. If you are, lose weight. Never mind the details of the best diet for heart disease, just get the weight off. Follow The Simple Weight-loss Diet.
- If your cholesterol is even slightly elevated then follow The Very Nutritious Diet. Make sure that you achieve the following dietary goals:
  - ◇ three pieces of fresh fruit daily
  - ◇ two portions of green vegetables daily
  - ◇ three portions of fish per week with two of these being mackerel or herring
  - ◇ use mainly soya, canola and walnut oil. This latter is good for salad dressings
  - ◇ use a polyunsaturated margarine rather than butter
  - ◇ allow yourself one or two drinks per day. Some say that red wine may be particularly good for the heart
  - ◇ if you can, include garlic, onions and some nuts—walnuts, almonds and pecans—into your diet
- If this is not effective enough then more specialised dietary advice may be needed. For example a vegan diet might appeal to some, but be too difficult for many. You could modify this and add in oily fish to make it a 'tunatarian' diet. Allow yourself one portion of mackerel, herring or salmon daily. A strict vegan diet has been used as part of a highly successful non-drug treatment for severe angina.
- Regular exercise is a good idea for all. Probably it is best to get some expert advice about this. Ask your doctor, or there may be a post-myocardial infarction exercise group at the local

hospital. Some sports clubs or gyms run specialised classes for heart patients.

◆ Nutritional supplements do have some value too.

   ◇ Vitamin E at high dose, 600 IU per day, has been shown recently to reduce the risk of a heart attack. Take it but don't think this means you don't have to do anything else. Those who are taking the blood-thinning drug Warfarin will need to check with their doctor first, as vitamin E influences the effects of this drug.

   ◇ Vitamin C as a supplement of around 1 g per day may help lower an elevated blood cholesterol but probably only if your diet is devoid of fruit and vegetables.

   ◇ Magnesium might be helpful. Some but not all studies have shown that very high doses help in the recovery from a heart attack. It is perhaps most useful for those whose blood level is low as a result of diuretic (water) tablets.

   ◇ Chromium is a curious trace element. It is required in tiny quantities and it helps insulin in its action of controlling blood sugar. Supplements have been shown to help correct a diabetic tendency and improve elevated blood cholesterol levels. Low levels of the mineral are associated with coronary artery disease. A supplement of 200 µg per day is worth considering. It will need to be taken long term.

   ◇ Multi-vitamins are worth a mention. Perhaps the simplest thing to take is a modest strength multi-vitamin with vitamin E, 200 IU, and vitamin C, 250 mg. Older patients, those with a restricted diet or those on many drugs may be the most suited to this.

◆ Make sure that there is good control of any possible blood pressure, diabetes and any blood stickiness problem.

◆ Avoid stressful situations at home and at work. These very often precipitate attacks of angina or even a heart attack. Relaxation techniques are appropriate for those for whom this is a particular problem.

## Complementary Therapies

These have not come to the fore for heart disease in the way that they have in other areas. Perhaps it is because of the life-threatening nature of ischaemic heart disease that no great emphasis has been put on these complementary approaches. Any de-stressing therapies are worth considering. They should complement, not replace, conventional treatment. Aromatherapy, massage and acupuncture would fall into this category. Herbalism may prove to have much to offer. The potential of plant products to provide a degree of chemical protection from heart disease is slowly being realised. Seek expert advice from a qualified herbalist on this last point.

# KIDNEY STONES

Urine is a chemically complicated fluid. It is obviously composed mainly of water, but dissolved in this are significant amounts of certain minerals including sodium, calcium, magnesium, potassium and phosphate. The yellow colour is due to breakdown products from blood and plant pigments, and sometimes vitamin B2, riboflavin. There is a limit to the amount of a mineral that can be dissolved in a given volume of fluid. If urine volume is decreased, the mineral concentration increases; as a result, some of these minerals may be precipitated out as crystals which then form stones. The stones normally form in the kidney and once released they try and travel along the thin tube connecting the kidney and the bladder, the ureter. If this becomes blocked or goes into spasm, then pain results. Renal colic, as it is known, is one of the most painful conditions known in medicine, and very often patients attend hospital as an emergency with severe gripping pain in the side of the abdomen which may pass down into the groin. The site of the pain changes as the stone passes along the urethra until it eventually passes out into the bladder and hopefully through the urine to the outside world. The stone can be collected using a tea strainer. This is important as chemical analysis of the stone indicates the type of stone and the best treatment for its prevention.

## What Causes Them?

As there is a variety of kidney stones, there is a variety of possible causes. Usually there are several at work together, and typically a combination of them in any one individual. The following are all possible factors:

- Infection in the urine. This leads to a change in the urine's chemistry and under certain circumstances can lead to kidney stone formation.
- Too much calcium in the urine, which is only rarely due to too much calcium in the diet. An important possibility is an excessive level of calcium in the blood becauses of changes in hormone chemistry. More usually there is an excessive leaking of calcium out into the urine and this is probably aggravated by a diet high in sodium, sugar and low in magnesium and essential fatty acids.
- Dehydration, which is an important cause of kidney stone formation in the tropics.
- Accumulation of oxalic acid. This comes from certain foods in the diet and some people excrete excessive amounts of this acid into the urine.
- An excess of uric acid in the urine. This compound is also the cause of gout. Again some of us pass larger than usual quantities out into the urine and, because it is hard to dissolve, it can easily lead to kidney stone formation.

## What Your Doctor Can Do

- Treat the acute episode with strong painkillers.
- Investigate the type of stone. This involves analysis of any stones captured, blood test and urine tests. These tests centre upon measuring the levels of the minerals and compounds previously mentioned.
- Test the urine for infection, which is a significant factor in stone formation.
- Give specific recommendation, depending upon the type of stone. This may require expert assessment but some general guidelines can be given.

## *What You Can Do*

The following recommendations will apply almost no matter what the type of stone is:

◆ Drink plenty of fluid—at least 1.75–2.75 litres of water daily.

◆ Eat a diet low in sugar, salt and refined foods, and high in fruit, vegetable and wholegrain cereals. This sort of diet reduces the loss of many minerals in the urine, but more specialised dietary advice may be required.

◆ Supplements of magnesium, which passes out into the urine and generally has stone-inhibiting properties. They are not very effective but is very safe and may be followed on a long-term basis. The reasonable dosage is 200–300 mg per day of elemental magnesium.

◆ Sometimes a low-calcium diet is recommended if there is continuing loss of calcium in the urine.

◆ Supplements of bran may inhibit the absorption of calcium from the diet and reduce the amount lost in the urine. They are not recommended if the person is at risk of developing osteoporosis.

◆ Supplements of evening primrose oil and fish oil, Efamol Marine, have an interesting and useful effect in recurrent kidney stone formation when these are high in calcium. They reduce the loss of calcium via the kidney, and together with the above simple dietary means, may even reduce the rate of stone formation. It is thought that they may do this by preventing the loss of calcium from bone.

◆ Follow a diet low in oxalate. This compound is found in a variety of foods notably tea, coffee, peanuts, chocolate, rhubarb and spinach. A reduced dietary intake may be required in some adults and children who have this type of kidney stone. Expert assessment is required before beginning this diet.

◆ Lose weight if you are overweight.

◆ Cut down on alcohol—particularly important if you have gout.

*See also*: References.

# LIBIDO, LOSS OF

In our youth, before the responsibilities of life settle on our shoulders, many of us take our libido, or appetite for sex, for granted, never dreaming that anything might influence it. However, the passionate nights of a new relationship live on in the dreams of most, but only the reality of a few. Childbirth, sleepless nights, the stresses and strains of life and general preoccupation, all contribute to a waning sex drive.

Over the years at the WNAS we have come to realise, from dealing with thousands of women of all ages, that women regard their loss of libido as their lot. They accept that it is all part of their fading youth, even if it happens in their late twenties! They don't discuss it with others through embarrassment as they assume they are suffering alone, and it doesn't occur to them that the situation is reversible.

There are no hard and fast rules about what is a normal level of libido, and there is no such thing as a 'normal' libido. What is normal to one couple may be abnormal to another. You can only judge your libido by your own standards, and if you feel that your sexual desire has diminished, for whatever reason, you will need to seek help to restore it.

## What Causes Libido to Diminish

Most of us have a natural interest in sex initially. That's the way we were designed. There are, however, a number of reasons why sex drive can decrease either over a period of time or suddenly following a particular incident.

Loss of libido can be due to physical or hormonal problems or mental stress and sometimes a combination of the two. Amongst the causes are:

- After childbirth, many women lose interest in sex because of their rapidly changing hormone levels, their disturbed nights and the fact that Mother Nature makes a woman treat her baby as a priority rather than her husband's needs.
- Excessive weight gain, weight loss, irregular periods, hair loss or excessive hair growth may all signify hormonal problems which can also result in a low libido.

- Other hormone disturbances like thyroid problems, or galactorrhea, a white milky discharge from the nipples, can cause low libido.
- Sometimes people are put off sex as intercourse becomes painful. The pain can be due to infection, vaginismus, when the vaginal muscles go into spasm, an enlarged or displaced womb or other conditions.
- Long-term illness and lack of energy.
- Psychologically distressing past experiences which still haunt you.
- Simply a lack of feeling for your partner.
- Stress, worry and depression often take their toll on sex drive. When you are mentally preoccupied with pressing problems the body naturally diverts its energy to helping you through the troubled times and sexual desire may take a back seat.

## What Your Doctor Can Do

If you feel that the cause of your loss of sex drive may be due to hormonal problems, or pain or discomfort, your doctor should be able to offer you some effective treatment. If there is an underlying psychological problem, or you are feeling overwhelmed with stress you will need to get some professional counselling to help overcome the problems before you can expect your libido to return. The doctor can:

- give you routine blood tests, including serum ferritin to check your iron stores
- give you a physical examination to eliminate any underlying physical cause
- refer you for some counselling if your relationship is under strain or if you are suffering the effects of past trauma

## What You Can Do

If, however, you feel that your libido has decreased for no apparent reason, particularly if the situation is worse before your period, then it is possible that you can gain some benefit by attending to your diet.

At the Women's Nutritional Advisory Service we have found that a programme of diet, exercise and nutritional supplements helps some 90 per cent of women get their sex drive back within four to six months.

The body depends on important vitamins and minerals in order to function properly. During and when under stress there is a significantly increased demand for essential nutrients. Because we lack education about the foods which contain these important nutrients, these increased demands may not be met. We know, for instance, that the mineral magnesium is necessary for normal hormone function, and that B vitamins and the mineral zinc are particularly important in sex hormone metabolism and maintaining your sex drive. So it stands to reason that if your diet does not provide you with a constant supply of good nutrients, the body will eventually stop functioning normally, and your sex drive may well be affected.

- Follow the instructions for The Very Nutritious Diet.
- Eat plenty of ordinary foods like bread, milk, eggs, meat, chicken, nuts, beans, dried fruit, green vegetables, and fish. Oysters long regarded for their aphrodisiac qualities, are extremely high in zinc, and are vital for sperm and male hormone production.
- It is important to avoid drinking too much alcohol as it knocks most nutrients sideways. Whist you are trying to consume lots of good nutrients through your diet it would defeat the object to wash them away with alcohol. Alcohol may initially increase the desire but usually reduces the performance. Try to limit yourself to no more than three drinks per week.
- If you are overweight it is important to get yourself back into shape. Apart from the health benefits of being trim, your self-esteem will improve and you are likely to feel more desirable. Losing weight can help improve hormone function in women in particular.
- You will also help your sex drive on its way by taking regular physical exercise. Ideally you need to do four or five good sessions of exercise per week to the point of breathlessness. Adequate exercise helps to elevate your mood is likely to have a positive effect on your hormones and your energy levels.
- If you lead a busy life and have children to care for it is important to take time out with your partner from time to time.

There is nothing like a few days away without any interruptions to rekindle the old flame.

◆ Watching a video together like 'The Lover's Guide' or referring to a book specially prepared to help you improve your sex life, might bring back that old familiar, tingling feeling.

◆ Plus, you might well speed things along by taking specific nutritional supplements such as Blackmores Active Woman formula. Extra supplements of zinc may be useful for those with a low intake.

Flagging libido does not signal 'the beginning of the end', it is simply your body's way of telling you that all is not well. Providing there is no underlying cause, self-help measures and patience will bring back the old sparkle! Patience is essential, as these recommendations are not a magic pill, you must expect to work at it over a period of several months.

## Complementary Therapies

Herbal medicine would be our first choice once nutritional deficiencies have been corrected.

## Diana's Story

Thirty-two-year-old mother of two, Diana had enjoyed her sex life until after the birth of their second child she suddenly went completely off sex and couldn't bear to be touched.

*I felt very guilty about losing interest in sex. I'd become very moody and depressed, and was irritated by any approaches from my husband. I didn't even want to kiss and cuddle which was so unusual for me. He used to creep up behind me and kiss the back of my neck when I was cooking or washing up, and I'd always enjoyed it. Now if I thought he was approaching I'd quickly move out of the way, and if he put his arm around me I would shrug him off.*

*In bed I'd curl up and pretend to be asleep before he could make a move. When I first pushed him away he looked so hurt and asked if he had done anything to upset me. I just made excuses about being tired or busy as I couldn't face telling him the truth—that I'd gone off him. It was horrible because I knew I still loved him, but I felt I was betraying him by not wanting to make love to him any more.*

*Once or twice I thought I would go through with it for his sake which was disastrous as my lack of response made him feel even more rejected. He eventually asked me if I wanted to separate. I tried to convince him that it was because my body felt switched off and not because of anything he had done. He was very supportive under the circumstances and suggested that when I felt ready for sex I should make the first move as he couldn't bear any further rejection.*

*By chance a couple of weeks later I read about a range of symptoms which I knew I'd been suffering from—including loss of libido, depression and a sore throat. I contacted the organisation mentioned which was the WNAS. I was advised to give up smoking and caffeine, sugar and salt. I didn't think I would manage without these vital lifelines, but I was so determined to succeed. I was also prescribed supplements of Optivite, zinc, vitamin C, and Normoglycaemia to help with my cravings for food premenstrually, which was also a problem. I took regular exercise as well and within a few weeks I could feel my symptoms begin to lift. My moodiness vanished and one afternoon I suddenly realised that I wanted sex again.*

*My first thought was how to break the news to Jeff after so many months without sex. I felt scared of being rejected too. I resorted to the corny old candlelit supper, and over a bottle of wine hinted that I was 'in the mood'. At the end of the evening I said to Jeff, 'I think I'll go to bed now', and with a twinkle in his eye, he said, 'I think I'll join you'.*

*That night was a great success, and a terrific boost for Jeff's flagging confidence. I've had the occasional relapse, especially if we've been out to dinner with friends and I've binged on all the baddies I'm supposed to avoid. But mostly, our sex life is great—in actual fact it's even better than before! A while ago a friend commented that Jeff and I rarely go out. Jeff told her that was because we always go to bed early. She didn't get the message, so he spelled it out 'We go to bed early, but we're awake for hours . . .'*

# LIVER DISEASE

There is a large variety of conditions that affect the liver, and they are the province of the hospital-based liver specialist. Some points are worth mentioning in a book of this sort, though. More will be heard of liver problems, as time passes, especially as some types become more commonplace and there is increasing recognition that some disorders of female sex hormones and related problems are due to liver conditions.

## What Causes It?

◆ Viral hepatitis. There are several types of these viruses, termed hepatitis A, B, C, D, or E virus. The first and last cause an acute hepatitis with a flu-like illness and jaundice in some, though not all. The middle three can produce a chronic inflammation of the liver. They are spread through contact with saliva, by sexual intercourse or from blood to blood transmission as in intravenous drug users. Worldwide there are several hundred million people infected with these viruses.

◆ Excessive amounts of alcohol. The risk appears in those drinking more than 4 units per day. The duration of alcohol excess is a risk factor, and there also appears to be a genetic component too.

◆ Exposure to many toxins. These include oil-derived and industrial chemicals, pesticides and many different drugs including anti-cancer preparations, some antibiotics, drugs used to treat psychiatric disorders, the oral contraceptive pill (rarely) and even regular high doses of paracetamol.

◆ A wide variety of infections and inflammatory conditions. These include arthritis, colitis, and Crohn's disease. One particular type develops almost only in middle-aged women, and can accompany heavy periods, skin itching, malaise, and prominent blood vessels on the chest and neck.

◆ 'Fatty liver'. A relatively mild disturbance in liver function easily develops in some people who are overweight, diabetic or drink too much. If tackled early, then this is completely reversible.

## What Your Doctor Can Do

Where liver disease is suspected, specialist treatment is essential.

◆ Remove the cause. Most usually this means stopping a drug and avoiding alcohol.

◆ Give drugs to control the inflammation. These include steroids and powerful immune-altering drugs.

◆ Correct nutritional deficiencies. Just about every nutrient can become deficient, so early recognition and treatment are important. Older women may be especially at risk, so calcium and vitamin D may need to be given to prevent osteoporosis and bone softening. The metabolism of the B vitamins is easily

disturbed, plus zinc deficiency and vitamin A deficiency are all
possible.

◆ Consider a liver transplant. Now becoming more commonplace
and with a good degree of success. For many the alternative is
death.

## What You Can Do

This is really most relevant to those with mildly disturbed liver
function which may have been detected on routine blood tests,
those with early liver disease or the increasing number who will
be found to be carriers of hepatitis C virus which is currently estimated to be many as one million people!

◆ Don't drink alcohol.
◆ Don't be overweight.
◆ Follow the recommendations for The Very Nutritious Diet.
Eating little and often may reduce the metabolic load of a meal
upon the liver.
◆ Do not take drugs unnecessarily, and avoid illicit drugs.
◆ Take supplements of vitamin B complex as there are a few
studies that have shown small improvements in liver function
within the normal population. It is possible that, as most of the
B vitamins are processed by the liver, this harmless approach
could help some of those with a mild disturbance in liver
function.
◆ Other supplements, especially vitamins C, E and beta-carotene
which have tissue-protecting properties, may be needed
depending upon the advice of your specialist. High doses of
vitamins A and D are to be avoided.

## Complementary Therapies

Herbalism probably holds the most promise, but you should seek
the advice of a qualified herbalist as some herbs are in fact toxic
to the liver.

## Angela's Story

Angela was a plump, pleasant, sixty-year-old woman. For many years she had
been troubled by fatigue and a general malaise. An underactive thyroid had

been diagnosed, but treatment for this had not helped entirely. Further investigation revealed that she had persistently abnormal tests of liver function. Specialist investigations had not revealed the cause, and she had refused the liver biopsy test offered. Blood tests showed that the level of various liver-derived enzymes were two to five times the preferred values. She was a non-drinker, but a little overweight at 73 kg, and the tests that had been performed suggested there was a degree of fatty infiltration in the liver.

Nutritional tests had shown that a number of nutrients were moderately low, including zinc, magnesium, selenium, vitamin E and some of the essential fatty acids. She took supplements of these together with vitamin B complex, biotin, choline and inositol. She began a weight-reducing diet though this only resulted in her losing 1–2 kg.

After a year her liver function tests had become nearly normal and there was some improvement in her fatigue. It was not possible to know exactly which nutritional factors contributed to the improvement in her liver function tests. It was probably a combined effect.

# MASTITIS

Mastitis may occur when you are breast-feeding. Mastitis is simply inflammation of the breast, which usually comes about when some of the milk ducts deep in the breast become blocked and in some cases infected. You may suddenly notice a red patch on the breast, which is tender to the touch, and have a headache, and/or feel weak and feverish. This can all have an extremely rapid onset, and be very dramatic, with fevers soaring to 40°C.

## What Causes It?

♦ Often the blockage occurs in the lower portion of the right breast of right-handed women, as it is more difficult to latch a baby on to the nipple with the left hand. Very often, because of the sitting position, the base of the breast fails to empty.

♦ An ill-fitting bra that is too tight.

◆ Cracked, sore nipples allow bacteria from the baby's mouth to enter the milk ducts and multiply.

## What Your Doctor Can Do

◆ Offer painkillers to help with the pain, which is sometimes very severe, and to bring the fever down.
◆ Prescribe antibiotics to combat the infection, especially if the fever becomes high.

## Danielle's Story

Danielle, thirty-two, was very keen to continue breast-feeding despite the problems she encountered.

*I was very keen on breast-feeding, and got off to a very good start after the birth of our son. I had plenty of milk which let down well, but Alex didn't seem to empty my breasts properly. Consequently I became susceptible to breast lumps— which repeatedly turned into mastitis. The first episode was very frightening as my temperature went up suddenly to 40 degrees. I felt very disorientated and nervous. I wanted to avoid using antibiotics if at all possible, and managed by using a combination of two homeopathic remedies, Belladonna and Phytolaca.*

*The mastitis recurred on ten or eleven occasions. I succumbed to antibiotics only once, as I felt too ill to manage without them. In the main I used hot water pads before feeding and a pack of frozen peas after feeding. I spent lots of time massaging my breasts and having warm baths to keep the flow of milk going. I took some vitamins and minerals, in particular vitamin E, which I understood would help prevent further episodes. I am so glad that I managed to continue breast-feeding Alex, despite the pain. It is such a precious time, I was determined not to let anything disrupt it.*

## What You Can Do

◆ Keep feeding your baby, no matter how painful it may be, as emptying your breast will help to resolve the problem.
◆ Feed your baby with its body nestled under your arm and legs tucked behind you, as it may be easier to get the baby's jaws in the proper position.
◆ Offer the inflamed breast to your baby first, and make sure you empty it fully.
◆ Use a breast pump to fully empty the breast if necessary.

◆ Massage the sore parts of your breast with your fingers, encouraging the milk out of the ducts.

◆ Have plenty of hot baths, with hot flannels pressed directly on to the breast.

◆ Alternatively, place packs of frozen peas on the breast to reduce the inflammation.

◆ Try some gentle arm movements to keep the circulation flowing in the area.

◆ Take plenty of rest in between feeds; you will need all your strength.

◆ Use a homoeopathic remedy, either Lachesis or Belladonna, every few hours until the inflammation and the fever subside.

◆ Remember that painkillers and antibiotics are there if you need them. If the breast becomes infected, and you feel really unwell, you owe it to yourself and your baby to speed the recovery. Neither the painkillers nor the antibiotics will harm your baby, and neither will the milk from an infected breast.

Some women never experience mastitis, whilst others seem to get it repeatedly, despite taking precautions. Do persist. Your baby gets a far greater start in life by being breast-fed.

*See also*: Breast Problems. Plus Recommended Reading List and Standard References.

# MENOPAUSE

For at least three-quarters of all women, the menopause brings with it rapid changes and unwanted symptoms which often disrupt life and result in utter misery. Frequent hot flushes during the day, and sweats at night leave them exhausted, disoriented and despondent. A dry vagina and reduced libido can wreck their sex lives, and repeated insomnia can leave women wondering whether life as they knew it is over.

The menopause is a transition which signals the end of a woman's monthly fertility cycle, and in order to have a smooth passage through it, women's bodies need to be in really good shape.

## What Is the Menopause?

The menopause itself is merely the day menstruation stops, which one can only usually be certain about with hindsight. Therefore many women will experience the actual menopause without really knowing at the time. Most of the symptoms experienced occur whilst in the perimenopausal stage, which means *around the time* of the menopause.

After the age of forty, the supply of eggs starts to run out, and the level of the female hormone oestrogen starts to fall. The dwindling number of eggs then mature irregularly, so that as the menopause approaches, the length of the menstrual cycles start to vary and periods become irregular.

Periods cease when eggs run out. As oestrogen levels fall, the lining of the womb loses its main source of stimulation, and periods stop altogether. The majority of women will have their last natural period somewhere between the ages of forty-five and fifty-five, with the average standing at just over fifty. In rarer cases women start an early menopause in their late twenties or early thirties, and sometimes women go on having periods until they are in their late fifties. However, statistics do show that smokers may reach the menopause as much as two years earlier than non-smokers.

## What Are the Symptoms?

From a survey of 500 women who had recently gone through their menopause, we at the WNAS discovered that there were three main groups of symptoms that occur at the time of the menopause, but only one group is directly related to the falling oestrogen levels. The other two groups of symptoms that we discovered were more to do with dietary and lifestyle inadequacies.

*Oestrogen withdrawal symptoms*
These are predominantly:

- hot flushes
- night sweats
- vaginal dryness

- loss of libido
- urinary symptoms
- skin changes
- difficulties with intercourse

*Physical symptoms*
These consist primarily of:

- aches and pains
- irritable bowel syndrome
- constipation
- fatigue
- migraines and headaches

*Mental symptoms*
These included:

- anxiety
- panic attacks
- palpitations
- irritability
- aggressive feelings
- mood swings
- depression and confusion

All of the symptoms listed are commonly experienced. What is not widely appreciated however, is that HRT is only aiming at the oestrogen withdrawal group, and not necessarily the physical and the mental groups of symptoms.

We know from research conducted on several groups of younger women suffering with premenstrual syndrome that minerals like magnesium, iron and the B vitamins are often in short supply, which affects the efficiency of brain chemistry and hormone function. The menopause is a great transition, which places extra demands on brain chemistry. If the body is not 'firing on all four cylinders' because of previous dietary inadequacies and lack of education, a bumpy ride can be expected. It is thought that approximately 75 per cent of women in the Western world will experience adverse symptoms at the time of the menopause.

## What Your Doctor Can Do

The favoured treatment for menopausal women is hormone replacement therapy, HRT. Oestrogen therapy was initially pioneered in the USA. Oestrogens alone were used for the first twenty years, but then it was discovered that women with an intact uterus had a greatly increased risk of cancer of the lining of the uterus, and so progesterone was added to make it safer.

## Types of HRT

### Oestrogens by mouth

This has been the commonest way of giving oestrogen (prescribed by more than three-quarters of the doctors in our survey), but as it goes via the liver it is more likely to cause feelings of nausea than other forms. It has to be taken every day in pill form, but the advantage is that the dose is under individual control.

### Oestrogen vaginal creams

These deliver oestrogen direct to the vagina and vulva and help with vaginal lubrication. They are considered useful for women suffering with a dry vagina, but the absorption can be erratic, and it is not therefore regarded as a long-term treatment.

### Oestrogen by skin patch

The patch releases a steady supply of oestrogen which by-passes the liver and avoids the slight adverse effects of some oral preparations. Although it is undoubtedly a clever innovation, which mimics our own ovaries, the levels of oestrogen released from the patch vary according to the climate and level of physical activity. It has to be accompanied by progesterone therapy in women who have their uterus intact. Skin irritation is also reported in 5 per cent of users.

### Oestrogen by implant

This is another method of delivering oestrogen without it going via the liver. The implant can provide a supply of oestrogen for up to six months. It is placed under the skin by means of a small operation under local anaesthetic. Occasionally the pellet is rejected or becomes infected. The advantage is that once given, you can forget about it, *unless* there are side-effects. Once again women with a uterus will need to take progesterone with it to induce a withdrawal bleed. The implant can deliver high levels of oestrogen initially, gradually decreasing as the effect wears off. Sometimes flushes become worse as the effect of the implant wears off, mimicking the failing ovaries.

### HRT without a bleed

The monthly bleed or irregular bleeding does put many women off taking HRT. New treatments coming on to the market have tried to conquer this problem. Tibolone (Livial) is a synthetic substance with mild oestrogen and progesterone effects. If taken continuously it controls oestrogen-withdrawal symptoms, without stimulating the lining of the uterus, so there is usually no withdrawal bleed. It can only be taken by women whose periods ceased more than a year prior to commencing treatment.

### Other products

Other products being developed and introduced to the market are numerous.

- The use of oestrogen and progesterone together given throughout the month in tablet form, which may cause little or no bleeding—again only suitable for those who haven't had a period for at least a year.
- IUD coil containing progesterone, which may help those who have heavy bleeding or PMS with other HRT preparations.
- Oestrogen gel that can be absorbed through the skin. It will need to be combined with progesterone tablets for women with a uterus in order to avoid developing cancer of the lining of the womb.
- Oestrogen and progesterone tablet combinations. A wider choice of these will soon be available, which may reduce the risk of nausea, headaches, mood changes and PMS-like symptoms.

## The Risk Factors of HRT

Some women swear by HRT, but these are greatly outnumbered by the women who cannot tolerate it. Research shows that up to two-thirds of women who try HRT come off it within the first year, due to either side-effects or dissatisfaction. Because doctors are not widely educated about alternative treatments to HRT for women experiencing symptoms of the menopause, women are often left on 'a medical scrap heap' to fend for themselves. A survey of 1000 GPs that we undertook at the WNAS shows that almost half the doctors experienced problems when prescribing HRT, and 43 per cent claimed that they experienced problems when treating menopausal women.

Large trials are underway to examine the actual risks attached to taking HRT. There are undoubtedly still recognised risks, and until these long studies are completed, which is likely to take another twenty years, the jury is still out. The most serious risk is an increased possibility of breast cancer—10–20 per cent after ten years on HRT.

Also don't take HRT if you have:

◆ a history of cancer of the womb or breast
◆ vaginal bleeding of uncertain cause
◆ endometriosis (where the womb lining grows and subsequently bleeds outside the womb)
◆ thrombosis (blood clots)
◆ severe cardiac, liver or kidney disease

HRT may also aggravate:

◆ migraines
◆ multiple sclerosis
◆ epilepsy
◆ diabetes
◆ high blood pressure (occasionally)
◆ gallstones

*Side-effects*
(Compiled from data supplied by the manufacturers of HRT preparations and from the UK doctors' guide to drug prescribing.)

## Less serious

◆ gastro-intestinal upset
◆ nausea and vomiting
◆ weight gain—usually slight

- breast tenderness and enlargement
- premenstrual syndrome symptoms such as mood changes
- breakthrough bleeding
- headaches or migraine
- dizziness
- leg cramps

**Minor problems**

- increase in size of uterine fibroids
- intolerance of contact lenses
- certain skin reactions
- loss of scalp hair
- increase in body or facial hair

The survey also showed a great inconsistency in prescribing alternatives to HRT, with some thirty-six different treatment approaches nominated; hardly surprising considering that 82 per cent of the GPs in the survey felt they had had inadequate training on the nutritional approach to health, and a further 8 per cent failed to answer the question.

## *What You Can Do*

There is a great deal that you can do to ensure a smooth passage through the menopause, and to prevent heart disease and the bone-thinning disease, osteoporosis, without taking HRT. The recommendations that we use at the WNAS are all based on published scientific papers. So, for example, did you know that:

- A group of Australian workers published a paper in the *British Medical Journal*, which showed that a group of women going through the menopause, regularly consuming foods and drinks that contained naturally occurring oestrogens, were able to bring about the same positive changes in the lining of the vagina, as women taking HRT.
- Practising relaxation techniques each day can reduce your hot flushes by as much as 60 per cent.
- Taking supplements of calcium, essential fatty acids and marine fish oils, can reduce the amount of calcium lost through the urine, increase the amount of calcium absorbed through the

gut wall, and improve the calcium balance in the bones.
- Taking regular low-impact aerobic exercise, like brisk walking, skipping, racquet sports or working out, is a good protection against both heart disease and osteoporosis.

## Dietary Recommendations

Consume regular amount of foods that contain plant oestrogen, called phytoestrols, which Mother Nature, in her wisdom, has provided us with. These include:

- soya beans and soya bean products like flour, tofu (soya bean curd), miso, tamari, soya bean oil
- linseeds
- the herb red clover (tablets, or sprouted seeds)
- alfalfa
- ginseng (dried to eat or as tea, or capsules/tablets)
- celery, fennel and other green and yellow vegetables
- anise and liquorice
- rhubarb
- the herbs dong quai and black cohosh

It is well established, for example, that Japanese women, who already eat a diet particularly rich in plant oestrogen, have far fewer problems at the time of the menopause, demonstrating once again that there is a lot we can do for ourselves.

- Reduce your intake of sugar and junk foods. This includes sugar added to tea and coffee, and that in sweets, cakes, biscuits, chocolate, jam, puddings, marmalades, soft drinks containing phosphates, ice cream and honey. Consumption of these may impede the uptake of essential nutrients and may cause water retention.
- Reduce your intake of salt, both added to cooking and at the table. Also avoid salted foods like kippers and bacon. Salt causes fluid retention and induces calcium loss from the body in the urine. Use potassium-rich salt substitutes such as garlic, onion, kelp powder, fresh herbs, sesame powder or other mild spices.
- Over-spicy food, hot drinks and alcohol can aggravate flushes. Let your hot drinks cool down and keep alcohol to a minimum

whilst going through the menopause. Alcohol tends to knock most nutrients sideways anyway, and this is definitely a time to conserve essential nutrients.

◆ Eat vegetables and salads daily. Three portions of vegetables and a salad should be eaten every day, as they contain plenty of essential nutrients. Where possible use organic, or grow your own.

◆ Eat plenty of fresh fruit, at least two servings each day, as these are good sources of nutrients.

◆ Concentrate on consuming foods that are rich in important nutrients, especially magnesium, calcium, B vitamins, essential fatty acids and zinc. You will need to refer to Appendix I, 'Nutritional Content of Foods'.

◆ Limit your consumption of red meat to one or two portions each week. Substitute meat with fish, poultry, peas, beans and nuts. You may like to refer to the Vegetarian, or Tunatarian diets (page 448), when you learn that meat eaters have a lower bone density than their vegetarian counterparts.

◆ Dairy products, such as milk and cheese, are excellent sources of calcium. Use low-fat versions if you need to watch your weight. Aim to drink 600 ml of milk per day, or eat other foods rich in calcium.

◆ Keep your consumption of animal fat down to 30 per cent of your total kilojoule intake. For most, this means reducing fat intake by at least one-quarter. Instead use cold pressed oils such as safflower, sunflower, olive, sesame, canola etc., and use soft polyunsaturated spreads instead of hard margarines or lard.

◆ Drink plenty of liquids, preferably the equivalent of six glasses of water daily. Use decaffeinated drinks, or better still alternatives, and keep carbonated drinks down to a minimum.

◆ If you smoke, try to cut down gradually, or stop completely, as smoking can aggravate some symptoms, especially hot flushes and night sweats. Stopping smoking at the time of the menopause can reduce your risk of hip fracture by as much as 40 per cent.

◆ Keep a supply of nutritious snacks to eat between meals if you get peckish. Nuts, raisins and fresh or dried fruit are fine.

## Other Useful Self-help Tips

◆ Aim to exercise for at least half an hour five times per week— you need to do weight-bearing exercise that is also aerobic. The benefits are a healthy heart, strong bones and a feeling of well-being.

◆ Try to spend 15–20 minutes relaxing each day to keep the stress levels down and the flushes at bay. Research shows that these simple measures will reduce hot flushes by as much as 60 per cent!

◆ Wear several layers of thin comfortable clothing during the day so that you can peel them off should the need arise.

◆ Use lightweight layers of bed clothes so that you can adjust them according to temperature. Wear cotton nightdresses instead of man-made fibres.

◆ Carry some cool wipes in your handbag until the flushes have abated.

◆ Take extra care of your hair, skin and nails: use rich hair conditioner, good moisturising lotions for your skin, and nail strengtheners.

◆ Do toning pelvic-floor exercises once or twice a day by repeatedly holding in the vaginal muscles to the count of ten and releasing slowly.

## Nutritional Supplements

At the time of the menopause we often have to put back into our bodies what time and nature have taken out. At the WNAS we successfully use a selection of scientifically based supplements which individually address the variety of common symptoms. The following chart will allow you to assess which supplements you should be trying according to your current symptoms. We usually aim at sorting out the short-term oestrogen withdrawal symptoms initially, and once under control move on to address the long-term business of maintaining a healthy heart and strong bones.

## Complementary Therapies

As well as dealing with symptoms on a nutritional level it is important to address the underlying problems that may well have accumulated over the years. Not meeting your nutritional needs at various stages in life, being pregnant and breast-feeding, coping with stressful situations and perhaps suffering premenstrual symptoms before your menopause, may well have left their mark. Your body may need some extra help in order to recover at the time of the menopause, which can be provided by some of the complementary therapies.

## MATCHING NUTRITIONAL SUPPLEMENT TO SYMPTOM

| PROBLEM | TYPE OF SUPPLEMENT | DAILY DOSAGE | AVAILABLE FROM |
|---|---|---|---|
| Hot flushes and night sweats | *Natural vitamin E | 200–400 IUs | Chemists, health-food shops |
| | Panax ginseng | 1–2 x 600 mg tablets | Chemists, health-food shops |
| | 45 Plus (herbs + nutrients) | 1–2 tablets | Chemists, health-food shops |
| Anxiety, irritability, mood swings, depression | Hypericum | 2–4 tablets | Health-food shops, chemists |
| Eczema, dry skin | *Efamol/evening primrose oil | 2–8 x 500 IU capsules | Chemists, health-food shops |
| Heavy periods | Vitex Agnus Castus | 1 tablet 3 x daily | Chemists, health-food shops |
| | Bio-Iron tablets | 2–4 daily | Chemists, health-food shops |
| Painful periods | *Bio-Magnesium tablets | 2–3 daily | Health-food shops, chemists |
| Breast tenderness | *Efamol/evening primrose oil caps | As above | Chemists, health-food shops |
| Constipation | *Bio-Magnesium | 2–4 tablets daily | Health-food shops, chemists |
| | Linusit Gold | 2 tablespoons | Health-food shops |
| Osteoporosis | Efacal, Total calcium tablets | 4 capsules | Chemists, health-food shops |
| | Calcium carbonate, gluconate or citrate | 1000 mg elemental calcium | Chemists and health-food shops |
| | *Magnesium amino acid chelate | 150–600 mg elemental magnesium | Health-food shops |

### Acupuncture and acupresssure

Many problems that occur at the time of the menopause—like hot flushes, night sweats, insomnia, depression, aches and pains, mood swings and headaches—may well respond to acupuncture or acupressure. Acupuncture will need to be administered by a qualified practitioner, and acupressure can be a useful self-help tool. The Acupuncture Association of Australia has a list of accredited members.

## Herbal medicine

The indication for herbal medicine at the time of the menopause is quite strong. Trials have demonstrated that herbs can help to reduce hot flushes, reverse the ageing process of the cells in the lining of the vagina, and speed up the healing process of broken bones. There are herbal preparations that can be purchased in the health-food shop like ginseng, dong quai and Agnus castus, which you can help yourself with. However, a qualified herbal practitioner may prescribe a combination of many different herbs. You may even be given herbs that are to be taken at different times of the day, or even different times of the month depending on whether you are perimenopausal or postmenopausal.

## Homoeopathy

Sepia and sulphur are just two of the many remedies that may be indicated for hot flushes and night sweats. There is also a wide choice of remedies for poor memory, depression, insomnia, anxiety attacks, irritability, headaches and confusion. To find a qualified practitioner in your area contact the Australian Association of Homoeopaths. *The Women's Guide to Homoeopathy* is an excellent reference book, see the Recommended Reading List, Appendix III.

## Cranial osteopathy

It is certainly worth paying a visit to a qualified cranial osteopath at the time of the menopause. Not only do they provide help for long-standing back, head and neck problems, but they have been shown to reduce hot flushes. The treatment for women suffering with menopausal symptoms is often aimed at improving pituitary function, the gland found at the base of the brain, and balancing the function of the adrenal glands and the pelvis.

The Australian Osteopathic Association has a directory of accredited practitioners. See Useful Addresses, Appendix V.

## Anna's Story

A forty-seven-year-old businesswoman and active grandmother, Anna started experiencing symptoms some five years before she contacted the WNAS.

*I'd had a hysterectomy where one ovary was removed when I was thirty-eight, and started getting menopausal symptoms a few years later. I had hot flushes at night, panic attacks when driving and my skin itched constantly to the point where my scratching would make me bleed.*

*My male GP was unsympathetic, but a woman doctor gave me blood tests and confirmed it was the menopause. I tried the patch version of HRT, but my skin came up in lumps. I tried another that was better, but I started getting headaches and nausea. I then tried HRT in pill form, but that was no better. I became very depressed, and was suffering with headaches that lasted a week. I used to look after my grandson as well as working, which was very difficult as I was constantly aching and had pains in my muscles, wrists and elbows.*

*Then I saw a TV programme about nutritional treatment for the menopause. I got in touch with the WNAS and was put on a wheat- and yeast-free diet, with no caffeine and lots of fruit and vegetables. I took supplements of Gynovite and Efacal and took up exercise and relaxation several times per week. My life has been completely transformed. I am now able to enjoy my time with my husband and help out with my grandchildren. I feel positive again and much more like my old self.*

*See also*: Osteoporosis, Sample WNAS Programme, Normal Menopause, High Calcium Menu. Plus Recommended Reading List (*Beat the Menopause Without HRT, Osteoporosis—the Invisible Killer*) and References.

# MIGRAINE HEADACHES

Migraine headaches are a common problem in both adults and children, and are often related to hormonal events like puberty, the onset of a period or the menopause. Migraines can be distinguished from other headaches because they are characterised by a severe, intermittent ache which is often accompanied by a variety of symptoms including nausea, vomiting, disturbance of vision, flashing lights, and other strange feelings, all of which may occur either before or at the start of a headache. Intolerance to light and noise are also common features of a migraine. The attacks can last anything from several hours to two to three days.

As many sufferers know, once an attack has begun, it is virtually impossible to stop it running its course. This is now thought to be due to a series of chemical or electrical changes that occur in the blood vessels of the head and the brain. It seems that there is a strong physical or chemical basis to many sufferers' migraine headaches, which may be triggered by a variety of factors.

## What Causes Them?
Potential triggers for migraine headaches include:

◆ Stress, such as family or work tensions, or lack of sleep.
◆ Often migraine headaches occur in relation to the menstrual cycle during the build-up to a period, or on the day it arrives.
◆ The oral contraceptive pill can also trigger migraine headaches in some people, as can hormone replacement therapy.
◆ Missing meals also seems to be a trigger for migraine, and children may be particularly susceptible to this.
◆ Doing without your regular cups of tea and coffee can certainly cause withdrawal migraine headaches and seems to occur particularly at the weekends, when you are out of the office, when going on holiday perhaps, or if there is a change in your daily routine.
◆ Additionally, there is a wide variety of foods that are known to trigger migraine headaches in susceptible individuals. The commonest foods include cheese, chocolate, most alcoholic beverages and particularly red wine, yeast extracts (for example Marmite), pickled herrings and soy sauce, which are all rich in certain types of chemicals called amines. Some migraine sufferers seem to be particularly sensitive to amines. Other less common triggers include certain fruits, in particular citrus fruits, bananas, plums and pineapples, broad beans, artificial colourings and monosodium glutamate, that favourite flavour-enhancer of many a Chinese meal and savoury snack. Some migraine headaches can also be due to a sensitivity to milk and wheat, even though they do not contain amines.

## *What Your Doctor Can Do*

◆ Measure your blood pressure, as occasionally migraine head-aches are due to the presence of high blood pressure or other conditions affecting the nervous system.

◆ Examine you, and if your symptoms are severe or persistent, refer you to a neurologist to determine whether there is an underlying medical cause.

◆ If severe migraines occur as a result of taking hormones or the oral contraceptive pill, then a change in treatment may well be needed. We often find that hormone replacement therapy, pre-scribed at the time of the menopause, produces more frequent and more severe migraine attacks.

◆ Suggest you take aspirin on a regular daily basis, as this may ease the mechanics of a migraine. Research shows that blood platelets of migraine sufferers clump together more than they do in non-sufferers, particularly between attacks. Aspirin has been shown to reduce the degree to which platelets stick together.

◆ Prescribe medications specially designed for migraine head-aches, like Migril or Migraleve, which often ease the symptoms, but do not address the root cause.

◆ Give you some dietary advice, as there is plenty of evidence to show that certain foods can trigger platelet stickiness, and thus precipitate an attack.

◆ Offer some other drugs which may be useful in preventing migraines. They include low doses of antidepressants, anti-arthritis drugs and beta-blockers used for high blood pressure.

## *Deborah's Story*

Deborah was fifty-two when she approached the WNAS. She had two grown-up daughters and was just beginning her menopause. She had suffered migraine headaches, for at least two weeks per month, for over twenty years.

*I was in a real state when I went along to the WNAS for the first time. My migraines were ruining my life, and no amount of Imigran or Migril seemed to control them. Things went from bad to worse when I was put on HRT eighteen months before the start of my menopause, as the frequency of the migraines accelerated until I was experiencing them daily. My doctor had no other suggestions, which made me feel very depressed, especially as both my mother and one of my daughters suffered with migraine as well.*

*I read about the work of the WNAS in a national newspaper and in desperation made contact. I was given lots of information about my body's requirements during my first consultation, and then sent off for a month to follow an exclusion diet, take gentle exercise and some supplements. I didn't get on very well with some of the supplements, as they seemed to make the headaches worse, but I continued with the others.*

*I had awful withdrawal symptoms for the first week, but after a month I realised that my hot flushes had gone, and so too had the giddy feelings and lack of energy. Within three months of starting the programme, I had two normal periods, which had been missing for several months, and no migraines for the first time in twenty years. It felt like nothing short of a miracle to me. I felt marvellous. It turned out that caffeine and chocolate brought the headaches on and I obviously avoid them like the plague now that I know.*

*My husband was so delighted that he had got his partner back, he booked a Caribbean cruise as a second honeymoon! It has been nearly four years now, and I haven't looked back.*

## What Your Dentist Can Do

Primarily, he can check to see whether you are grinding your teeth or clenching them at night, as this can send the jaw muscles into spasm. Also the jaw can sometimes be out of alignment (this can be corrected by wearing a plate designed by a dental specialist).

Just how spasms trigger headaches is not clear. One theory is that the exhausted muscles build up waste products, and instead of draining into the circulation they flow up the venous system into the head, irritating the brain. Another theory is that the muscles and jaw joints are sending a continuous stream of unconscious messages to the brain that they are not 'comfortable', and in an attempt to block out the flood of information, a migraine is started. Ear aches, neck aches and even sore throats can also be triggered by temporo-mandibular (jaw bone) joint dysfunction.

## What You Can Do in the Short Term

If you feel a migraine headache coming on:

◆ The first thing to do is to rest and avoid stress, if at all possible.
◆ Take a simple painkiller, such as paracetamol or aspirin; certain

special forms of these are available for migraine sufferers. There is also a variety of other stronger drugs which can be taken and these can switch off a migraine attack. You will need to ask your doctor about these as they are available on prescription only.

◆ Sometimes taking one or two teaspoons of sodium bicarbonate in a glass of water can help to relieve a migraine. This loads the system with carbon dioxide.

◆ Another way of loading your system with carbon dioxide is to place a large paper bag over your mouth and breathe in and out of it slowly for 5–10 minutes.

◆ Massage your temples, forehead, ears and skull gently whilst breathing regularly and deeply.

◆ The herb, feverfew, has been shown to be helpful with migraine headaches. You can buy feverfew pills in health-food shops.

◆ Another very simple but useful remedy is to chew on some crystallised ginger and use root ginger in your cooking. Ginger helps to dilate the blood vessels that have constricted during a migraine attack.

## What You Can Do in the Longer Term

◆ If you suffer with migraines it would be a good idea to eliminate the foods associated with migraine from your diet, and also to limit intake of tea and coffee. Reduce your intake gradually, eat regularly, and avoid stress where possible. Follow the recommendations and Menu for Migraine suggestions. The success of diets excluding these and other foods can be very high. Reduction rates of 90 per cent of migraines have been recorded, but this does vary a lot from individual to individual.

◆ If after a few weeks that doesn't seem to do the trick, then follow The Simple Exclusion Diet, for four weeks.

◆ If you smoke, cut out cigarettes.

◆ If you take the Pill, try another method of contraception for a few months to see whether there is any relationship between this and your migraine headaches.

◆ Never miss a meal—make sure you eat wholesome food little and often to maintain your blood sugar levels.

◆ Take plenty of aerobic exercise, at least three times per week, as studies have shown that this will reduce the number of migraine attacks.

◆ Get out into the fresh air when possible, and make an effort to look at distant scenery, to give your eyes a different perspective to your everyday chores, particularly if you are doing lots of close-up intricate work.

◆ Learn to manage your stress with regular relaxation.

### Complementary Therapies

Herbs like feverfew and ginger are particularly helpful, and can be tried without advice. Your herbal practitioner will prepare a prescription for you which may well relieve your symptoms. There are many homoeopathic remedies to try, which may also be of help, both in the long term, and in the shorter term, when you feel an attack coming on.

Acupuncture, acupressure, Alexander technique, massage and cranial osteopathy are all likely to be of help in relieving and managing the symptoms of migraine. It is very much a personal choice, and a question of assessing what suits you.

*See also*: Stress, Allergy, What's Wrong with Present-day Diet and Lifestyle?, The Simple Exclusion Diet, The Caffeine-Free Diet, Menu for Migraine. Plus Recommended Reading List and References.

# MISCARRIAGE

The definition of a miscarriage is the loss of any pregnancy before twenty weeks' gestation. Approximately 15 per cent of all recognised pregnancies miscarry. However, a pregnancy which miscarries within the first two weeks of conception is unlikely to be recognised as such. As many as 60 per cent of conceptions may miscarry within days of fertilisation and the rate of spontaneous miscarriage in the general public is 25 per cent.

The majority of women who miscarry once go on to have a successful pregnancy next time around. However, there are others, approximately 1 per cent, who suffer recurrent miscarriages, three or more failed pregnancies before twenty weeks' gestation. Even so, over half of these women do go on to have a successful pregnancy, despite their frustration and disappointment along the way.

## *What Causes It?*

There are many factors that can be the underlying reasons for miscarriage:

- Genetic problems. Defects in chromosome or material from either partner is probably the main cause of sporadic or one-off miscarriages, accounting for 55 per cent. It is Mother Nature's way of deciding not to continue with a pregnancy that might have resulted in a handicapped or significantly deformed child. The risk of miscarriage increases if there is a history of genetic illness in either partner's family.

- Increasing age of the mother is associated with an increase in miscarriage rate, possibly because of the greater likelihood of chromosomal damage to the eggs, which occurs in Down's syndrome, for example.

- Environmental factors, including smoking and drugs. Smokers are 25 per cent more likely to have a pregnancy end in miscarriage than non-smokers. It is the commonest environmental hazard associated with miscarriage. Passive smoking might also increase the risk. If you want a successful pregnancy, live in a smoke-free environment.

- Alcohol and illicit drugs carry a similar risk. Those who smoke heavily and/or consume excessive amounts of alcohol or street drugs are far more likely to have a lower intake of good nutrients, which can be a contributory factor to a miscarriage. It's as if Mother Nature knows that the body is not in good enough shape to nurture a baby. The importance of adequate levels of nutrients should not be underestimated. Some women with recurrent miscarriage have recorded a relative lack of a chemical called prostacyclin, necessary for the growth and development of the growing baby. Adequate supplies of zinc, B vitamins, magnesium and other nutrients may also be necessary for the right biochemical environment for the developing embryo.

- Toxic metals. Abnormally high levels of cadmium, present in cigarette smoke, and lead from petrol have been found in the tissues of still-born babies. These metals are more toxic if the diet lacks essential nutrients like calcium, iron and zinc, and a poor intake of these nutrients is associated with an increased risk of miscarriage.

◆ Hormonal abnormalities. Severe hormonal imbalances, often associated with infertility, can also result in miscarriage. Additionally obesity, poor diet and lack of essential nutrients that contribute to normal hormone function, might also disturb the delicate hormone chemistry required for the survival of a pregnancy. Disturbances in thyroid function can also increase the risk of miscarriage, but the risk is minimised when the thyroid is treated.

◆ Pre-existing disease. Diabetes, high blood pressure and rare diseases that affect metabolism, may be associated with increased risk of miscarriage, which makes careful control of these conditions essential.

Blood abnormalities associated with arthritis contribute to the rate of miscarriage, as does a condition known as SLE—systemic lupus erythematosus—that causes arthritis, skin disorders and other problems in young women. The blood of female sufferers, who may be identified only because they have recurrent miscarriages, may contain what are known as antiphospholipid antibodies. Anyone who has endured three consecutive miscarriages should be tested for SLE, or related blood abnormalities as these may lead to disturbance in the blood formation in the blood vessels in the placenta, and result in miscarriage or still-birth later in pregnancy. If the tests are positive, specialist treatment prior to conception would be necessary.

◆ Anatomical problems. Abnormalities of the genital tract like a soft weakened cervix (neck of the womb) will allow a miscarriage to occur. Surgical treatments before attempted conception, or a stitch in the cervix once pregnant, may be needed.

◆ Infection. It is acknowledged that a variety of infections, including rubella (German measles) and listeria, an infection from 'live' soft cheeses, if contracted during early pregnancy can lead to miscarriage or congenital deformity. Low-grade mild bacterial infection of the vagina has also been linked to recurrent miscarriage more recently.

## What Your Doctor Can Do

◆ Examine you to determine whether you have any anatomical abnormality that needs attention.

◆ Check your hormone levels, as recent research has shown that increased levels of the pituitary hormone LH (luteinising hormone) close to conception, and a low level of the ovarian hormone progesterone shortly after conception, may reduce your chances of a successful pregnancy.

◆ Take a vaginal swab to assess the possibility of infection.

◆ Investigate the possibility of an hereditary genetic defect.

◆ Following three consecutive miscarriages, measure your anti-cardiolipin antibodies, and lupus anti-coagulant.

◆ Give you some reassurance.

## What You Can Do

◆ Try not to worry unduly.

◆ Follow the instructions for 'A Preconceptual Plan' (see Preconception). This will mean ensuring you are eating a good diet, taking regular exercise, living and working in a wholesome environment, and keeping away from the 'social poisons'.

◆ Give your body a rest and recover after miscarriage, before trying to conceive again. It is preferable to give yourself at least four to six months between pregnancies.

◆ Take the opportunity to have any medical problems checked by your doctor or a specialist.

## Complementary Therapies

It is worth investigating what herbal medicine has to offer, especially if you have had more than one miscarriage. Acupuncture may be able to help your body back to normal function, and to speed the recovery process from the last miscarriage. Certainly an appointment with a cranial osteopath will be useful, and aromatherapy massage will help to soothe away your anxiety.

Whilst investigating what these complementary therapies have to offer, it is important to have any medical investigation that is indicated, especially if you have suffered recurrent miscarriage. Don't despair, the chances of you having a live baby after a single miscarriage are 80 per cent, only falling to 74 per cent after three miscarriages.

## Danielle's Story

Danielle is thirty-two and has had four miscarriages between her two successful pregnancies.

*I had the first miscarriage ten years ago. I was three months' pregnant at the time and we had not really planned a baby. It wasn't until after I had miscarried that I realised how much I would have liked a baby. My husband felt ready for children three years later, and we then spent three years trying to conceive without any luck. We both had investigations and everything seemed to be normal. As luck would have it, as the investigations finished I fell pregnant naturally, and although I bled through the first part of the pregnancy, I managed to produce a healthy baby boy.*

*I had subsequent miscarriages when Alex was eighteen months old and again at two and a half, and again when he was three and a half. Usually I was between nine and twelve weeks' pregnant when I lost the baby. I would always start with spotting and gradually I would miscarry. Twice I ended up having a D & C, and on another occasion I managed with scans to ensure that I had fully miscarried. I was then given a laparoscopy to check to see why I kept miscarrying and the only thing the doctor found was a slightly misshapen uterus which was apparently somewhat flat on one side. Whilst investigating he also found adhesions on the ovaries and on my tubes which he removed after the fourth miscarriage.*

*I was advised to ask my GP to test my anti-cardiolipin antibodies and lupus anti-coagulant as this might throw some light on the underlying reason for the miscarriages. The doctor would not conduct the tests as he said I had already been investigated for inflammation. I felt pretty desperate about having another baby which obviously was affecting my relationship with my husband.*

*I heard about the work of the WNAS on the radio and wondered whether I might be nutritionally deficient after so many miscarriages. I went along to the clinic and was given a dietary programme to follow with nutritional supplements and a recommendation to do lots of exercise, which I used to do regularly. I enjoyed the programme immensely and managed to get myself back into really good shape within four months. I felt like a different person.*

*The following month I managed to fall pregnant again. Although I did experience some spotting, I rested a great deal and managed to carry the baby to full term. She was a beautiful, wide-eyed little girl, and was well worth waiting for.*

*See also*: Recommended Reading List (*Healthy Parents, Healthy Baby*) and Standard References.

# MOUTH DISORDERS

The most common diseases in the world are those of the mouth, such as dental caries or tooth decay, and periodontal or gum-disease.

Dental health problems are among the health conditions most frequently reported in Australia and New Zealand. Dental decay and loss of teeth are the two major problems. Historically, there has been a comparatively high rate of teeth loss, but this is now rapidly declining. However, most people still have substantial experience of dental decay.

## *The Mouth*

Each tooth in the mouth contains a crown, which is the part visible in the mouth, and the root, which is anchored in a socket in the jaw bone and covered by the gums. Teeth are composed of a number of different layers, which each serve a function.

Enamel covers the crown of the tooth and is the hardest structure in the body. It reaches to just below the edge of the gum, and joins the cementum, which is the thin layer of bone-like tissue covering the root of the tooth and which helps to secure the tooth in its socket. Dentine is the hard, bright yellow, primarily non-living tissue that forms the bulk of the tooth. It reaches from the crown down through the roots. Finally, the pulp is the living centre of the tooth, which contains the nerves and blood vessels, and is therefore the part of the tooth that registers pain or thermal changes.

The supporting structures of the teeth are known as the periodontium, and comprise:

- part of the jawbone which surrounds and supports the roots
- the membrane which acts as the attachment between the cementum and the socket in the jawbone
- the gum, known as the gingiva
- the pink membrane and underlying tissue that covers the bone
- the cuff of gum around the tooth, which is an important feature in gum disease

## Saliva

This is the watery fluid that is produced by salivary glands within the mouth. It is Mother Nature's own mouthwash. There are three pairs of glands in the mouth from which saliva is secreted. Amongst its other functions, saliva dilutes the amount of sugar-produced acid present in the mouth because of the calcium and phosphates it contains. Both these minerals in the saliva act to repair some of the damage done by dental decay.

## Plaque

We all have a thin, sticky film, composed mainly of bacteria, called plaque, covering our teeth. It continually forms in the mouth and sticks on rough surfaces on the teeth. It is most comonly found in the little crevices between our teeth, on the backs of our teeth, and at the gum margin, where gums and teeth meet. Plaque feeds on sugary deposits from our diet, and the by-products of this cause both tooth decay and gum disease.

# Tooth Decay

When plaque is exposed to sugar from the diet, the bacteria contained in it convert the sugar into acids, which attack enamel on the teeth. After repeated acid attacks a cavity forms which becomes deeper as more acid is released from the plaque. The cavity eventually works its way through the enamel and the dentine and into the pulp chamber, which then becomes infected with bacteria. The pain of toothache is generated from the pulp, and if nothing is done the pulp dies, and the infection then infiltrates the root of the tooth, forming an abscess in the bone surrounding it.

# Gum Disease

There are a number of stages to gum disease, the most minor of which is gingivitis.

### Gingivitis

Plaque accumulates around the margins of the gum and the teeth, and between the teeth in the crevices, and if left to stagnate, produces poisons which in turn cause inflammation of the gums known as gingivitis. The gums become red, swollen and shiny and have a tendency to bleed easily. If you notice blood after you brush your teeth, you should consult your dentist.

### Periodontitis

When plaque is left to stagnate it gradually absorbs calcium salts from the saliva and hardens to become calculus, or tartar. This sits around the gum margin and is a constant source of inflammation to the tissues. As the disease progresses, the calculus works its way down between the gum and the tooth into a pocket, and this stage is known as periodontitis.

### Periodontosis

As the pockets surrounding the teeth become deeper the calculus gradually wears away the bone that supports the teeth in their sockets. In the final stages, pus forms, the tooth becomes loose, there is soreness, pain and a bad taste in the mouth, and eventually the tooth falls out.

Younger people experience gingivitis when they are being careless with their oral hygiene, and this is how the disease process begins. An improved oral hygiene regime can reverse the disease process, until, with age, the gums recede and bone is lost. Neither of these tissues, gums or bone, can be replaced once lost, and so it is vital to remove the plaque thoroughly each day in order to prevent diseases of the mouth.

### Acute Ulcerative Gingivitis

This is an infection of the gums which is possibly bacterial in origin, but it seems it can also be attributed to some underlying nutritional cause. It was given the name 'trench mouth' following widespread outbreaks amongst soldiers who were sharing utensils in the trenches during both the First and Second World Wars. However, it is acknowledged that many of these soldiers were also suffering from scurvy, the result of severe vitamin C deficiency. The gums become infected, turn a greyish colour, the top surface often rubs away leaving sore, painful patches, and it feels like something is wedged between your teeth, particularly the back teeth. As the surface of the gums is attacked and the cells die, a tremendous odour is created. This condition needs to be treated urgently with Flagyll, a special form of antibiotic. You would be feeling unwell enough to seek dental or medical advice if you were suffering, and not able to enjoy a meal because of the pain and soreness.

# Herpes Simplex

This is the commonest virus of the mouth. The initial infection, which often affects young children, appears as blisters and ulcers on the gums, lips and soft tissue inside the mouth, and often remains undetected by the mother. It can cause a fever and make the child feel lethargic for up to fourteen days. This initial phase of herpes is called 'herpetic stomatitis', which simply means herpes in the mouth. This same virus can also cause genital herpes in children, but more commonly in adults.

## What You Can Do

- Give a soft liquid diet, as it may be too uncomfortable to eat normally.
- Analgesics, such as paracetamol, will help to reduce the discomfort.
- Chlorhexidine-based mouthwashes or dental gel will help to reduce the accumulation of plaque at a time when toothbrushing is too uncomfortable.
- Vitamin and mineral supplements should be given, with extra vitamin C and zinc to help promote healing.

# Cold Sores

Following an initial attack of herpes in the mouth, the individual is likely to develop cold sores on the lips or face, which are secondary outbreaks of herpes simplex. They can be precipitated by numerous external factors:

- excessive sunshine
- emotional stress
- fatigue
- inadequate diet
- periods of ill health

# Herpes Zoster

This form of herpes may affect the tissues in the mouth during a primary episode of chickenpox. Subsequent attacks can appear in the form of shingles, and may affect the nerves in the head, face and any part of the trunk, chest or abdomen, causing an outbreak of a typical rash with small blisters, which may ulcerate and crust with blood. Ulcers may also form on one side of the mouth.

## What You Can Do

- Make sure you are well nourished—follow the recommendations for The Very Nutritious Diet.
- Get adequate sleep.
- Don't spend long periods of time sunbathing.
- Protect your lips with petroleum jelly in the sunlight, or other herbal creams.
- Avoid oral sex completely whilst you are infected.
- Try supplements of lysine, which is an amino acid found in foods and which can replace the chemically related amino acid arginine, needed by the virus to replicate itself.
- Follow a diet rich in lysine and low in arginine. This means avoiding nuts, chocolate, carob, oats, wholewheat, and soya beans. Instead eat more fish, chicken, meats, milk, cheese, mung and other beans (but not soya).

## Acute Thrush

The digestive tract is like a hose-pipe that leads from your mouth to your tail end. If thrush is present in one part of the tube, it can travel to other areas. Thrush can be found in the mouth, appearing as soft white masses on the surface of the tissue, which when scraped off, leave a red or bleeding patch. Occasionally it is a feature of diabetes, or can occur in a patient whose salivary glands are malfunctioning. It can be treated with antibiotics and you would be advised to follow the instructions given in Candida and Thrush.

## Mouth Ulcers

Approximately 10 per cent of the population experience aphthous ulcers (mouth ulcers) at some time. They are little sores that have a yellowish white appearance, and can appear singly or in crops. They also vary in size, but as a general rule the larger they are, the more pain they seem to cause. There is no recorded pattern to their occurrence, except that many women seem to get them in their premenstrual phase.

## What Causes Them?

Although there is no specific agreed cause, there are a number of precipitating factors:

- Undue stress.
- Fluctuating hormone levels. The vast majority of the women we see with ulcers have outbreaks in the two weeks before their periods. The conclusion is that a relationship exists between hormone levels and aphthous ulcers. However, in our experience hormone levels may fluctuate abnormally when brain chemical metabolism is disturbed.
- Nutritional deficiencies. In the absence of adequate nutrients, brain chemistry is often disturbed and the immune system may become impaired, rendering the body more susceptible to conditions like mouth ulcers. In our experience when the deficiencies are corrected the outbreaks of ulcers diminish.
- Food allergies. We have observed a relationship between food sensitivities and mouth ulcerations. We very often find that women sensitive to wheat get a recurrence of ulcers when they try to reintroduce it into their diet.
- Accidental trauma to the tissue. Sometimes hitting yourself with a toothbrush or knocking into something can result in ulceration.

## What Your Doctor Can Do

Prescribe an antiseptic or zinc-based mouthwash, or hydrocortisone pellets or cream, which can be placed over the ulcerated areas to reduce the inflammation.

## What You Can Do

- Get your diet in order. If you have PMS as well, follow the recommendations on pages 478–9. If you suspect you may have some food allergies, follow the recommendations for The Simple Exclusion Diet. If neither of these apply, then follow the recommendations for The Very Nutritious Diet.
- Take multi-vitamin and mineral supplements, and perhaps extra zinc and vitamin C.
- If the ulcers continue for more than four weeks, get your doctor to examine them as it is possible to get cancer in the mouth, and it is obviously better to be safe than sorry.

## Susan's Story

Susan was a fifty-one-year-old women with two grown-up children. She had been experiencing problems with her periods, constipation, general lack of vitality and lichen planus, which is a chronic inflammatory disease of the mucous membranes and usually affects the mouth.

*I had not been feeling well in myself for some time, and had put on 9.5 kg in weight and was experiencing hot flushes. My cravings for food, particularly sweet food, had begun to get out of control and I found myself bingeing on biscuits, cakes, chocolates and sweets, which was particularly worrying as my parents were diabetic and obese. I had an outbreak of very sore ulcers in my mouth but instead of clearing up in the usual way they seemed to spread and become more extreme, to the point where my eyes were affected too. They felt painful and swollen, irritated and sore.*

*I went to my doctor for some advice. He was somewhat mystified and wondered at first whether it was thrush. He tried me on various different types of medication, but the symptoms did not respond at all. My daughter, who is a chiropodist, suggested that I visit my dentist, which I did and he diagnosed lichen planus. He referred me to the local district hospital. The diagnosis was confirmed and it was suggested that I either take steroids or learn to live with the problem. When I went back to my dentist and told him I didn't really want to take the steroids, he told me that he had heard that diet might help. By this time I felt that my nerve endings had become hypersensitive too, so I stopped drinking coffee and approached the WNAS for some help.*

*After thorough examination I was given a programme consisting of modifications to my diet, daily relaxation, regular exercise and supplements.*

*I followed the advice I was given by the WNAS and within a matter of a few weeks the lichen planus had calmed down, and my eyes were no longer affected at all. I am not in any pain now. I still have the lichen planus mildly, but it does not hurt at all or bother me. In addition to overcoming the chronic mouth problem, I also managed to sort out my constipation, food cravings and flushes and lost the excess weight. I feel very well and have sufficient energy to cope with life.*

# Burning Mouth Syndrome

A burning sensation from the oral tissues is a fairly common complaint. It is not usually present in the morning, but seems to get worse as the day goes by, and may be relieved by eating or drinking or removing dentures.

## What Causes It?

There are, once again, numerous factors associated with burning mouth syndrome:

- problems with dentures
- deficiencies of the blood
- diabetes
- dry mouth
- the menopause
- candida or thrush
- anxiety
- fear of cancer
- depressive conditions
- sensitivity to a mouthwash or over-use of mouthwashes
- oesophageal reflux—where partially digested food is brought back

One factor not given much attention is that a significant proportion of people who suffer burning mouth syndrome are likely to be suffering from a vitamin B1, B2, or B6 deficiency. In a Scottish study of those who were deficient, replacement therapy produced a resolution of symptoms in the majority of cases.

## What Your Doctor Can Do

- Offer a routine check-up to eliminate the possibility of diabetes, thrush, blood insufficiency or depression being the underlying cause.
- An enlightened doctor would hopefully check your B vitamin levels, and prescribe the appropriate B vitamins if the results indicated a need.
- If you wear dentures your dentist should check to make sure they are not causing an adveaction in your mouth.

## What You Can Do

- Follow the recommendations for The Very Nutritious Diet, unless you feel your symptoms are associated with the menopause, thrush, or anxiety, in which case refer to appropriate dietary recommendations.
- Take strong multi-vitamin and mineral supplements daily, and possibly extra vitamin B complex.

◆ Get regular exercise and relaxation.
◆ If you have your own teeth, follow The Good Oral Hygiene Plan outlined below.

## The Good Oral Hygiene Plan

◆ Keep your breath fresh by brushing your teeth and gums carefully, twice a day, for at least three minutes each time. If your gums are really inflamed and sore, you can start by using a soft-headed brush, aiming to change over to a medium-headed brush to maintain the health of the gums. Gums need to be massaged to create a hard skin layer on the surface, a bit like that on the palms of your hands. Massage in little circles on the spot at the place where the gum and teeth meet, the gingival margin. If you are not sure about brushing techniques, check with your dentist or hygienist.

◆ You also need to floss between your teeth each day, in front of the mirror to ensure you don't damage the gums. This disturbs the plaque and food debris which build up between the teeth, and are out of the reach of your toothbrush.

◆ Use a mouthwash to loosen the plaque before cleaning your teeth.

◆ Rinse your mouth with water after meals, taking care to swish the water around your mouth to loosen any remaining particles of food.

◆ Eat raw vegetables and fruit regularly as snacks as these exercise your gums, and unlike sweet processed carbohydrates, don't feed the plaque in your mouth.

◆ Drink lots of fluid to keep the saliva in your mouth flowing freely.

◆ Have routine checks with your dentist and hygienist at least every six months.

◆ Follow the recommendation for The Very Nutritious Diet, or if you suspect you may be suffering food intolerances, follow the recommendations for The Simple Exclusion Diet.

◆ Take supplements of multi-vitamins and minerals and additional vitamin C, at least 1 g, per day.

# MULTIPLE SCLEROSIS

This is a common and well-known disease which affects the nervous system. It is primarily a disease of northern Europeans, and occurs infrequently in other races. It is rare in Afro-Caribbeans unless they are born and raised in the United Kingdom, and is rarely diagnosed in Australian Aborigines or Maoris. There can be strong family tendencies, with the risk rising as high as one in three for the partner of an affected identical twin. The prevalence is also less in areas remote from Europe. White South Africans and Australians of European origin have only half the rates of those found in many parts of northern Europe. It is sometimes linked with virus infections including measles, mumps, rubella and the Epstein-Barr virus (causing glandular fever), but the link is not proved.

## *What Causes It?*

Multiple sclerosis (MS) is due to a loss of the insulating fatty sheath around nerves. This fatty material, known as myelin, facilitates the rapid conduction of impulses along the nerves. Its loss in either the brain or spinal cord means that messages do not get through, with consequent disturbances in sensation, movement and vision.

Typical features include:

- loss of vision affecting one or both eyes
- weakness in an arm or leg
- spasm in the major muscles of the arm or leg
- loss of sensation almost anywhere in the body
- disturbance in bowel or bladder function
- double vision
- a variety of other unusual neurological symptoms
- depression and mood changes

In four out of five patients the disease waxes and wanes. In each attack a different part of the nervous system may be affected producing new problems. These may last for several weeks or months, with slow and sometimes complete, sometimes incomplete, recovery. After many years, ten or twenty, there may be slow but progressive deterioration. In young women the disease is often very mild, and disabling events occur only very rarely. However, up to 15 per cent become severely disabled within a short time due to aggressive disease.

## What Your Doctor Can Do

◆ Refer you to a specialist for a variety of investigations in order for the diagnosis to be made. There is a variety of other possibilities in patients who appear at first glance to have multiple sclerosis.

◆ Exclude vitamin B12 deficiency by measuring its level in the blood or performing specialised tests of vitamin B12 usage.

◆ Treat the symptoms, which may involve a variety of medical basics to aid with constipation, incontinence and reduction of muscle spasm, and drugs to control tremor and to minimise feelings of giddiness.

◆ There have been a number of attempts to influence the course of the disease using drugs that alter or influence the immune system, as this is involved in the initial episode of tissue injury. Preliminary evidence suggests that these powerful drugs may be useful but at present they tend to be used in those who have rapidly progressive MS. Just recently, beta-interferon, a naturally occurring immune-altering chemical, showed a one-third reduction in new episodes, but without any measurable reduction in disability or overall course of the disease. This is now available for some patients within the United Kingdom and the United States of America.

## What You Can Do

◆ Change your diet. There is some preliminary evidence that diet changes may help. This is taken from pulling the results of three trials where increased doses of linoleic acid, the parent Omega-6 series essential fatty acid, was given in substantial amounts to MS sufferers. This essential fatty acid and its biochemical by-products are found in high concentrations in the nervous system and influence its structure and function. Not all patients benefited but there is a suggestion that those with early disease and relatively mild disability could benefit from a diet rich in these fats (see The High Essential Fatty Acid Diet).

◆ Take supplements of evening primrose oil. This, with or without fish oil, may assist the above diet. Unfortunately, there are no large published trials and the effects are likely to be slow. A reasonable dosage of 4–6 x 500 mg capsules daily will probably need to be taken for many years.

◆ Take supplements of vitamin B and multi-vitamins. These nutrients are involved in maintaining the chemistry of the essential fatty acids. It is conceivable that some patients with MS lack nutrients involved in fatty acid metabolism. A supplement of 400–600 IU of vitamin E together with a moderately strong multi-vitamin supplement should ensure adequacy of these factors needed for normal essential fatty acid metabolism.

◆ Limit exposure to environmental toxins. This means not smoking, and drinking moderately. Rarely, assessment for environmental poisons, such as lead, cadmium and mercury, is needed. Some researchers have linked the presence of mercury amalgam fillings in teeth with increased risk of multiple sclerosis in some communities, but this is not certain. Similarly no firm link has been made between food allergy and multiple sclerosis.

### Complementary Therapies
A number may produce symptomatic relief, but it is difficult to give firm guidance. Aromatherapy, massage, physiotherapy, acupuncture, and reflexology will all have their advocates. Try them and see.

*See also*: Standard References.

# NAIL PROBLEMS

A number of minor nail problems are worth mentioning. Sometimes they indicate a nutritional imbalance.

- Brittle nails can be due to iron deficiency.
- Spoon-shaped or upturned nails can be due to iron deficiency or to repeated trauma.
- White spots on the nails were thought to be due to zinc deficiency. Repetitive minor trauma such as housework or use of a keyboard are more likely.
- Ridging of the nails can be due to eczema, psoriasis or other skin problems. Mild forms are quite common in normal individuals and have no nutritional significance.
- Fungal infections of the nails are common and respond well to the use of modern anti-fungal agents given either as local applications in the form of paint or as tablets. Additionally a supplement of zinc taken for three to six months might be helpful.

## SKIN, HAIR AND NAIL VITAMIN AND MINERAL DEFICIENCY

| SIGN OR SYMPTOM | CAN BE CAUSED BY DEFICIENCIES OF |
|---|---|
| Cracking at the corners of the mouth | Iron, vitamins B12, B6, folic acid |
| Recurrent mouth ulcers | Iron, vitamins B12, B6, folic acid |
| Dry, cracked lips | Vitamin B2 |
| Smooth (sore) tongue | Iron, vitamins B2, B12, folic acid |
| Enlargement, prominence of taste buds at the tips of the tongue (red, sore) | Vitamins B2 or B6 |
| Red, greasy skin on face, especially sides of nose | Vitamins B2, B6, zinc or essential fatty acids |
| Rough, sometimes red, pimply skin on upper arms and thighs | Vitamin B complex, vitamin E or essential fatty acids |
| Skin conditions such as eczema, dry, rough, cracked, peeling skin | Zinc, essential fatty acids |
| Poor hair growth | Iron or zinc |
| Dandruff | Vitamins C, B6, zinc, essential fatty acids |
| Acne | Zinc |
| Bloodshot, gritty, sensitive eyes | Vitamins A, B2 |
| Night blindness | Vitamin A, zinc |
| Dry eyes | Vitamin A, essential fatty acids |
| Brittle or split nails | Iron, zinc, essential fatty acids |
| White spots on nails | Zinc |
| Pale appearance due to anaemia | Iron, vitamin B12, folic acid, essential to consult your doctor |

## Martine's Story

A forty-five-year-old mother of three, who worked part-time as a secretary, Martine had been neglecting herself since her mother's death nine months earlier, eating largely junk food, and had put on 12.5 kg in weight. She was unhappy, had dry spotty skin and her hair was in poor condition. She also had dry rough red pimples on her upper arms and thighs, split brittle nails and cracking at the corners of her mouth.

*I hadn't been feeling brilliant for some time, so having to cope with my mother's death on top of that was probably the final straw. My eating got out of control and over a period of nine months my weight gradually went up to nearly 75 kg. My normal weight was around 60 kg, so I felt so uncomfortable, and obviously couldn't fit into any of my clothes, which was very depressing. I also noticed that my breasts became incredibly sore each month before my period.*

*As well as being overweight, I experienced mood swings and noticed that my skin, hair and nails had deteriorated. My nails were split and brittle, my skin became very dry and spotty, and my hair become very dull and split. I felt like a walking wreck. I tried dieting, but found I couldn't stick to a diet for more than a few days which was very demoralising.*

*I read that cravings for food may be a physiological problem in a report on some research conducted by the WNAS, in Here's Health magazine. I contacted them for advice and was given a programme to follow that involved eating good food little and often, exercise and nutritional supplements. I started in December, which was difficult because of Christmas. But once the new year came, I found I was able to stick to my programme, in fact I was surprised how much I enjoyed it.*

*I lost weight gradually, without counting kilojoules, and my vitality returned. Within four months I had lost 6 kg in weight, my skin was clear, my nails had grown beautifully and even my hair had got its old shine back. The breast symptoms had cleared up too. I felt like a new woman and totally in control. I've had some ups and downs since, but I feel that I now know what my body needs, so it's much easier for me to get back on the right road again.*

*See also*: Standard References.

# OBESITY

In January each year the media attempt to seduce women with even more 'new' methods of restricting their intake of food in order to look more like super-models, and an international effort to halt the worldwide tendency towards obesity has recently been launched. According to the World Health Organisation, 'obesity is rising sharply and the current management or prevention strategies are not capable of arresting this epidemic'.

- ◆ In the USA and Canada one-third of the adult white population is judged to be obese, and one estimate is that on present trends the entire population of America will be obese by the year 2234!
- ◆ Australia and New Zealand follow in the polls, European countries also scored highly, and obesity is even becoming a problem in developing countries.
- ◆ According to the Risk Factor Prevalence Study Management Committee Report prepared in Canberra in 1989, obesity in Australia increased between 1983 and 1989 by 15 per cent for women and slightly more for men, bringing the totals to 11.1 per cent for women and 9.3 per cent for men. Additionally, the overweight population increased by between 5 and 7 per cent to 22.4 per cent for women and 36.8 per cent for men.
- ◆ The Australian Institute of Health & Welfare's unpublished report of 1993 estimated the direct costs of obesity in 1988–89 at $672 million, with obesity-related coronary heart disease and hypertension accounting for 62 per cent of that amount. The cost of treatment of obesity within the health-care system was $393 million.

One could be forgiven for wondering how these trends have come about when millions of people begin weight-loss diets each year all over the world. Booksellers fill their shelves with new diet books which they hope will catch the wave of New Year resolutions, and millions of hopeful, unsuspecting people will fall for the hype.

The majority of people who start a diet this month will be starting new diets again this time next year, hoping that their new shape will make them feel good. Fitting into a new outfit may be the goal of many, but the 'feel good' factor does not necessarily follow, and the lost kilos all too soon return. It is acknowledged that weight-loss diets slow down our metabolic rate, which then makes it difficult for us to return to our normal way of eating without putting on more weight than we started with. It follows that after several episodes of 'yo-yo' dieting we will be restricted to consuming very few kilojoules and insufficient nutrients in order to maintain either our weight loss or our sense of well-being.

## What Is Obesity?

In developed countries, obesity is now probably the most common diet-related disorder, while in developing countries obesity is usually a mark of prosperity. Being overweight may be a distinct advantage in a country or community that is used to food shortages; those who are thin and lean may fare less well than their plump counterparts at times of shortage. Unfortunately, we cannot use such excuses for ourselves, and so let's get down to some hard facts; facts which we think will give you an understanding of why you are overweight, and how this can best be tackled, in the short and long term.

First of all, how is obesity defined? The graph opposite gives measurements for height and weight. It is divided up into five sections, -1, 0, 1, 2, and 3. These are grades of obesity based on weight and height taken from the formula originally devised by a Belgian scientist, Quetelet. Quetelet's Index, which is more usually known as Body Mass Index—BMI—is widely used in the assessment of obesity. The formula is derived by multiplying the weight in kilos by itself and dividing by the height expressed in metres. The categories are as follows:

-1: less than 20
0: 20–25
1: 25–30
2: 30–40
3: greater than 40

Normal or ideal weight is grade 0. Grade 1 is overweight, usually between 10 and 20 per cent above the ideal weight; grades 2 and

3 are regarded as obese—more than 20 per cent above the ideal weight.

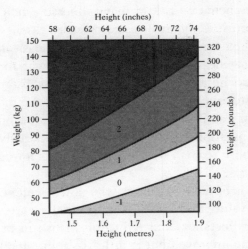

As measured by Body Mass Index, the range associated with the greatest life expectancy and lowest death-rate is 20–25. There is a very slight rise in death rate in those who are mildly over-weight, grade 1, but this low rise is so small as to be insignificant. It is grade 2 and especially grade 3 obesity which carry the greatest risk to health. An adult with a BMI of 40 has three times the risk of dying in a year than someone whose weight is ideal. An individual with a BMI of 35 has approximately twice the death-rate of his or her ideal counterpart.

For the majority who are just slightly overweight, grade 1 obesity, the major reasons for dieting are cosmetic and a sense of well-being. Not being overweight, and having a slim, attractive shape, is highly desirable in current fashion. Many of us feel better psychologically when that spare tyre has been whittled away, and if the diet is combined with an exercise programme, there can be a very real improvement in feelings of overall fitness. Medically, there is little change in factors such as blood pressure, and risk of heart disease, though there could be a moderate fall in blood cholesterol level if this is elevated at the start of the diet.

For those with grade 2 or 3 obesity, the potential benefits of losing weight are very real, and the effects on psychological state of a successful weight-loss programme can be dramatic. For example, normal employment may be very difficult for those who are grossly overweight, grade 3 obesity.

## The Health Risks of Obesity

Those who are obese, grades 2 and 3, have a shorter life expectancy, and an increased risk of many illnesses, including diabetes, high blood pressure, heart disease, osteoarthritis, gout, gallstones, reduction in exercise tolerance/level of fitness, and depression. Furthermore, general medical problems may be more difficult to treat in those who are obese. Gastrointestinal disorders, including indigestion, heartburn and constipation, may be more difficult to assess in an obese individual, as the information obtained from a medical examination may be limited. Additionally, the survival rate of the obese woman with breast cancer is lower than her slim counterpart.

The young obese individual who loses weight to normal or near-normal value may have a substantial improvement in life quality and expectancy, and reduction in risk in practically all of the above. The improvement in arthritis, gout, blood pressure, diabetes, or blood cholesterol level may be dramatic, and evident within a few weeks or months of a dietary programme.

## What Causes It?

Genetic factors are involved. Analysis of families shows that if both parents are obese, 70 per cent of the children will be obese. If one parent is obese, 40 per cent of the children will be obese, and if both parents are lean, then only 10 per cent of the children will be obese. The predisposition of the parents is thus carried down partially to the children, but of course, we could argue that obese parents eat too much, and thus are likely to over-feed their children, making them obese in turn, and that this has nothing to do with genetics or inheritance. However, in studies of children who have been adopted, the adopted children take after the weight characteristics of their biological parents, rather than those of their adoptive parents. This and other work lends substantial support to the idea that the tendency to obesity is to a large degree genetic.

Environmental factors are significant as well. By environment is meant all the factors that occur around us and potentially influence our internal metabolism which we have already seen is initially determined by genetic make-up. With regard to obesity, the most important environmental factors are the food supply, level of exercise, lifestyle and social pressures.

If the food supply, for example, is so meagre that there is barely enough to go round, or starvation conditions exist, then obesity will obviously disappear from the community at large. In such a situation, with a limited food supply, environment is more important than any genetic factor. However, when there is an abundance of food, this allows the obesity tendency to express itself fully. When food is plentiful, some 25 per cent (or more as we have seen for countries like Australia and the USA) of the population may become obese.

The majority of obese individuals will have one parent who is overweight, and only a minority would be the offspring of two obese or two thin parents. At this point you might feel like shooting your mother and father, but this isn't very practical! Nor could one forbid the obese to reproduce. The effect of this would be surprisingly small and it would take several generations of extremely unpopular enforced birth control to even halve the rate of obesity in the population, or to restrict the food supply to the whole population, punishing lean and obese alike. Again, this is unlikely to win any favour with the population at large. The only practical solution is in some way to limit the kilojoule intake of those who are overweight, while taking other steps to improve their rate of weight loss.

In conclusion, it does seem that some people were born to be fat, but are only able to be fat because of the relatively affluent society in which they live.

## What Your Doctor Can Do

- ◆ Check your thyroid to see whether it is underactive.
- ◆ Check to ensure that you are not suffering with diabetes.
- ◆ Take your blood pressure to determine whether it is high.
- ◆ Offer you a simple diet, or refer you to the local dietician.

At the Women's Nutritional Advisory Service we have been treating and giving advice to women, many of whom were failed dieters, for some twelve years. We have come to understand that finding the right programme for each individual is the key to both long-term weight-loss and, more importantly, good health. Without kilojoule-counting, we have managed to help thousands of people to understand their body's needs, and as a result to lose weight and reclaim their health. Using our methods people have not only lost weight, but have also overcome common symptoms like migraine headaches, irritable bowel syndrome, fatigue, acne, premenstrual syndrome, eczema and a whole host of other ailments, as well as feeling fitter. The WNAS programme is not just about diet, it encompasses lifestyle, exercise, nutritional supplements when appropriate, and relaxation.

## Josephine's Story

Josephine, a forty-six-year-old mother of three, moved with her husband to Geneva thirteen years ago. Her main problem was an extra 16 kg gained in 1979.

*I found it difficult to cope in Switzerland in some respects, as our children were still in school in the UK and I think the depression concerning that led me to comfort-eat. My usual weight was around 60 kg until 1979. We moved house and in that year I suddenly gained 16 kg. Ever since then I have been struggling with my weight. I managed to lose the weight again, a year after I had put it on. Then unfortunately it crept back on again, and I have been saddled with it ever since.*

*I contacted the WNAS for help and made an appointment for my first telephone consultation. I was given a programme aimed at keeping my blood sugar level constant, so that I did not get cravings for sweet food and cheese, as I had done previously. I followed the Vitality Diet, which is a plan written by the WNAS, which involved cutting out all sorts of things initially and then adding them back gradually.*

*During the first week of the programme I felt half-drugged and had an awful headache. This gradually wore off until I suddenly felt as if I had come out the end of a tunnel. I lost 5 kg in the first month. The weight seemed to fall off me, and then the weight loss slowed down to a more gradual pace. As a result of the diet I found that I could not tolerate chocolate or vinegar, and alcohol made me feel as if I had a hangover. I had also been suffering with irritable bowel syndrome for four years and cutting out wheat, oats and coffee seemed to sort all those symptoms out as well. I reached my target weight and everyone commented on how well I looked, and I certainly felt brilliant.*

## What You Can Do

Follow the instructions for The Simple Weight-loss Diet.

Start the diet when you are ready to do so. You will need time, this is not a diet to do in a hurry. You need to plan and set aside time for shopping, preparation and consumption of meals. Go shopping before beginning your diet, preferably after you have eaten so that you are not starving hungry and tempted to cheat. Take a list with you, and make sure you stick to it.

◆ Eat regular meals, at least three meals a day, preferably with two small snacks in between.

◆ Never miss meals: irregular eating leads to less healthy weight loss and increased feelings of hunger.

◆ It is useful to eat from a small plate, not a large one. A well-stocked medium-sized lunch or breakfast plate looks more satisfying than a large dinner plate only half filled.

◆ Chew your food well and savour each mouthful. Try not to hurry your meals.

◆ Eat fresh foods whenever possible. If at all possible, prepare one meal at a time. If this is not practical, try cooking a chicken, for example, to eat cold over a period of several days.

◆ Grill food rather than fry, to keep your fat consumption low and to preserve the nutrients.

◆ Do at least four sessions of exercise per week to the point of breathlessness, which will help to speed up your metabolic rate, and thus burn the fat off! If you haven't been exercising regularly for some time, take it easy to begin with.

◆ Consider spending a week at a health retreat to get yourself started—perhaps as part of your annual holiday. Having the appropriate food handed to you literally on a plate, and spending your time being pampered, will undoubtedly help you to focus on a new sense of well-being.

◆ If you have tried endless diets without success, and feel you have a psychological block about losing your weight, ask your doctor about the possibility of some counselling.

## Complementary Therapies

If your problem is related to an underactive thyroid or sluggish metabolism, it may be worth investigating what our recommended therapies have to offer. The acupuncturist would be our first port of call, as unblocking the energy channels will help you back to optimum metabolism.

The nitty-gritty on overcoming obesity, though, is to eat less and exercise more.

*See also*: What's Wrong with Present-day Diet and Lifestyle?, The Simple Weight-loss Diet. Plus Recommended Reading List and References.

# OSTEOPOROSIS

As a result of osteoporosis one in three women and one in twelve men will suffer fractures of the hip, spine or wrist. Apart from the obvious pain and disability, osteoporosis often brings with it a loss of height and curvature of the spine, known in the UK as 'dowager's hump'. Within six months of sustaining a hip fracture it is estimated that some 20 per cent of patients will die. However, osteoporosis is both preventable and treatable.

## What Is Osteoporosis?

Osteoporosis is literally a thinning of the bones. The bones are composed of a 'skeleton' or scaffold of connective tissue around which minerals in crystalline form are laid down, rather like bricks being built up on a steel framework. The framework has a certain flexibility as well as great strength, and the minerals give the structure resistance to pressure or crushing. So the structure of bone is rather similar to that of reinforced concrete.

We have two types of bone: trabecular, which accounts for about 20 per cent of our bone mass, and cortical, which accounts for the other 80 per cent. Trabecular bone is found mainly in the spine, pelvis and ends of the long bones, such as the head of the femur. It is the type of bone most quickly lost after the menopause. Cortical bone is found in the shaft of long bones and the skull, and is lost more gradually. We are continually losing small amounts of bone throughout our adult life, but about 10 per cent of our skeleton is remodelled during the space of a year.

In osteoporosis an imbalance develops between bone loss and the rate at which new bone is deposited. There is a reduction in both the amount of connective tissue and the mineral content of the bone. The loss of bone mass reduces its strength and increases the likelihood that the bone will break when pressure is brought to bear on it.

You are at risk of osteoporosis if you have or have ever had or suffered from:

◆ poor diet, low in calcium, especially dairy products
◆ an early menopause, spontaneously, or following surgery
◆ thyroid or other hormonal problems
◆ low body weight, or anorexia
◆ petite build
◆ cigarette smoking
◆ regular and excessive alcohol consumption
◆ lack of exercise and sedentary lifestyle
◆ excessive physical activity, as in athletes or ballet dancers
◆ steroid drugs
◆ more than one fracture since the menopause
◆ a close relative with osteoporosis
◆ chronic illness affecting digestion, kidney and liver function

*Bone density*
There are a number of dietary, lifestyle and environmental factors that influence the strength and density of bones. The mineral content of a woman's bones at the time of the menopause is not so much influenced by her current dietary intake, but by her past intake of calcium over the previous forty or fifty years.

The strength of bones is determined by:

◆ diet, especially the intake of calcium during the growing years
◆ physical activity, particularly weight-bearing exercise
◆ hormonal factors, particularly the balance of oestrogen
◆ genetic factors, which determine the size of bones and muscles

Modern diet has much to do with the risks of developing osteoporosis in the same way as it influences heart disease and cancer. Many of us consume a diet which, though adequate in the short term, does not provide a good or optimum intake of nutrients in the longer term, thus predisposing us to diseases such as osteoporosis.

## Calcium

Calcium is particularly important. About 70 per cent of women have an inadequate calcium intake. This means that they reach middle and old age with a low bone mass and a high risk of osteoporosis. A study published in the *British Medical Journal*, by Professor John Kanis, from the Medical Research Council in Leeds, showed that long-term doses in excess of 1000 mg of calcium per day decreased hip fracture rate by 25 per cent.

Up to two-thirds of our calcium intake may never reach the bone because of certain dietary factors. Common foods such as bran and fizzy drinks contain high amounts of phosphates and can interfere with the absorption of calcium from the diet. A diet rich in salt and animal protein can increase the loss of calcium from the urine.

It is vitally important to concentrate on a diet rich in calcium. You will note from the calcium list of foods (Appendix I) that Cheddar cheese contains ten times more calcium than cottage cheese, for example. You will need to take a close look at the list and choose the foods that you enjoy, knowing that they are rich in calcium and other important nutrients.

Calcium in bone also needs phosphate, another mineral, which is abundantly supplied by both healthy and convenience foods.

## Vitamin D

This is mainly derived from the action of sunlight on our skin, and only small amounts come from the diet. It is needed to enhance the absorption of calcium from the diet.

## Essential fatty acids

Recent research suggests that the essential fatty acids, EFAs, which are part of a healthy diet, also influence the balance of calcium in our bodies, especially in our bones. There are two types of essential fatty acids, the Omega-3 series and the Omega-6 series. The Omega-3 series are derived from fish oils, oily fish including mackerel, herring, salmon, pilchards and sardines, as well as from some cooking oils such as rapeseed, from linseed, soya beans and walnuts. These oils may help to reduce the risk of heart disease and benefit arthritis, and also may slow the natural loss of calcium in the urine, which includes some lost from our bones.

The Omega-6 series of EFAs are found in sunflower and corn oil—and margarine made from them—almonds, green leafy vegetables and wholegrain cereals. These help maintain healthy skin and influence the risk of heart disease. They also seem to help in the absorption of calcium from the diet. The body's ability to make full use of them declines sharply with age.

In addition to this, smoking, alcohol, a poor diet and some conditions such as eczema and diabetes, disturb the metabolism of these essential fats and can lead to deficiency states.

It appears that a number of connected minor nutritional deficiencies have resulted in many of us being at increased risk of osteoporosis from middle-age onwards. For healthy bones it is worth noting the following.

- The best sources of calcium are dairy products, white bread, bony fish and hard water.
- Vitamin D may be obtained from sunlight, fortified cereals, margarine, butter and eggs.
- Regular exercise is an excellent way of helping to increase the uptake of calcium by bones.
- To help achieve a healthy calcium balance in the body, it is best to eat a broadly based healthy diet, limiting the intake of sugar, convenience foods, salt, alcohol and excessive amounts of animal protein.
- Daily supplements of calcium, evening primrose oil and fish oil provide additional calcium and essential fatty acids which are necessary for healthy bones.

### Oestrogen

An important part of oestrogen's role is to maintain bone mass and help with the constant process of bone remodelling. When oestrogen levels are optimum our bones are constantly regenerating, but when levels fall calcium is no longer directed to our bones and the net result is bone loss. Bone mass is at its peak during the early thirties, and from then on it declines, with an annual bone loss rate of approximately 1 per cent per year. However, for most women the bone loss increases at around the time of the menopause, and for up to ten years afterwards, with a further loss of 2–3 per cent per year. By the age of seventy, approximately one-third of bone mass will be lost.

Women who experience an early menopause, or who stop menstruating because of excessive dieting or exercise, will have depressed levels of oestrogen, and as a result will be at greater risk of osteoporosis.

## What Your Doctor Can Do

Interest in osteoporosis has increased considerably during the last decade because of the more widespread use of detection methods. The density of bones can now be measured by scanning the hips and the vertebrae of the spinal column. There are a number of tests available that help to determine the degree of bone loss or fracture risk.

Ordinary X-rays are used to detect existing fractures, but a measure of bone mineral density, using a specialised form of X-rays, is needed to measure bone mass and to monitor the results of treatment. Those with a high risk, or with established osteoporosis, should be scanned at regular intervals, of between one and two years.

Simple blood and urine tests are being developed to help identify those who are likely to be 'fast bone losers'. This will not replace bone mineral density scanning, but may prove to be a useful screening test. The blood tests are for calcium and bone chemistry; blood and urine tests are for hormones.

There are a number of very different treatments available for those with osteoporosis. Your own doctor will need to assess which of these options is the most appropriate for you. Those undergoing treatment from their doctor or specialist will need to be monitored, as no treatment is universally effective or free from side-effects.

### Hormone replacement therapy

Although until recently HRT was thought to have been the great bone saver, and indeed after ten years it seems that women taking HRT have a considerably greater bone mass than women who have not, this does not appear to be sustained in the longer term. After twenty years of taking HRT it seems that there is a tailing off effect, and the women who took HRT may only have a 3 per cent greater bone mass than women who for their own reasons did not.

The usage of HRT in the first ten or more years of the menopause is associated with a significant reduction in the hip fracture rate in women. However, up to two-thirds of women who take HRT come off it within the first nine months because of side-effects or dissatisfaction. (See The Risk Factors of HRT, on page 309.)

For women with an early menopause (before the age of forty-five) and for some of the others in the high-risk groups, it is probably advisable to discuss with your doctor the risks and benefits of taking HRT. Those women who start their menopause in their mid-forties onwards will be well advised to help themselves to better bone health, certainly if they are unable or unwilling to tolerate HRT. Indeed, research shows us that there are many tools which will help us to preserve our own bone mass.

## June's Story

June, a thirty-eight-year-old mother of three grown-up children, was keen to stop taking HRT even though she had found she had osteoporosis.

*I served in the police force for many years, and was 165 cm tall on my inception. Following a prolapse I had a hysterectomy five years ago, and although my ovaries were intact, my doctor prescribed HRT in the form of Premarin. I persevered with this for a few years, but was put off by the awful side-effects of nausea, depression and weight gain. I put on 7 kg which took me from a trim size 12 to a large size 14. But I was afraid to stop taking the HRT as I noticed from comparing height with other family members that I had lost 5 cm in height. Additionally I knew that my mother had lost 15 cm off her height and my father had osteoporosis after long-term use of steroids.*

*I eventually came off the HRT two years ago because I felt so awful, and the night sweats and flushes that followed were flattening. My skin became very dry and the condition of my hair deteriorated. One year later I read a magazine article about the WNAS's holistic approach to the menopause, and as the case history in the article sounded just like me I decided to book an appointment at their clinic.*

*During my consultation a programme of diet, exercise, relaxation and nutritional supplements was devised for me, and I got started straightaway. I adjusted to the programme quite quickly and soon noticed that I was feeling better in myself. Within two months the flushes calmed down, my libido started to return, and I generally felt more positive.*

*A year on, I have gone from strength to strength. I feel well, I no longer suffer with symptoms of the menopause, and the condition of my skin and hair has improved. I have continued to take the multi-vitamins and the Efacal the WNAS suggested, and am managing my health myself. I never did have a bone density scan so I have nothing to compare, but I haven't lost any more height and I feel more agile than I have for years.*

### Calcium supplements with Etidronate or Alendronate

Etidronate (Didronel PMO) and Alendronate (Fosamax) are two synthetic compounds based on phosphorus which combine with calcium in the bones and help to prevent its loss. They reduce bone loss in the spine, and in the case of Fosamax, in the hip and the forearm. Fracture rates may also be reduced. These treatments are usually combined with calcium or a calcium-rich diet. They are available on prescription and need to be taken for a two- to three-year period in order to reduce established osteoporosis.

### Calcium supplements alone

At a dose of 1000 mg per day by itself, these are mildly effective for some men and women with osteoporosis, and have been shown to reduce hip fracture risk by 25 per cent. It is a cheap, simple and safe treatment, but nowhere near as effective as HRT. Calcium absorption varies greatly from person to person, and is influenced by many dietary factors.

### Calcium supplements with vitamin D

These are a useful treatment for the very old and those with poor sunlight exposure. Low levels seem common in elderly Europeans, especially if they are housebound. Although vitamin D is necessary for the absorption of calcium from the diet, most of us synthesise enough from sunlight. Giving strong vitamin D supplements to those who are not deficient can actually cause bone loss due to excess stimulation of the bone-dissolving cells. Supplements containing vitamin D should therefore be taken with caution unless there is a proven deficiency.

### Calcitonin

This is a hormonal treatment given by injection, which can be quite effective. This hormone influences the movement of calcium around the body. It is not a sex hormone. Its inconvenience limits its popularity.

## What You Can Do

Do not underestimate the benefits of self-help measures. Each of the diet and lifestyle changes will, by themselves, make little difference in the short term, but over a period of years are likely to be of substantial benefit. Many of the measures will help not just osteoporosis, but also help reduce the risk of heart disease and stroke. What you have to do is:

- change and improve your diet
- take regular weight-bearing exercise
- make lifestyle changes
- consider taking nutritional supplements
- see your doctor if you are a high-risk case to discuss assessment and other treatments

*Dietary and lifestyle tips*
- Concentrate on eating foods rich in calcium.
- For those women around the time of the menopause and beyond, consume foods that contain naturally occurring oestrogens.
- Make sure your diet contains a variety of foods rich in essential fatty acids.
- Limit your consumption of alcohol to a maximum of three to four drinks each week.
- If you smoke, try to cut down gradually or, better still, give up altogether.
- Consume foods rich in vitamin D if you do not get much sunlight exposure. They include dairy products, margarine, reduced fat milk, reduced fat cheese, fortified cereals like Cornflakes and Rice Krispies or take cod liver oil capsules.
- Try the menopause menus (pages 488–92).

*General health tips*
- Avoid excessive consumption of sugar and foods rich in sugar such as fizzy drinks, sweets, cakes and biscuits. Such foods are low in essential nutrients, especially calcium, and high in kilojoules.
- Reduce your intake of salt, both added to cooking and at the table and avoid salty foods like bacon and kippers.
- Eat vegetables and salads daily.

- Eat at least two servings of fresh fruit per day.
- Limit your intake of saturated animal fats by consuming leaner cuts of meat, reduced-fat dairy products, and avoiding fried foods. This is particularly relevant if you are overweight.
- Reduce your intake of tea, coffee, cola and chocolate which all contain caffeine, and use alternatives now available in most supermarkets and health-food shops.

### Regenerating lost bone?

A diet rich in essential nutrients and regular exercise can affect bone mass, and so too can a relatively new supplement called Efacal, a specially formulated product produced by Efamol. A number of studies suggest that combining calcium with essential fatty acids from evening primrose oil and marine fish oil may be an effective way of treating osteoporosis. A recently published study, conducted by Dr Kruger and her colleagues from the University of Pretoria, South Africa, tested the effect of these oils on calcium balance in a group of women with osteoporosis. After a four-month trial period there were a number of changes which suggested increased absorption of calcium from the diet and increased uptake of calcium by the bone. Efacal has been shown to:

- improve the uptake of calcium from diet through the gut wall
- decrease the amount of calcium lost through the urine
- help direct calcium to sites of deposition in the bone and may thus help prevent the bone-thinning process. It is effectively the stamp on the envelope that makes delivery far more likely

Each capsule of Efacal contains 400 mg of Efamol pure evening primrose oil, 44 mg of marine fish oil and 100 mg of calcium. Those at risk of osteoporosis should take 4 capsules every day with the evening meal. For preventative purposes, 4 capsules should be taken every day for an initial twelve-week period, followed by a daily dose of 2 capsules per day.

### Exercise

Exercise is a valuable tool at all stages of life to promote good health, and is an acknowledged way of helping to protect against heart disease and to help keep bones strong. Plenty of exercise in childhood, including sport at school, helps to build up a high peak bone mass.

From the time bones reach their peak mass, which is approximately in the mid-thirties, the destiny of bone health for many rests in their own hands. It is influenced by diet, as you have seen, and also by lifestyle. At the time of the menopause, when women are most at risk of bone loss, exercise must become a vital part of the everyday schedule. Research has shown that weight-bearing exercise, in other words anything that involves putting weight through your bones, helps to stimulate the regeneration of bone tissue by reducing calcium loss.

The consensus from studies is that you need to exercise moderately three or four times each week, for 30–45 minutes each time, so long as you do not suffer with cardiovascular disease. The pay off, apart from helping to strengthen your bones, will be that within twelve weeks you can expect to feel more energetic, cope with stress more effectively, sleep better, have increased resistance to infection and feel a lot better generally!

Anything that involves putting pressure on your bones is classed as weight-bearing. Examples are:

- jogging
- brisk walking
- playing racquet sports
- lifting weights
- a workout
- skipping
- press-ups
- even squeezing tennis balls

Walking helps to preserve the hips and the spine, but hand and wrist exercises, which consist of gripping and rotating, are necessary to strengthen the wrist bones. The disabled, the bedbound— even if it is only for a few weeks—and the housebound are very much at risk, as are astronauts because of the weightlessness.

However, too *much* exercise can be damaging. It is now known that young female athletes, gymnasts and ballet dancers are high risk groups for osteoporosis. Their intensive training and low body weight often prevent them from menstruating, resulting in lowered levels of oestrogen, which subsequently affects their bone mass.

It is important that those who exercise vigorously have an adequate and nutritious diet in order to maintain their body weight. Failure to do so will further increase the risk of osteoporosis. Some performance athletes and young ballet dancers may need nutritional supplements in order to ensure dietary adequacy.

*Avoid smoking and alcohol*
Smoking and drinking alcohol to excess are two of the easiest ways of increasing your risk of osteoporosis.

- Women who stop smoking and drinking at the time of the menopause may reduce their hip fracture rate by as much as 40 per cent
- Both smoking and drinking alcohol have a broad spectrum anti-nutrient effect, and accelerate the loss of nutrients.
- Smokers and those consuming lots of alcohol usually have different diets and different essential fatty acid levels too, but it's never too late to stop!

*See also*: Menopause, Thyroid Disease, What's Wrong with Present-day Diet and Lifestyle?, Sample WNAS Programme: Prevent Osteoporosis, High Calcium Menu. Plus Recommended Reading List (*Beat the Menopause Without HRT, Osteoporosis—the Invisible Killer*) and References.

# PAINFUL OVULATION

Painful ovulation, or *Mittelschmerz*, as it is also known, is quite common and isn't usually severe. The pain is usually on one side of the abdomen and in many cases only lasts a few hours. Slight mid-cycle spotting may also accompany the pain.

*Mittelschmerz*, literally 'middle pain', can occur in women of all ages. At its most severe, it can feel like a needle-piercing pain combined with severe cramp, as if someone is squeezing your insides, and this can last for several days. The pain often starts as a gnawing sensation with an ache in the groin, which then builds up to a crescendo.

First, let us look at the process of ovulation. It's a natural process that takes place in any fertile woman. It's the body's way of preparing for pregnancy, and it occurs once a month. An ovum or egg is produced by a follicle in the ovary approximately halfway through a regular menstrual cycle. The common signs of ovulation include an increase in body temperature, and changes in the amount and constituency of cervical mucus.

When an egg grows each month it develops inside a small cyst. By the time it is ready to be released, it will have reached about 2.5 cm in diameter. If you are examined on an ultrasound scan immediately prior to ovulation, the cyst would show up on the ovary, and this would be entirely normal. When the cyst ruptures, the fluid from it leaks into the abdominal cavity. Often some blood will escape from the cyst as well, and this too spills into the abdomen. Under normal circumstances the body deals with these fluids through its natural wastage system. Both the fluid, and the blood, are capable of irritating the lining of the abdominal cavity and it is this irritation that causes the *Mittelschmerz* pain in some women.

Why some women suffer ovulation pain, and others don't remains a mystery to doctors. Sometimes the ovulation pain signals the beginning of the unpleasant symptoms of premenstrual syndrome, but ovulation pains can just as easily occur in women who do not suffer with PMS. In some cases women suffer with ovulation pain for several days, followed by nearly two weeks of awful PMS symptoms which takes them into a heavy and painful period. This only leaves them with one normal week per month in which to recover!

If you suffer with excruciating pain mid-cycle, and it occurs on a regular basis, you should consult your doctor to ensure that there is nothing more sinister involved. It's a good idea to chart your symptoms to ensure that they do occur mid-cycle, and are not being confused with a grumbling appendix, for example, or another abdominal problem.

As these cycles differ from month to month, the pains may start by themselves, or they may begin *after* childbirth, but then again they can occur for the first time after childbirth. So there is no hard or fast pattern.

## What Your Doctor Can Do

◆ Examine you to determine whether the pain is related to ovulation or something entirely different, like an inflamed appendix or bowel. As everything is so close together it is sometimes difficult to tell, unless you chart your symptoms over a few months, to confirm a mid-cycle pattern.

◆ Most doctors will recommend the contraceptive pill as a solution, as this usually prevents the body from ovulating. When this happens, the cyst that causes the pain when it erupts isn't able to develop, and as a result *Mittelschmerz* doesn't occur. So the Pill may be a good solution if you are looking for contraception as well, and if it suits you.

◆ The only other solutions your doctor is likely to suggest are either painkillers or, in very severe circumstances, when you have had your family, a complete hysterectomy with the removal of the ovaries. As you will see from our piece on Hysterectomy, this would not be our preferred method of treatment by a long way.

At the Women's Nutritional Advisory Service, we have been treating women with period-related problems since 1984. Initially, we set out to help women over their premenstrual problems but as an added bonus we discovered that we were also helping to lighten and regulate periods as well as helping to overcome period pains and mid-cycle ovulation pains.

Low levels of nutrients, particularly magnesium, iron and B vitamins can affect brain chemistry, and thus the ability to deal with ovulation and the muscle contractions of the uterus. Pregnancy and breast-feeding place substantially greater nutritional demands on women's bodies, and often, as they are under-educated about foods that are rich in the important nutrients, these nutrients are not replaced.

We know from experience that by improving diet, taking specific nutritional supplements and exercising, you stand every chance of overcoming menstrual symptoms, including mid-cycle ovulation pain.

## What You Can Do

◆ Try to reduce the number of teas and coffees you drink to no more than a total of four per day. Try decaffeinated varieties and the herbal alternatives. One particular herbal tea, which is a tea lookalike, called Rooitea, has been shown to decrease muscle spasm, so may well be worth trying.

◆ Have a salad and three portions each of fruit and vegetables daily. Include green leafy vegetables like broccoli, cabbage or spinach as these are potentially high in magnesium.

◆ Cut down on sweets, cakes, biscuits and chocolate and eat more wholesome snacks instead, like nuts and raisins, Ryvita and spreads, or fresh fruit and yoghurts.

◆ Avoid animal fat and use lean cuts of meat.

◆ Reduce your alcohol consumption to no more than three or four glasses of wine or the equivalent per week.

◆ When the pain occurs, place a heat pack or hot water bottle over your abdomen, and try to rest, lying face down on your tummy, for 10–15 minutes.

◆ As well as making dietary changes you may be helped by taking some specific vitamins and minerals which are rich in magnesium.

◆ You may also need to take some extra magnesium supplements around mid-cycle.

◆ Regular exercise is helpful throughout the cycle as it will help to keep your muscles toned.

◆ Yoga and other methods of relaxation are useful tools, especially around the time of ovulation, as they will help you to relax.

◆ Massage is another effective way of helping to reduce muscle spasm. Try self-massage using aromatherapy oils.

## Complementary Therapies

Acupuncture and cranial osteopathy would be top of our list of therapies to try, both of which are good ways of unblocking the energy channels. Herbal and homoeopathic remedies would be worth a try too. If you are self-medicating you could try Colocynth, Naja, Lycopodium or Palladium, all of which are homoeopathic remedies. Herbal medicine prepared by a qualified practitioner would also be worth trying. If you would like to consult an expert, you will find the addresses of the relevant associations in Appendix V.

*See also*: Standard References.

# PALPITATIONS

The term palpitations is used to describe rapid or irregular heart-beats. They are felt as a thumping or fluttering sensation in the chest and may last just for a few moments or persist for hours or days depending upon their cause. Associated symptoms include shortness of breath, giddiness or sudden blackout, chest pain or an urgent desire to pass water.

The heart has its own clock which keeps the heart beating at around seventy beats per minute. An impulse is generated at the top part of the heart called the atrium and this is spread to the other parts of the heart by a conducting system which is distinct from the muscles of the heart. The pacemaker or its conducting system may be at fault.

## What Causes Them?
- ischaemic heart disease
- disorders of the heart pacemaker system itself
- disease of the valves of the heart
- an overactive thyroid gland
- infection
- side-effects to drug therapy
- nutritional problems
- alcohol excess
- caffeine sensitivity

## What Your Doctor Can Do
- Assess the type of palpitation and its possible cause. This always needs an ECG (electrical heart tracing), blood tests and often specialist examinations if the palpitations are severe.
- Treat the palpitations with a variety of drugs. Occasionally this means using powerful drugs with significant side-effects. These may be minimised by some of the self-help measures.
- Treat any underlying heart problem or other cause.
- For some types of palpitations, treatment with aspirin or another anti-clotting drug is needed as there can be an associated risk of a stroke.

## *What You Can Do*

- Avoid alcohol.
- Avoid caffeine, which is found mainly in tea, coffee, cola-based drinks and some painkillers.
- Exercise regularly if possible and appropriate. This can help to establish a more normal heart rhythm and over-ride the tendency for certain types of palpitations.
- Try and cut short an attack of rapid heartbeat with the following manoeuvres:
  - Lie down, take a deep breath in, pinch your nose and close your mouth and try to breathe out but do not let any air pass.
  - Massage the mid-point at the front of the neck at the level of the Adam's apple. This is where nerves that control heart rate and blood pressure are situated.
  - Close your eyes and press quite firmly with your fingers on them.

These measures all help to send a certain signal to the heart which can help switch off certain types of usually non-serious palpitations.

- Supplements of vitamin B and magnesium might be helpful. A strong B complex and about 300 mg per day of magnesium would be appropriate. Check with your doctor first before trying this. It should be combined with The Very Nutritious Diet. You will need to follow this routine for three to four months before any real benefit can be seen, but the result is unlikely to be powerful enough to control palpitations of a serious nature.

# PANCREATIC DISEASE

The pancreas is a large gland situated just below the stomach, and has two main functions. The bulk of the gland is involved in producing digestive enzymes needed for the breakdown of fats, and its other responsibility is the production of the hormone insulin.

## What Are the Symptoms?

Poor function of the pancreas causes diarrhoea due to the poor absorption of fats. The stools are typically pale, offensive smelling and associated with abdominal bloating and wind. Abdominal pain usually occurs at some stage, and can be severe; typically it is situated in the upper abdomen and may pass through to the back.

## What Causes It?

The main causes are:

◆ alcohol excess
◆ an association with gallstones
◆ following certain infections including mumps virus
◆ an association with a variety of rare conditions
◆ after radiation therapy for cancer

## What Your Doctor Can Do

◆ If possible, remove the cause.
◆ Give digestive enzymes to replace those usually provided by the pancreas.
◆ Consider surgery if the structure of the pancreas is very distorted.

## What You Can Do

◆ Do not drink alcohol.
◆ Do not smoke cigarettes—they reduce pancreatic function.
◆ Follow the recommendations for The Very Nutritious Diet.
◆ Eat little and often, avoiding very fatty foods. Regular snacks between meals of fruit with small amounts of nuts, bread with small amounts of nut or seed spreads, or milk-based beverages should be tried.
◆ Nutritional supplements are often needed. Multi-vitamins with vitamins A and D are likely to be an appropriate supplement. Supplements of zinc and selenium may also be necessary. Vitamin C can help relieve the pain from this condition.

❖

# PELVIC PAIN

Pain in the pelvis can vary from fleeting mild discomfort to severe gripping pains that take your breath away. These can prevent you from taking another step, and they can wreck the quality of your life. The pain may pass up into the abdomen or up into the buttocks and down into the legs. There is a variety of under-lying causes for the pain, some of which are more serious than others.

- the presence of fibroids
- cysts on the ovaries
- infected Fallopian tubes
- endometriosis or adenomyosis (endometriosis growing within the muscular coat of the womb)
- an ectopic pregnancy
- pelvic inflammatory disease
- appendicitis or other non-gynaecological condition

We have covered the conditions that cause pelvic pain that we can influence with self-help measures. They are listed in the following order: fibroids, endometriosis, pelvic inflammatory disease, ovarian cysts and polycystic ovaries.

## *Fibroids*

Between 20 and 25 per cent of women over the age of thirty-five have fibroids. They are benign (non-cancerous) tumours or fibrous lumps, which grow in the muscle lining of the uterus wall, and are the commonest reason why women experience regular heavy periods. One-third of women with fibroids bleed so heavily that they become anaemic. The fibroids are composed of a combination of smooth muscle and connective tissue. Their size can vary from that of a small pea to that of a large orange, or even larger, which would greatly increase the volume of the uterus.

Fibroids grow slowly, and can cause heavy bleeding, back pain, pelvic pain and, when large, place pressure on nearby organs or structures like the bladder, bowel or rectum. When there is pres-sure on the bowel, constipation can occur, and when pressure is placed on the rectal or pelvic veins, haemorrhoids or varicose veins in the legs can develop. Only very rarely do fibroids develop into cancer.

## What Are the Possible Symptoms?

◆ long heavy periods
◆ infertility
◆ pressure in the abdomen which may press on other organs like the bowel, and cause constipation, or the bladder and cause frequent urination
◆ swollen abdomen
◆ backache

## What Causes Them?

◆ Fibroids are thought to depend on oestrogen, as they do not occur prior to puberty and become smaller after the menopause. Just why they occur in some women and not others is not fully understood.
◆ There is a higher incidence of fibroids amongst obese women who have above average levels of growth hormone and blood glucose.
◆ It is thought that genetic factors may also play a part in the predisposition, as black women in the USA, for example, are three to nine times more likely to develop fibroids than their white counterparts.

## What Your Doctor Can Do

◆ Eliminate the possibility of you being pregnant by testing your urine and examining you.
◆ Perform a cervical smear to eliminate the possibility of cancer of the cervix.
◆ Give routine blood tests to check for anaemia, any underlying infection or sinister growth.
◆ Prescribe a supplement of iron (to be taken with fruit juice) if you are anaemic.
◆ Give a vaginal ultrasound to check the appearance of the uterus and other related structures. This is easy to perform and is an excellent test.
◆ Refer you to a gynaecologist for a laporoscopy, a minor investigative operation that, with the use of a laporascope inserted through the abdominal wall, examines the pelvic structures.

The surgeon may suggest removing the fibroids if they are potentially troublesome, and this procedure is called myomectomy. Laser therapy is sometimes used also these days.

In the main small fibroids are not troublesome, and are best left alone. It they do become large, and there is fear of them pressing on a nearby organ or blocking the cervix or the fallopian tubes they will need to be removed. Women with fibroids are often advised to have a hysterectomy. If you receive this advice, and you are not too troubled by your symptoms, then you should certainly question it.

## What You Can Do

◆ Waiting to see whether the fibroids cause symptoms that affect the quality of your life is a reasonable policy. If not, they are probably best kept away from the surgeon's knife.
◆ In theory a diet that prevents oestrogen surges may help to control fibroids. Concentrate on eating a high-fibre, low saturated fat diet; including some of the foods that naturally influence oestrogen activity, like linseeds and soya products, may be a good idea.
◆ Lose weight if you need to.
◆ Vitamin B and magnesium may also help to regulate oestrogen metabolism, so you could try supplements of these. Any response to these treatments is likely to take months if not years. So be patient!

## Complementary Therapies

Herbal medicine may have quite a bit to offer. It will take an experienced herbal practitioner to work out the right prescription for this condition. Homoeopathic remedies are worth a try, and so too is acupuncture.

# Endometriosis

Endometriosis, where the tissue forming the lining of the womb grows outside the womb, around other organs, is the most common cause of chronic pain in women of child-bearing age. The pain nearly always coincides with the menstrual period, and may also be experienced at the time of ovulation, approximately mid-cycle. The pain can also be triggered by sexual intercourse, a bowel motion or emptying the bladder, and sometimes causes spotting between periods.

The extraneous endometrial cells (womb lining) not only grow outside the uterus, but they also mimic the function of the endometrium, in that they have a monthly bleed. In mild cases the blood is reabsorbed by the body, but in more severe cases cysts form, which then weep and cause pelvic irritation. The length of time a woman suffers varies from person to person. Some women only suffer for a few months, whilst others suffer all their menstruating lives. It is often better during pregnancy, which is why becoming pregnant may be offered as the solution.

Endometriosis can be very painful, restricting your lifestyle and physical abilities. It is associated with infertility, but it seems that many sufferers do manage to conceive without too much difficulty. Reports of just how common this condition is are varied probably because it is difficult to assess precisely. The diagnosis has to be made during a laporoscopy, a telescopic look into the abdominal cavity, which is not something most well women would undergo just to pass the time of day! Therefore, it is impossible to assess how many women without symptoms may or may not be suffering to some degree. The current medical view is that some women are born with a predisposition to endometriosis.

## What Are the Symptoms?
◆ period-like cramp pains which may be quite severe
◆ heavy bleeding
◆ inability to conceive
◆ painful intercourse

## What Your Doctor Can Do
To some degree the cause of endometriosis is still somewhat of a mystery, and the choices doctors have at their disposal are limited to drugs and surgery.

◆ Eliminate the possibility that anything other than endometriosis could be causing the pain, by taking a careful history, examining you and doing routine blood screening. Infection causing PID (pelvic inflammatory disease) must be excluded.
◆ Drugs such as progestogens and Danazol are able to cause the endometrial tissue to shrink. They work by blocking the action

of oestrogen, which seems to be an important factor in the multiplication of endometrial cells. The treatment would need to be continued over several months, and would only mask symptoms. Most of the drugs used do have a list of side-effects, so it is often a question of making a choice between existing symptoms or the drug-induced symptoms. The success rate using drug therapy is in the region of 40 per cent.

◆ More powerful drugs called gonadotrophic release hormone agonists. These hormone-suppressing agents switch off the whole menstrual cycle, producing an artificial menopause. They are very effective, but can only be used in severe cases and for a limited period of time. Hot flushes and osteoporosis are inevitable side-effects.

◆ A skilled surgeon may be able to remove the endometrial cells and cysts from the unwanted places in the pelvic cavity by laporoscopy. Laser treatment seems to be equally good at destroying these unwanted cells as the scalpel. The success rate following surgery is in the region of 80 per cent, double that for drug therapy, but surgery is not without risks.

## What You Can Do

There is no clear benefit from the many branches of complementary therapy, although it is always worth trying new options as research evolves.

◆ Try following a diet high in fibre and low in animal fat, as this may prevent oestrogen surges.

◆ Take supplements of multi-vitamins and minerals, with extra magnesium, 300 mg, and evening primrose oil with marine fish oil, for their hormone-regulating and anti-inflammatory potential.

# Pelvic Inflammatory Disease

This is a term used to describe inflammation caused by micro-organisms to any of the female organs, including the fallopian tubes, ovaries, vagina, cervix, endometrium or uterus. The discomfort it causes can vary from none or very little to, in extreme cases, substantial pain and a life-threatening situation. It often causes scarring around the organs, and repeated episodes can cause irreversible damage to the fallopian tubes, a major cause of infertility.

Pelvic inflammatory disease (PID) is common. It is estimated that 10 per cent of women up to the age of forty-five have experienced it, and in three out of four of the cases it affects women who are under twenty-five. There are two separate organisms that have been isolated, *Neisseria gonorrhoeae* and *Chlamydia trachomatis*, present in 80 per cent of the cases of PID in women under twenty-five. This clearly means that this condition is sexually transmitted. It is far more common in promiscuous women who smoke, drink and take drugs, than it is in a celibate spinster!

## What Are the Symptoms?

- dull continuous pelvic pain varying from mild to severe
- fever or chills with flu-like symptoms
- increased or changed vaginal discharge in two-thirds of cases (meaning that in one-third of cases there may be no discharge and very few symptoms)
- bleeding between periods, or spotting
- painful periods
- backache
- painful intercourse
- infertility

## What Your Doctor Can Do

- Exclude the possibility of any other acute problem like an ectopic pregnancy, where the embryo grows in the fallopian tube, or appendicitis, through physical examination, urine and blood tests.
- Question you about your sexual behaviour to determine whether you are a likely candidate for PID.
- Perform a cervical smear to determine what sort of organism is growing.
- Treat you with any one of a number of antibiotics, depending on the organism.
- Insist that anyone with whom you have had recent sexual contact be screened too.
- In severe cases where an abscess has developed emergency surgery may be necessary.

As one in four women with proven pelvic inflammatory disease will suffer from either infertility, ectopic pregnancy or chronic pelvic pain as a result of PID, it is vital that treatment be started as soon as it is diagnosed. Remember, in extreme cases PID is a life-threatening condition.

## What You Can Do
◆ Take the medication prescribed by your doctor religiously.
◆ Make sure your partner is screened.
◆ Use a condom.
◆ If the infection is not clearing with the antibiotics, try taking strong multi-vitamins and minerals, plus 30 mg of zinc per day, for between three and six months.
◆ Follow the recommendations for The Very Nutritious Diet.

## Complementary Therapies
This is one of the times when there is no substitute for a drug. By all means try homoeopathic remedies and herbs, but do not rely on them.

# Ovarian Cysts
An ovarian cyst is a balloon-like structure with a thin wall of cells or fibrous material which contains a liquid jelly-like material. Normally, at the time of ovulation, the follicle containing an egg is designed to burst so that the egg can be released. Sometimes, instead, the follicle continues to grow, accumulating fluid and other tissue, and like the ovary itself, it becomes oestrogen-producing. Ovarian cysts vary in size, from pea-sized to the size of large oranges, or larger. Some cysts disperse themselves, but others linger on and eventually become surrounded by ovarian tissue.

Single small cysts on the ovaries come and go, usually without being noticed. A large cyst, however, will cause the abdomen to swell, and can be felt on external examination. The majority of cysts are benign (non-cancerous) but approximately 5 per cent of cysts do become malignant, and your chances of having a malignant cyst increase with age. When a large cyst is present it usually disrupts the menstrual cycle in some way. Apart from the swelling of the abdomen, which could be mistaken for a little too much good food, you may notice a change in your menstrual pattern. Either periods become irregular, or disappear completely, and when the cyst is large it is likely that it will put pressure on organs and structures in the vicinity, causing further discomfort, and in the case of the bladder, a desire to urinate frequently.

## What Your Doctor Can Do

♦ Feel your abdomen externally, and give you an internal examination. An ultrasound scan will confirm whether one or more cysts are present.

♦ If the cyst or cysts are small, a wait and see policy may be adopted, in the hope that they disperse themselves anyway. If a large cyst is detected, you will be referred to a surgeon, with a view to having it dispersed or surgically removed.

♦ If the cyst is found to be malignant, and it is thought that the cells may have penetrated other structures, it is likely that the fallopian tube and ovary it is attached to will be removed also as a precautionary measure (see Cancer of the Ovary, page 120).

## What You Can Do

♦ Follow a high-fibre and low animal fat diet, as this will help to control oestrogen surges.

♦ Keep your weight in the normal range, as women who are overweight are more prone to ovarian cysts.

♦ Possibly take daily supplements of multi-vitamins and magnesium, together with evening primrose oil and marine fish oil. These nutrients have the potential to influence the ovary's response to hormonal signals from the pituitary.

## Complementary Therapies

Herbal medicine and homoeopathic remedies are worth a try. See a qualified practitioner, as well as consulting your doctor.

# Polycystic Ovaries

This is a syndrome in its own right, and is characterised by a necklace-like structure of at least ten cysts surrounding each ovary. On an ultrasound scan the ovaries would appear on average to be three times the size of normal. This syndrome was originally associated with women who were of child-bearing age but whose periods had ceased, with an overgrowth of hair in unwanted places, and with a tendency to be considerably overweight, known as Stein-Leventhal syndrome.

It is now thought that up to 90 per cent of women with

infrequent periods and 30 per cent of women whose periods have ceased prematurely have this syndrome. It has also been suggested that as many as 20 per cent of the normal population have mild polycystic ovarian disease, which can be detected by ultrasound, although in women whose periods are regular it is thought to be in the region of only 7 per cent.

## What Causes It?

◆ There is undoubtedly an hormonal disturbance in women with polycystic ovaries, with an excess of LH (luteinising hormone) from the pituitary and androgens (male hormones).

◆ The development of obesity is thought to be a precipitating factor.

◆ Medical conditions where there is an over-production of other hormones may stimulate the ovaries to develop this condition.

◆ Binge-eating as in bulimia nervosa (see Eating Disorders) has also been found to be associated with polycystic ovaries. In one study, published in the *Lancet*, it was discovered that it was rare for bulimics to have a normal ovarian picture on ultrasound. It is thought that the fluctuating levels of the hormone insulin, brought about because of the bingeing, may also stimulate the underlying tendency to polycystic ovaries.

## What Your Doctor Can Do

◆ Examine you physically to determine whether there is any other underlying problem.

◆ Arrange for you to have an ultrasound scan.

◆ Suggest that you lose weight, if you are overweight.

◆ Prescribe the oral contraceptive pill or other hormonal therapy depending on whether you are hoping to conceive or not.

◆ In severe cases surgery is performed. The current favoured approach is laser or diathermy during a laparoscopy, which aims to pepper the ovarian surface, and is less likely to cause adhesions (fibrous tissues that stick to other organs).

## What You Can Do

◆ Lose weight if you are overweight by following The Simple Weight-loss Diet. This is vital. One study from St Mary's Hospital in London revealed that even modest weight loss from a low-fat high-fibre diet can correct the hormonal abnormalities, reduce the hirsutism and improve the chances of conceiving. Don't worry if you do not reach an ideal weight. A 6.3 kg weight loss can produce a real change in body chemistry.

◆ Possibly cutting down on wheat (bread, cakes, biscuits and pasta) and relying upon rice, green vegetables and fish, might help hormonal balance.

*See also*: Standard References.

# PEPTIC ULCERS

Ulcers in the stomach and duodenum are referred to as peptic, duodenal or gastric ulcers. In both conditions there is a break in the important protective lining of the stomach, or the first part of the duodenum. Once breached, the acid from the stomach, the digestive juices and bile from the liver can all irritate the exposed tissues and contribute to the development of a chronic peptic ulcer.

For much of this century the treatment consisted of dietary change, a variety of antacid medications and surgery. The last ten years has seen nothing short of a revolution in the treatment of peptic ulcers which precipitated a breakthrough in identifying their cause. This work was led by a young gastroenterologist, Dr Barry Marshall, from Perth. As a consequence, highly effective treatment programmes have been developed making surgical treatment nearly a thing of the past.

## What Are the Symptoms?

The symptoms of a peptic ulcer are shared by many other common digestive problems including irritable bowel syndrome and gallstones.

Typically there is pain in the upper abdomen, which may be worse after eating, or worse when the person is hungry. Loss of appetite and weight are more a feature of ulceration in the stomach. Either type of ulcer may bleed, with the person vomiting bright red or processed blood. Alternatively processed dark or blackish blood will be passed in the stool. Occasionally the whole illness is silent until the ulcer actually perforates when severe abdominal pain is experienced.

## What Causes Them?

The research of Dr Barry Marshall led to the discovery that peptic ulcers are virtually always associated with the presence of the bacterium *Helicobacter pylori*. The eradication with antibiotics and other drugs leads to resolution of the ulcer and, unlike many other treatments, there is a greatly reduced chance of the ulcer recurring! Approximately 80 per cent of peptic ulcers are complicated by the presence of this bacterium. The infection is often acquired in childhood and may lie dormant for years. Its presence is also associated with a number of other less common types of inflammation of the stomach.

However, important though Helicobacter might be, it is not the only factor and the other long understood one is acid production by the stomach. Very high levels occur in association with duodenal ulcers, and moderately elevated levels with gastric ulceration. If no acid is produced, then ulceration of this type is not a problem. A number of factors either stimulate acid production or damage the protective layer of cells and mucus lining the stomach and duodenum.

- Smoking, alcohol and, to a lesser extent, coffee and soft drinks are all associated factors.
- Lower socio-economic status is also a risk factor, and this may simply reflect standards of hygiene or intake of essential nutrients.
- Ulcer-causing drugs like anti-arthritis drugs, aspirin and steroids. They certainly can encourage an existing ulcer to bleed and may contribute slightly to the development of an ulcer in the first place.
- Stress is often blamed, but whilst it may aggravate symptoms it does not cause them.

## *What Your Doctor Can Do*

- Assess your symptoms and try to determine the likelihood of there being an ulcer. A chronic ulcer in an older patient requires rather more active treatment.

- Prescribe simple treatment of antacid medicines based upon magnesium or aluminium salts. These may produce rapid relief of pain, but the dose often needs to be repeated very frequently. If the symptoms truly subside with this and other simple measures, then it is unlikely that it was a chronic peptic ulcer.

- Arrange for definitive investigations, usually examination of the upper part of the gut by use of a specialised flexible telescope (endoscopy) or a barium meal.

- Test for the presence of *Helicobacter pylori* either from a biopsy at the time of endoscopy, or by a blood test or a new breath test. Its presence alone is not indicative that there is an ulcer present.

- Treat you with powerful antacid medicines called H2 receptor antagonists of which Cimetidine and Ranitidine are two examples.

- Treat Helicobacter infection with a mixture of antibiotics and H2 receptor antagonist drugs, and sometimes a drug containing bismuth is added.

- Make sure that this germ has been eradicated by repeating the endoscopy or the breath test but not the blood test. This is particularly important if there was a gastric ulcer or if the ulcer had bled.

- Consider surgical treatment for unhealing gastric ulcers or ulcers that have bled repeatedly.

## *What You Can Do*

Your role is still important, but the advances in medical care have meant that the emphasis on diet for treatment of ulcers has rightly lessened. This doesn't mean you can eat what you like, instead simple sensible measures are worth following, especially in the early stages. Many cases of non-ulcer indigestion may benefit from a change in diet and prevent the need for further investigations.

- Stop smoking as this will greatly improve the response to medical treatment and reduce the chance of recurrence.

- Only consume moderate amounts of alcohol and never on an empty stomach.
- Eat little and often, to minimise the surge of acid with a meal.
- Avoid large amounts of coffee and sugar as there is some evidence that they may stimulate acid production.
- Avoid foods that you feel make it worse. There is too much individual variation, and no set diet is universally successful. It is better to trust your own judgement. Foods to which the odd individual is genuinely allergic could stimulate the production of acid because of the action of histamine released at the time of an allergic reaction.
- De-stress. If symptoms are severe, some time off work or away may be needed. Take time to consider what lifestyle changes need to be made.
- Chew some liquorice. It contains chemicals that may promote the healing of ulcers. The effect is small and it should not be used by the elderly, those with high blood pressure or kidney problems or fluid retention as it promotes salt and water retention.

## Complementary Therapies

Again there may be benefit from acupuncture, homoeopathy and herbalism, but if you have a proven peptic ulcer make sure you tell your medical specialist what you are doing.

## Kay's Story

Kay was a happy-go-lucky, thirty-four-year-old play-group leader. She really came looking for a diet to help her lose weight. Even though she was very petite, her weight had crept up to 76 kg, about 18 kg over her ideal weight. She made light of her other problems which included irregular periods, excessive facial hair growth, fatigue and indigestion. Three years earlier she had been admitted as an emergency because of stomach pains. Investigation then found that she was bleeding from a duodenal ulcer which had been treated with acid-suppressing drugs but not antibiotics.

Clearly she was likely to benefit from a weight-reducing diet, but it was likely that there was more than this going on. Blood tests showed a high level of antibodies against the germ *Helicobacter pylori*, suggestive of active or recent infection. There were also mild deficiencies of vitamin B and zinc. Her irregular periods and hair growth were very suggestive of polycystic ovaries.

She began on a weight-reducing, low-fat diet, antibiotics for her Helicobacter infection, and supplements of zinc and multi-vitamins.

Her 'indigestion' cleared up and she was referred on to a hospital gastroenterologist to make sure that the infection was fully resolved. Falling weight and improved nutritional status may well help her irregular periods but these too may require investigation.

# PERIOD PROBLEMS

## *Painful Periods*

Period pains commonly affect younger women mainly, but not exclusively, as older women may sometimes experience them as well. When periods first begin in early teens, they are usually not painful, but may become so in mid to late teens or later depending upon the reason for the onset of the pain. The development of pain with menstruation is usually taken to indicate the presence of ovulation, the time when the egg is released, within each menstrual cycle.

## *What Causes Them?*

Period pain or to use the medical term, dysmenorrhoea, most often occurs because of excessive muscle contractions of the uterus with each period. Four common gynaecological problems may, however, cause the periods to become painful and they include:

- infection of the tubes or ovaries
- fibroids
- endometriosis, where the lining of the womb is found in other tissues such as the wall of the uterus or around the ovaries
- a deficiency of the mineral magnesium, the most commonly deficient nutrient in women of child-bearing age, which is needed for optimum muscle function

Any woman with excessively painful or heavy periods, in particular if there is pain throughout the month or an irregular menstrual cycle, should see her general practitioner for a gynaecological check-up. A simple examination would normally determine if one of these problems is present.

Often no cause is found and simple dysmenorrhoea is diagnosed. In this situation periods are often painful for the first 24 or 48 hours and perhaps even for the day before the onset of menstruation. Period pains are often felt as mild to severe cramp-like pain or discomfort in the lower abdomen. It can also be felt as low back pain or aching down the legs and, when severe, can be accompanied by giddiness, faintness, nausea and even occasional vomiting. These other symptoms are probably due to the hormonal and chemical changes that occur with menstruation.

Symptoms of premenstrual syndrome such as irritability, mood swings, depression or breast tenderness may also be present, but are not particularly related to the presence of period pains.

## Ilana's Story

Ilana, a thirty-year-old barrister, had endured severe period pain and vomiting every month for seventeen years.

*It was like someone jerking a knife into my stomach. I'd be doubled over with pain and I'd always have to spend the first day of my period in bed. I experienced nausea and bloating and found it very difficult to function properly at work. I'm a barrister, so I have to be able to think clearly. Taking time off every month was affecting my reputation and career prospects adversely. I had so many symptoms before my period that I was really only normal for seven days each month.*

*I read about the WNAS and went along to their London clinic. I was asked to follow a very restricted diet initially, which was pretty tough, and to take supplements and to exercise. Within the first month, to my utter amazement I had no pain. The nausea went as well as the bloating, I just couldn't believe it. That was nine years ago, and I haven't had any period problems since. I am able to relax my diet, but I know if I go back to my old ways my symptoms will start to return. This programme was a complete cure for me, it totally revolutionised my life. I feel healthy and stable and am extremely grateful to the WNAS.*

## What Your Doctor Can Do

A variety of treatments already exist that may be helpful, and could be suggested by your doctor when you seek advice.

◆ Magnesium check. Measure your red cell magnesium, to see whether you have a deficiency. This is a simple blood test, and should be readily available.

◆ Painkillers. Your doctor may recommend the use of certain types of painkillers or hormonal products. Some mild painkillers may not be very effective for severe pain but a more powerful sort which are either prescribable (*mefenamic acid-Ponstan*) or are available on the advice of your pharmacist can be particularly useful. It may be necessary to try a number before finding the most effective one for you.

◆ The contraceptive pill. A number of hormonal preparations are available but often the most useful, particularly in young women who require contraception, is to use the oral contraceptive pill. The more modern low-dose pills have much fewer side effects than older preparations.

◆ Iron. Your doctor can prescribe iron supplements if you are anaemic as well.

## What You Can Do

There are a number of avenue you can explore to help reduce painful periods:

◆ Physical exercise may sometimes be helpful with a variety of gynaecological problems, and may help your tolerance of pain. Try to exercise three or four times per week. During a painful period try to do some gentle yoga exercises instead of strenuous exercise.

◆ Heat seems to have a soothing effect. Applying a hot water bottle or a thermal heat pad can be very soothing.

◆ Changing and improving your diet can help also with minor hormonal abnormalities some of which are thought to underlie such gynaecological problems. Ensuring a well-balanced diet without excessive consumption of fatty foods, and with a good intake of fibre from fruit and vegetables may help control hormone metabolism and can reduce some of the excessive hormonal swings that occur during the menstrual cycle.

- Eat a diet rich in essential fatty acids, especially fish oils. Women with period pains are known to have a lower intake of these oils, which may have anti-inflammatory, and painkilling properties.
- Some minerals may also be helpful. Magnesium is particularly important in muscle and hormonal functions. Its balance with calcium influences the contraction of uterine muscle and one study suggests that taking supplements may help reduce period pains. Good dietary sources of magnesium include all vegetables, especially green ones, nuts, seeds, beans, peas and lentils. Sugar, sweets, cakes and biscuits are low in this important mineral.
- If your periods are heavy, ensuring a good dietary intake of iron is also important, and this is found in meat, fish, chicken, eggs, nuts, seeds and vegetarian protein.

Magnesium supplements can be obtained from health-food shops. At the WNAS we tend to use magnesium amino acid chelate, to gut-tolerance level. In other words if you take too much you will get diarrhoea. A magnesium rich multi-vitamin, multi-mineral supplement might also be helpful.

Remember if your period pains do not respond to these self-help measures or painkillers you must consult with your general practitioner or family planning clinic.

## Complementary Therapies

When period pain is due to muscular spasm, acupuncture and cranial osteopathy will be obvious choices as they both help to free up pockets of blocked energy in the body. Herbal and homeopathic remedies are also worth a try. If the pain is caused by an infection, this will need to be dealt with by conventional medicine, however, complementary therapy will help to boost the immune system which increases your resistance to infection in the long-term. Often when nutritional deficiencies have been addressed, particularly low magnesium levels, and the muscles are functioning normally, the period pains subside. It may therefore be worth following the advice given in this chapter for a few months before seeking further advice.

# Heavy Periods

The average blood loss for each menstrual period is approximately 35 ml, or just over 2 tablespoons. A heavy period, or menorrhagia as it is technically known, constitutes a loss of 80 ml of blood loss per period, which is considerably more than average (just over 5 tablespoons). It is enormously difficult to assess the actual loss of blood during a period. Even studies that counted the number of sanitary towels or tampons that women get through were inaccurate, as it was discovered that women change after collecting differing amounts of blood.

Generally women find that their periods get heavier as they grow older, particularly those that have had children. Flooding can occur in the years leading up to the menopause, resulting in soiled top clothes, as well as underwear. Apart from the sheer embarrassment and hassle of dealing with heavy periods, they can also result in iron deficiency anaemia.

## What Causes Them?

Excessive blood loss at period time is a problem for approximately 10 per cent of menstruating women. Once again there are many possible underlying causes.

◆ Approaching the menopause, the lining of the uterus can become thicker, resulting in heavier blood loss.
◆ The presence of fibroids in the uterus can increase the flow of a period.
◆ A recently fitted IUD can result in heavy periods, which usually settle down after the first few months.
◆ A hormonal imbalance in the body.
◆ According to our experience, heavy periods can be caused sometimes by nutritional deficiencies.
◆ An early miscarriage. Sometimes a woman may conceive without realising, but because it is an unviable pregnancy Mother Nature terminates it, in the form of what appears to be a very heavy period.

## Alison's Story

Alison, a thirty-six-year-old proprietor of a fashion business and mother of three, had experienced irregular, heavy and painful periods all her life.

*My periods had always been irregular heavy or painful, but they became even worse after I gave birth to my third child. I hated taking painkillers and dreaded the thought of each period. As I was unable to function for several days each month I couldn't keep my mind on my work. I was embarrassed to go out of the house in case I flooded. My GP suggested a hysterectomy, which I wanted to avoid if possible.*

*I read about the WNAS in Prima magazine and in desperation contacted them for help. I went on an elimination diet, which involved cutting out certain foods and then gradually re-introducing them to see if I had a bad reaction to them. I discovered that what upset me most were things I ate a lot of, such as wholemeal bread and muesli, and drinking fresh coffee. I was also advised to exercise and to take Optivite, a magnesium-rich multi-vitamin and mineral supplement, and Efamol evening primrose oil.*

*Within four months of following this regime my periods were back to normal, in fact better than they had been for years. No more heavy bleeding and clots, and regular—I could hardly believe it. That was six years ago and my periods have remained regular. I still follow a modified version of my programme and feel extremely well generally. I don't think my success was due to any one thing, but to a combination of diet, supplements and increased exercise that worked. I am very grateful to the WNAS for their help as is my husband who says I am more like my old self again, the girl he married twenty-four years ago.*

## Delia's Story

Delia, a forty-two-year-old mother of two, and a practising osteopath, had been complaining of extremely heavy periods for nine months. She had been diagnosed as having a substantial fibroid, and was advised to have an emergency hysterectomy.

*I first experienced heavy periods after being sterilised three years ago. I was prescribed hormone therapy and transamic acid, which seemed to increase the symptoms, and the gynaecologist diagnosed a large fibroid at the time. The bleeding eventually settled down, and I thought little more of it. In March 1984 the heavy bleeding began again, and I bled every day for nine months. I felt so ill and washed out as a result.*

*I went to visit my doctor in desperation, and it was arranged that I should be admitted to hospital the next day, as an emergency patient, for a hysterectomy. I thought long and hard about it, as I was not keen to have the operation unless it was absolutely necessary. That night I made the decision to try to resolve the problem by alternative means, and telephoned the hospital to cancel the booking.*

*Being a cranial osteopath myself, I decided to ask a colleague for some treatment. I also received some homoeopathic treatment and went to the Stewarts' clinic. From blood tests it was discovered that I had low iron levels, and reasonably low zinc and magnesium levels as well. I was asked to take specific strong multivitamins and minerals, plus extra supplements of nutrients I was short of. In addition to this I was asked to make specific dietary changes, and to exercise gently when possible.*

*Within six weeks the bleeding had stopped, and I was back to having regular periods. One amazing event, which I know my doctor finds hard to believe, is that during that time I passed what I thought was an unusually large lump, much bigger than a usual clot. When I was eventually re-examined, there was no sign of the fibroid, so I can only assume it came away naturally.*

*My periods were relatively light after that episode, and I felt so much better in myself. I had gained 9 kg in weight during my troubled year, which went during the following year. I persisted with the supplements, until I began my menopause, at which time I was advised to take other supplements, and make other changes to my diet.*

*It has been twelve years now, and I look and feel so much better. People say that I look younger now than I did then, and I certainly feel a great deal healthier, and have a much more positive outlook. I am currently doing a postgraduate course and enjoying every minute of my life.*

## What Your Doctor Can Do

If your periods become unmanageably heavy, or you have a sudden episode of flooding you should consult your doctor for advice. After taking a history of the problem, your doctor will:

◆ Examine you to determine whether there are any fibroids present or any other physical abnormalities—in which case you would then be referred to a gynaecologist who would decide whether you needed minor surgery.
◆ Take some blood for a serum ferritin test to check whether your iron stores are in fact low, in which case you would need a course of iron.

◆ Remove your IUD, if you have one, to see whether that alters the flow.

◆ Prescribe hormone pills to reduce the flow. The first choice for a younger woman might be the oral contraceptive pill, failing that, Duphaston, a progestogen preparation; and if that fails to work, then Danazol, which has considerable side-effects.

◆ Prescribe tranexamic acid, a drug that helps excessive bleeding. It can be more effective than hormones.

◆ Suggest a hysterectomy, which should be regarded as a last resort.

## What You Can Do

◆ Eat plenty of green leafy vegetables, liver, free-range eggs and other foods rich in iron.

◆ Take a good strong multi-vitamin and mineral supplement, with extra B vitamins, vitamin C with bioflavonoids, and magnesium.

◆ Rest when the flow is heavy, and avoid important social engagements until the bleeding has reduced.

## Complementary Therapies

Try herbal medicine or homoeopathy. If your periods are exceedingly heavy, it is better to consult an expert rather than attempting to self-treat.

# Irregular or Absent Periods

Women were designed to have regular periods, somewhere between every twenty-three and thirty-five days, which end a cycle or 'failed conception'. Each month the body should release eggs whose job it is to find a sperm to merge with. When this fails, a period arrives, approximately some two weeks later. After the first year, periods usually establish a pattern, which become the normal cycle, and for many this continues until they reach their menopause. Others experience irregular periods, or an absence of periods altogether, which means they are not releasing eggs (see Painful Ovulation).

## What Causes Them?

The medical term for an absence of periods is amenorrhoea, and there are two types. Primary amenorrhoea is when no period ever arrives, which is rare, and secondary amenorrhoea, is when periods have 'disappeared' for in excess of four cycles. Primary amenorrhoea may be associated with late puberty or a defect in the hormone and reproductive system, and there is little that can be done to correct that. There are many underlying causes of secondary amenorrhoea though, most of which can be addressed. Your periods can become irregular or disappear because of:

◆ pregnancy and breast-feeding—but this is perfectly normal. Very often when fully breast-feeding, periods will not return for between six months to a year
◆ sudden weight loss due to any illness, including the slimmers' disease, anorexia nervosa
◆ over-exercising. Athletes and ballet dancers often develop amenorrhea, and as a result, decreased oestrogen levels, which greatly increase their chances of developing osteoporosis later in life
◆ episodes of extreme stress, e.g. bereavement or divorce
◆ undetected and therefore untreated thyroid disease
◆ anaemia and monitored deficiencies, especially of vitamin B
◆ long-term medication

## Susan Wightman's Story

Susan Wightman, formerly Tooby, was the first woman in Britain to break 70 minutes for the half marathon, in 1988. She is a well-known Olympic marathon and cross-country runner who, with her twin sister Angela, has been training since the age of twenty. Her periods stopped for ten years as her diet did not meet her energy requirements.

*Both Angela and I have discovered that we were at risk of having osteoporosis. When we began our training, long-term damage didn't really seem relevant to us then. We felt fit and healthy and had the chance of going to the Olympics. At that time it would have been hard to persuade us about a possible risk in thirty years time.*

*I was conscious that I was a little on the plump side for a runner, and as I ran better when I was lighter I paid far too much attention to dieting. Looking back I realise that I was not eating an adequate diet to meet my energy output, and was certainly not consuming anything like enough calcium in my diet. I'm quite petite, and at one point weighed as little as 46 kg. My weight was so low that my periods stopped for ten years, which I now know would have reduced my oestrogen levels, and increased my chances of getting osteoporosis. I used to eat fruit only for breakfast, a scone for lunch and a slice of quiche and salad with fruit for my evening meal.*

*I sometimes felt pretty weak, and became very susceptible to injury. In my career I have experienced three stress fractures in my legs, with a fourth suspected. Because of this record the British Olympic Association included both myself and my twin sister in a bone-scanning survey that they were conducting. We were both found to be at risk of osteoporosis and put on a course of HRT and calcium. My sister came off the HRT after the first course, but I stuck it out for six or eight months before giving up. I felt bloated and moody and my running was impaired whilst on the HRT, but once off it my performance improved again.*

*I was due to compete in the Commonwealth Games in Auckland in 1990, but had to pull out because of a stress fracture, and at that point I realised that I would have to call a halt to my running career.*

*I got married in 1991 to Geoff who is also an international marathon runner and after eating a better diet, my periods returned and we managed to produce twins. I am delighted to say that a recent test showed that my bone mass has improved, and I no longer have signs of osteoporosis.*

*If I had my time again I would undoubtedly have eaten more sensibly, and I would not encourage a young female athlete to diet as we did.*

*I still run 64 kilometres per week, and work as a PE teacher in Nottingham. I have improved my diet, and I now take Efacal with the hope that I can maintain my new bone mass.*

## What Your Doctor Can Do

If your periods haven't arrived by the age of sixteen or seventeen it is time to ask your doctor for some advice. You will need to be investigated by your doctor initially, and subsequently by an endocrinologist.

If you had established periods but they have since disappeared, there are a number of things your doctor can do:

◆ Check to see whether you are pregnant.
◆ If you are taking prescribed drugs—assess your programme to see whether they are interrupting your cycle.
◆ Take blood to check your thyroid and iron levels.
◆ Assess the function of your pituitary gland, which is responsible for hormone function.

◆ Refer you for gynaecological investigation to check that your ovaries are functioning, and that there are no other obvious problems.

## What You Can Do
◆ Follow the recommendations in The Very Nutritious Diet.
◆ Take regular vitamin and mineral supplements.
◆ Get some help with sorting out any stressful situations that face you or counselling if you are bereaved or recently separated or divorced.
◆ If you are an athlete, a professional dancer or an exercise addict, work hard to ensure that you are meeting your kilojoule requirements.
◆ If your weight is low for your height and frame, actively work to increase your weight to the optimum range.

## Complementary Therapies
Many complementary therapies would be worth investigating. Consult a qualified homoeopath or medical herbalist, as they will certainly have numerous remedies for you to try. A burst of acupuncture wouldn't go amiss, as acupuncture is very good at unblocking the energy channels in the body.

*See also*: Recommended Reading List and Standard References.

# PERIPHERAL VASCULAR DISEASE

Just as the blood vessels supplying the heart muscle can become narrowed, so can the main arteries to the legs. The blood vessels in the upper limbs are almost never affected in this way, consequently all the symptoms relate to below the waistline.

## What Are the Symptoms?
The first symptom is usually pain in the calf on exercise. The pain is often severe, causes the sufferer to stop walking or to walk with a limp, and clears after a few minutes' rest. This clinical picture

is called intermittent claudication (limping). Cold feet, changes to the skin colour, loss of hairs on the legs and in men loss of the ability to have an erection are other features.

## What Causes It?
Essentially much the same factors as for ischaemic heart disease and atherosclerosis apply. Smoking, an elevated blood cholesterol and diabetes are the three most important and treatable factors. Increasing age is also important too.

## What Your Doctor Can Do
Anyone presenting with intermittent leg pains on walking, that clears with rest, should be assessed for the main risk factors for atherosclerosis.

Examination of the legs and abdomen will give a good idea of the severity of the disease. Those with severe symptoms, absent pulses in the feet, and younger patients may need specialist assessment. Surprisingly accurate assessment of the degree of atherosclerotic narrowing can be made from measuring the blood pressure levels in the leg, and from the use of an ultrasound pulse detector.

In those in whom major disease is suspected then specialist X-rays to look at the blood vessels can be undertaken. From this the appropriateness of surgical correction can be ascertained.

Drug treatments are not very effective at all. More important is control of elevated blood fats, both cholesterol and triglycerides. These latter can contribute to atherosclerosis and are more important in peripheral vascular disease than in coronary artery disease. Being overweight, drinking alcohol or consuming sugar to excess, or being diabetic raises this type of fat greatly. Combined drug and dietary treatment is known to control the elevated fats and can even reverse the atherosclerotic process if followed assiduously.

## What You Can Do
◆ Stop smoking completely.
◆ Walk, walk, walk! Painful though exercise might be, it helps to keep open the existing blood vessels. Daily walks to the limit of exercise tolerance are mandatory.
◆ Lose weight if you are overweight.

- Follow The Very Nutritious Diet, keeping the total fat content very low.
- Take supplements of vitamin E, at least 300 IU per day.
- Other supplements might be helpful but this is not certain. Multi-vitamins, anti-oxidants such as vitamin C and selenium and the trace element chromium look like the best bets.

## Complementary Therapies

Acupuncture and herbalism might be able to encourage the opening up of blood vessels. Worth a try, but don't rely on it.

# PRECONCEPTION

When a couple decide to have a family they are taking on one of the most important jobs in the world, so they must be in good health to ensure a healthy baby.

The ova, female eggs, and sperm may be adversely affected by inadequate diet, and by social and environmental factors. The egg is at its most vulnerable for about 100 days leading up to ovulation, the time when it is released, and sperms are also particularly vulnerable for approximately 116 days before they mature. So eating well, having a wholesome lifestyle and environment will contribute to the health of the next generation. It's an awesome task, and one that requires careful planning *at least four months* before conception.

## What Your Doctor Can Do

- Check your serum ferritin levels if you suffer with fatigue, have pale skin and heavy periods. This will determine whether you have low iron stores.
- Check to see whether you are up to date with your rubella immunisations. It is important to be immune to german measles because it can cause so much irreversible damage to an unborn child if contracted in the first few weeks of pregnancy.
- Arrange for you to have a thorough check up to ensure:

◇ your blood pressure is in the normal range
◇ you are free of diabetes
◇ you have no pelvic problems
◇ you have no vaginal or bladder infections
◇ you are not an HIV carrier
◇ you do not have any sexually transmitted disease

◆ Remove an IUD if you have one. This needs to be done at least six months before you plan to conceive. An IUD can also increase the risk of vaginal infection.

◆ Advise on medication. Ideally you should not be taking any medication during pregnancy that is not absolutely necessary. If you are taking prescribed drugs, discuss the situation with your doctor to see whether there is any need for you to reduce your medication or to switch to an alternative prior to trying for a baby.

◆ Prescribe supplements that contain folic acid and vitamin B12 to help prevent neural tube defects.

## What You Can Do

Here are some simple dietary recommendations which should be followed in order to help achieve an adequate intake of all the essential nutrients. This is especially important in the preconceptual phase and in the first twelve weeks of pregnancy as it determines the growth and development of your baby.

◆ Eat three regular meals a day. Doing so will give you the best chance of obtaining a balanced intake of all essential nutrients. Do not miss meals.

◆ Eat one cooked main meal per day. Cooked meat-, fish- or vegetable-based meals will again allow a good intake of essential nutrients, especially protein.

◆ Eat at least one portion (120 g) of meat or fish or vegetarian protein, such as beans, peas or lentils. Many convenience or prepared meals are low in protein, vitamins and minerals.

◆ Ensure a good intake of foods rich in folic acid, especially green leafy vegetables, fortified breakfast cereals, oranges and orange juice, eggs, almonds and sweetcorn. You can eat cooked liver once a month if you wish until you are pregnant, when you should stop.

◆ Enjoy good sources of calcium, including dairy products, milk (whole, skimmed or semi-skimmed) and cheese, but avoid soft cheese and cottage cheese. Soft cheese may contain the infecting organism listeria, and cottage cheese is low in protein and B vitamins.

◆ Eat at least three portions of fruit per day, and two portions of green leafy vegetables or green salad per day. This is in line with the latest recommendations for healthy eating for the general population, and will help maintain a good intake of fibre, vitamins and minerals.

◆ Eat two or three slices of wholemeal bread per day. White bread may be acceptable if the rest of the diet is well balanced. Some will need more bread than others, and those on weight-reducing diets may need to consume less.

◆ Use good-quality vegetable oils, which are high in essential fatty acids, especially sunflower, safflower, canola and walnut. Olive oil is not rich in essential fatty acids. Use margarines based on these oils, e.g. sunflower, or you can use a small amount of butter. Again cut down on these if you need to lose weight.

◆ Eat from a selection of foods rich in essential fatty acids. These include oily fish like mackerel, herring, salmon, pilchards and sardines, and spinach, walnuts, almonds, hazelnuts, pecans (peanuts are not so nutritious in this respect) and beans, especially pinto beans.

◆ Trim the skin and fat from meat and poultry. These tend to be high in the less helpful saturated fats, and most of the environmental toxins, if present, will be found in the fatty portions of them.

◆ Get your partner to follow the same dietary recommendations. The health of the father-to-be can also be a factor in the health of your future offspring.

## Current Thinking on Nutritional Supplements

Many multi-vitamins from chemists are not suitable for the pre-conceptual phase as they contain animal vitamin A (retinol) and inadequate amounts of folic acid (not enough to prevent neural tube defects). However, in recent years, research demonstrating the need for extra folic acid and vitamin B12 during the preconceptual phase, and the first trimester of pregnancy, has resulted in a number of new products arriving on the shelves.

- Folic acid alone, at a strength of 400 µg, is now widely available, and is recommended to be taken by all women prior to conception. The research shows that when this is taken with vitamin B12, the protection against developing a neural tube defect is even greater.
- A much higher dose of folic acid, 4 mg, is recommended for those women who have already given birth to a child with a neural tube defect and wish to conceive again.

## A *Preconceptual Programme*

- If you have been taking the contraceptive pill you will need to stop six months before you plan to conceive. The pill can interfere with essential vitamin and mineral levels.
- Use natural methods of contraception during your preconceptual programme. Getting to know your body and learning to recognise when you are ovulating will help you in the long term to know when it is right to conceive.
- Follow the diet plan outlined above for at least four months before conception, and get your partner to follow a similar diet, perhaps eating extra quantities if he is larger than you.
- Take care to avoid all the foods and drinks which have been shown to impede the absorption of good nutrients or might harm your chances of a healthy baby.
- Do not consume any alcohol. This is probably the best advice, though it is obviously hard for some to follow. You should not drink from about day ten of your cycle until when your period begins, when your egg is at its most vulnerable. Ideally both you and your partner should avoid drinking alcohol. At most, consume no more than 3 units per week.
- You should spend at least four months in a smoke-free environment. That means that neither you nor your partner should be smoking, and you should avoid smoky atmospheres.
- Take a multi-vitamin and mineral supplement that contains 400 µg of folic acid and vitamin B12 but not vitamin A (as retinol). The pharmacy or health-food shop will be able to advise you on the range of products now available.
- Take three or four good sessions of exercise per week, and try to get outdoors as often as possible, especially when it is sunny.
- If either you or your partner use street drugs you will need to stop, either with the support of each other if it's a social habit,

or with the help of a clinic if you are addicted.
- ◆ Avoid chemicals wherever possible. You should:
  - ◇ use lead-free petrol
  - ◇ use ecologically safe cleaning creams at home
  - ◇ avoid using aerosols
  - ◇ avoid using any chemicals if you are a keen gardener or grow vegetables
  - ◇ avoid sitting for too long in front of a VDU on a regular basis
  - ◇ not use copper or aluminium saucepans
  - ◇ only use the microwave for reheating or defrosting
  - ◇ keep away from busy main roads—if you live on one, try to move
  - ◇ not spray pets with chemicals to prevent fleas
  - ◇ avoid paint which contains lead, and should not sleep in a freshly painted room
  - ◇ not use a sunbed whilst you are pregnant
  - ◇ use a hot water bottle to heat your bed rather than an electric blanket
  - ◇ sort out areas of stress in your personal and work life before you conceive

Once you have conceived, you will need to continue with a healthy regime throughout your pregnancy. Refer to Pregnancy, for extra help and advice. Additionally, we now know that the type of diet our babies are fed during the first year of life will also play a major role in determining their long-term health prospects, so adopting a sound weaning plan thereafter is advisable.

*See also*: What's Wrong with Present-day Diet and Lifestyle?, Nutrition is the Key to Health. Plus Recommended Reading List (*Healthy Parents, Healthy Baby*) and References.

# PREGNANCY

The effect that diet, environment and lifestyle before and during pregnancy have on our unborn children should never be underestimated. Research shows quite clearly that we can 'programme' the health of a baby and influence its growth and development, at least four months before it is even conceived (see Preconception), and during the first three to four months of pregnancy. We can affect the shape and size of the baby, the health of its important little organs, its intelligence in later life, and even its fingerprints!

Examples of how our diet and lifestyle can influence the unborn are many.

◆ Babies who are small for dates are likely to have high blood pressure in later life and have a different fingerprint pattern to normal weight babies.

◆ Low birth-weight babies are seven times more likely to develop blood sugar problems or get diabetes than babies whose weight is in the normal range.

◆ Impaired lung growth during the developmental stages and early infant life, due to inadequate nutrition and environmental conditions, point to potential abnormal lung function and increased chances of suffering bronchitis, asthma and chronic chest infections.

There is enough new evidence to convince even the most sceptical amongst us that diet and environmental factors influence the well-being of the unborn child not only in infancy, but also in adult life.

From the time of conception, each minute bodily system has its own timetable for development, and the supply of essential nutrients and timing of contact with a toxin, will determine the type of damage that results.

According to relatively recent research data, babies who are undernourished in the first four weeks of development stand a much higher chance of developing heart disease, a major cause of death in middle age, and brain disorders, present from birth, which show up later in life in one in eight adults.

Low birth-weight babies, those born at term who weigh under 2.75 kg, if they survive, suffer higher rates of childhood illness, and stand a greater chance of being mentally retarded, of suffering from cerebral palsy, behaviour disorders, impaired vision or deafness.

## Dietary Requirements

Despite the fact that many us feel incredibly hungry during pregnancy, our actual requirement for extra kilojoules does not increase significantly in the first six months, and only by an additional 10–20 per cent during the last three months of pregnancy. What does increase is our need for good-quality, nutrient-dense foods, which are rich in folic acid, vitamin B12, essential fatty acids, and the mineral zinc and iron in particular (see below).

You experience the largest demand for nutrients during pregnancy and breast-feeding. Besides looking after yourself, you have the needs of a growing baby to meet, as well as the increased tissue of the uterus, placenta and blood. All this new tissue requires more kilojoules, proteins, vitamins and minerals.

It is normal to gain nearly 12.5 kg during pregnancy, but weight gain can vary depending on individual metabolic rate. Some women hardly notice any change in appetite, whilst others feel like they are eating for an army! Studies show that women who gain in excess of 13.5 kg during pregnancy have significantly more healthy babies. Slim women, who only experience a small weight gain, can have babies with a low birth weight. You should be eating enough to gain weight at the rate of 225–450 g per week, unless you are overweight.

- Folic acid deficiency and vitamin B12 insufficiency are now clearly linked to neural tube defects.
- Zinc deficiency during pregnancy has been linked with low birth weight, under 2.75 kg.
- Vitamin A is another nutrient linked to growth, and in fact it is recommended that all pregnant and breast-feeding mothers take supplements of vitamin A as beta-carotene the non-animal source (not as retinol), as well as vitamins D and C, in order to build up vitamin stores that can then be passed across the placenta.
- Essential fatty acids (EFAs) are vital for growth and

development of the baby, particularly for the brain and the central nervous system. Recent research suggests that a deficiency of these long-chain polyunsaturated fatty acids in the tissues of growing babies results in low birth weight, which may have life-long implications. We now know too that adequate intakes of EFAs in the new-born infant seem to influence vision and subsequent intelligence.

Babies born after an apparently normal pregnancy often have borderline levels of EFAs, as do premature babies. Breast milk, from a well-nourished mother, is a good source of EFAs, which probably explains why some breast-fed infants make better progress than bottle-fed ones. Trials feeding Efamol Marine—a combination of evening primrose and marine fish oils—to pregnant women during the final three months of pregnancy are underway. Good sources of essential fatty acids can be found in Nutritional Content of Foods, Appendix I.

Sadly, many of these important medical facts, which undoubtedly affect the welfare of our unborn children, are kept almost as trade secrets. The health and well-being of your growing baby is undoubtedly in your hands and, with a little knowledge, there are many positive steps that you can take to ensure your baby has the best possible chance in life.

## What Your Doctor Can Do

◆ Give regular checks to ensure that the growth of the baby is on target, and that you are in good health.
◆ Prescribe iron supplements, should your levels drop below the normal range.
◆ Offer screening facilities for prospective mums who are either at risk or over thirty-five years of age.
◆ Refer you to a specialist if there are any concerns during your pregnancy.

## What You Can Do

◆ Eat a wide variety of nutritious foods. The best are those rich in protein, such as lean meat (preferably additive-free or organic), fish, free-range chicken, nuts, seeds, peas, beans and lentils. Foods that are particularly nutritious and should be consumed regularly through pregnancy are listed in the following table:

```
··············································································
NUTRITIOUS FOODS TO EAT REGULARLY DURING PREGNANCY
────────────────────────────────────────────────────────────────
Lean meat                         Nuts
Eggs, preferably free-range       Wholemeal bread (up to 3 slices per
                                  day)
All green vegetables              Fortified breakfast cereal
Wheatgerm
··············································································
```

- ◆ Choose vegetable rather than animal fats. Use polyunsaturated margarines and cold-pressed oils, rather than animal fats which are high in kilojoules and low in essential nutrients. Trim any visible fat from meat or poultry, and don't eat the skin.

- ◆ Eat plenty of foods containing calcium and other good nutrients. Dairy products such as milk, yoghurt and cheese are all important sources of calcium. So too are the small bony fish like whitebait and sardines, and nuts, seeds and green vegetables. Aim for 300–600 ml of milk and yoghurt per day, and 175–225 g of cheese per week.

- ◆ Feast on salad, vegetables and fruit. Aim to eat a salad daily, plus three portions of vegetables, including one green leafy vegetable, and at least two portions of fruit each day. These are important sources of vitamins, minerals and fibre.

- ◆ Don't use pregnancy as an excuse to pig out on sweet food. Many women develop cravings for sweet foods during pregnancy, and use their lost waistline as an excuse to indulge. Sweet food, like puddings, cake or chocolate are permissible, but only in addition to nutritious food. Sweet foods are normally a very low source of good nutrients, and should never replace wholesome food. As long as you are not overweight to start with, have your treats after meals.

- ◆ Increase the fruit juice, and reduce the tea. It is vital to make the most of all the dietary iron during pregnancy, as your growing baby will be steadily stocking up on iron to last through the first few months of life. Drinking tea, which contains tannin that binds with iron from vegetable protein, will reduce the amount of iron that you are able to absorb by about half. By choosing citrus fruit juices, like orange or grapefruit, which are rich in vitamin C, you will approximately double the iron that is available to both you and your baby. Other foods and drinks rich in vitamin C are listed in Nutritional Content of Foods, Appendix I.

◆ Use tea and coffee substitutes. There are many different varieties to try. It is worth noting that one caffeine-free tea look-alike has shown positive results in South African trials on babies with colic. It contains a mild muscle relaxant. Raspberry tea could be consumed before delivery to relax the perineum.

◆ There's nothing better than regular exercise  Sticking to a regular exercise routine during pregnancy will help to keep you feeling healthy and will tone your body for the delivery. The endorphin release which results from exercise not only raises your mood, but also that of your baby. Research has shown that endorphins cross the placenta, and the baby is therefore able to share your sense of well-being!

◆ Continue with all the relevant steps in the preconceptual advice starting on  Avoid alcohol, cigarettes, street drugs plus environmental chemicals and hazards.

## *Potential Dangers in Pregnancy*

There are a number of bugs which can be very dangerous, particularly during pregnancy. Avoid them and the foods that might harbour them at all costs.

### *Listeriosis*

Even in a mild form, listeriosis can cause miscarriage, severe illness in a new-born baby, or a still-birth. It presents as a flu-like illness that is caused by the *Listeria monocytogenes* bug, found in some common foods. It is therefore imperative to avoid:

◆ Roquefort, Stilton and other blue-veined cheeses
◆ unpasteurised cheese such as Camembert and Brie or dairy products including goat and sheep products
◆ liver pâté of any type
◆ meals that are ready-cooked, and kept cold, but not frozen, and are designed to be eaten cold or reheated at home. Preferably avoid them altogether, or cook them until they are piping hot to kill off the listeria
◆ undercooked meat of any description
◆ pre-prepared salads

- soft ice-cream from a machine
- food that is past its use-by date

### Salmonella

This is a bacteria responsible for more food poisoning than any other, and manifests itself in sickness and diarrhoea. Poultry and eggs are probably the most common foods to be contaminated with salmonella, but thorough cooking often eliminates it.

- Don't eat anything that contains raw or uncooked egg, and don't forget less obvious foods like mousse and mayonnaise.
- Only eat eggs that have been cooked so thoroughly that the egg yolk is hard.
- Always wash your hands thoroughly if you have been touching raw meat, especially poultry.
- Don't let raw meat come into contact with any other food. This includes any spillage that may occur in the fridge.
- Use a special board to prepare meat and poultry, kept only for that purpose. Scrub it very thoroughly with hot water after use, and do the same with any surface touched.
- Cook all meat and poultry thoroughly so that the bacteria are destroyed.

### Toxoplasmosis

This is again a flu-like illness, which is caused by an infection by the bug called *Toxoplasma gondii*, sometimes found in raw meat, especially lamb, and also in cat faeces. As it can affect the unborn child it is important to take precautions.

- Never eat undercooked or raw meat.
- Wash your hands thoroughly after preparing meats.
- Wash all food preparation surfaces with very hot water or bleach.
- Clean and scrub all vegetables thoroughly to ensure that all soil and dirt is removed. If cats have soiled the earth, food can be contaminated.
- Don't let your cat have kittens at the time you plan to be pregnant, as kittens carry toxoplasmosis.
- Clear up cat mess with boiling water or bleach.

## *Current Thinking on Nutritional Supplements*

There is broad medical agreement that supplements containing 400 µg of folic acid and possibly vitamin B12 should be taken for four months prior to conception, until the end of the twelfth week of pregnancy, in order to prevent neural tube defects. However, opinions vary about what to do after that.

If you are eating an exceptionally healthy diet, which includes organic produce, and drinking very little tea, coffee or alcohol, then the chances are that you will be getting many of the nutrients that you and your baby need. However, if you have a poor appetite, have an unplanned pregnancy, or have not been eating very well, then as a precaution it would be advisable to take a multi-vitamin and mineral supplement, without animal vitamin A (retinol), each day anyway. It is far better to err on the side of caution.

Additionally, recent research shows that it may be advisable for some women to take supplements of evening primrose oil and marine fish oil for the last three months of pregnancy and during breast-feeding. Another study on breast-feeding mothers using Efamol evening primrose oil from between two to eight months of feeding, showed improved levels of essential fatty acids at a time when the natural supply in the milk would be tailing off.

Knowing that you can influence the health prospects of your new child may be rather daunting. There are countless rewards, though, to be had if you prepare your body for pregnancy and look after yourself to the best of your ability whilst pregnant. Creating a new little person is such a miracle, it's important to ensure that you are well enough to savour it, and that you do all in your power to enhance the miracle rather than damage it inadvertently.

*See also*: Recommended Reading List (*Healthy Parents, Healthy Baby*) and References.

# PREMENSTRUAL SYNDROME

Premenstrual syndrome, or PMS as it is more commonly known, is a collection of symptoms that occur up to two weeks before the menstrual period and tail off as bleeding begins. For many women it brings with it fear, misery and incapacitation. Sufferers often describe it as the Jekyll and Hyde syndrome, which comes upon them relentlessly at a similar time each month.

One of the difficulties of PMS is that it is not a syndrome which shows up under the microscope. Furthermore, despite the fact that women have been suffering for centuries, to this day doctors are unable to agree on the cause. Whilst some schools of thought class it as a hormone imbalance, others feel that it is associated with brain chemical metabolism, or indeed is actually all in the mind!

The WNAS has spent many years researching the premenstrual syndrome, and our conclusions show that although all of these hypotheses are partially correct, the underlying factor is related to nutritional and lifestyle inadequacies which, once corrected, result in relief from symptoms within a matter of months for over 90 per cent of sufferers.

## What Are the Symptoms?

The symptoms of PMS are always cyclic, and there are some 150 variations. The most common 'mental' symptoms include anxiety, irritability, mood swings, nervous tension, depression, confusion, forgetfulness, crying and loss of libido. Some of the most common physical symptoms include breast tenderness, headaches, cravings for sweet food, abdominal bloating and fatigue.

According to one WNAS survey, 73 per cent of women of child-bearing age suffer with PMS, and over half of all sufferers have experienced suicidal feelings at some time premenstrually. In addition many women report feeling violent and aggressive during their premenstrual phase, lashing out physically, and verbally abusing their partners and children. Productivity at work is affected by as many as five days per month, and working sufferers often organise their calendar around this monthly nightmare.

## Judy's Story

Judy, a thirty-six-year-old mother of two, had been working part-time as a secretary until she was knocked sideways by her uncontrollable PMS.

*I didn't suffer from PMS until my second child was born. I didn't realise what* the problem was. I knew that PMS could cause bloating and breast tenderness, but I thought the other symptoms were in my head—I thought I was going mad.

I'm normally a calm person but for two or three days a month I became a madwoman—especially at night when I couldn't sleep. I'd scream, swear, smash milk bottles and slam doors. My physical strength was frightening. I'd rip towels apart, and once I tied a nylon comb into a knot. I felt my brain was going to burst. I'd even punch and kick my husband, Robert, when he was asleep. I tried to slash my wrists and, when I took an overdose of tranquillisers, I bit right through Robert's thumb as he was trying to get them out of my mouth. I just couldn't control my emotions. I'd pinch myself until I was bruised, cut my skin with glass and bang my head against the wall, then spend hours crying.

I felt ugly and worthless, convinced my husband didn't love me. But he didn't know what to do with me. Confused, he'd just sit and stare into space while I was ranting. When I yelled the kids huddled in bed together, crying, and sometimes my husband had to take them out at night to get them away from me. Then when my son Steven was eleven he developed pains in his stomach and a twitch in his eye. He was referred to a child psychologist. During the fifth visit Steven announced, 'I'm scared Mummy's going to kill herself, or leave me!' I felt awful. I thought 'I've done this to him'. I knew then I needed help.

By chance, a few days later I read about a woman with PMS who'd stabbed her husband and for the first time I realised just how extreme PMS could be. When I read she was cured by diet I was disappointed, as I'd tried the popular remedies like evening primrose oil and vitamin B6 and they hadn't helped. I didn't see a doctor as I didn't want to admit I wasn't in control, but Robert urged me to try the diet, so I contacted the WNAS. They told me I was one of the worst cases they'd had—I had every symptom of PMS.

They put me on a diet of fresh fruit and veg, meat, fish, corn and rice, plus nutritional supplements. I could drink only mineral water or herbal tea. It was tough but worth it. At the end of the third month I wrote in my diary: 'No PMS!' I was finally free after ten years of hell.

I began re-introducing foods to check my reaction and that's when I found caffeine had been the culprit. I used to drink six to eight cups of coffee a day, and I craved chocolate before a period.

I haven't had PMS since. I feel I've been reborn—the diet saved my marriage and my kids. We're all so close now, but I really believe if I hadn't had help, Brian would have left with the kids and I'm sure I'd have committed suicide. PMS would have killed me one way or another. I've taken up amateur dramatics again. I'm now writing a book about my experiences in the hope it'll save other women from the same nightmare.

## What Causes It?

A hormonal cycle requiring production of oestrogen and progesterone by the ovaries is necessary for the development of PMS.
However, contrary to early theories, there is rarely a lack of either
of these two hormones in the average PMS sufferer.

Research has shown us that over 50 per cent of women with
PMS have low levels of magnesium, which is a mineral vital for
normal brain chemical metabolism, hormone function and smooth-
muscle control (the uterus and the gut are both smooth muscles).
Other nutrients like B vitamins, zinc and essential fatty acids may
also be in short supply.

Women often go through episodes in their lives that place extra
nutritional demand on their bodies. Pregnancy and breast-feeding
are two classic examples, where Mother Nature has deemed that
the baby is served with nutrients first in order to develop and the
mum is second in the queue. Therefore symptoms of PMS commonly get worse after pregnancy or weaning, or indeed may occur
for the first time in a mother who is suffering with nutritional
depletion.

Our bodies have very specific nutritional requirements. Just as
our cars would not run well lacking oil or petrol, the brain will not
be able to send out correct messages, and hormones will not be
produced in adequate amounts at the appropriate time of the cycle,
when levels of important nutrients are at a low ebb.

The WNAS programme, which successfully helps the majority
of women over their PMS, is designed to redress the balance, by
putting back into the body what time and nature have taken out.
In the short term it will undoubtedly involve making certain
dietary sacrifices until nutritional levels have been restored and
symptoms abated, but the general consensus is that the medium-
to long-term plan is immensely enjoyable.

In addition to making dietary changes, the WNAS programme
consists of taking regular exercise, and scientifically based supplements (at least in the short term) that act as a nutritional prop.

# What Your Doctor Can Do

Although many experts now believe that the nutritional approach to PMS is the best first-line treatment, the majority of doctors remain uneducated. According to a WNAS survey, 92 per cent of general practitioners have little or no nutritional training. Therefore what is on offer from your doctor is likely to be more drug or hormone oriented.

## Hormone treatments

Many of the hormone treatments for PMS were designed on the premise that this syndrome was associated with a lack of a particular hormone, but research over the last decade had shown that this is not so. However, when artificial hormones either abolish or suppress normal hormone function, it is likely that they may influence PMS symptoms. Whilst some hormone treatments may suppress symptoms, they do not address the root cause and thus alleviate symptoms in the long term. Additionally, most hormone treatments produce significant side effects, presenting the sufferer with additional hurdles.

- ◆ **Progesterone.** This is one of the two main hormones produced by the ovaries, and is used by many doctors as a pessary inserted into the vagina. It was once one of the commonest medical treatments for PMS, and yet only one of many studies on progesterone suppositories has shown only a small benefit in PMS.
- ◆ **Synthetic progesterone.** Known as progestogens, this is taken by mouth and has been shown to have modest success in two out of four clinical trials.
- ◆ **Oestrogen implants.** These are inserted under the skin of the abdomen by a small surgical procedure. Implants are not without side-effects, however, and in cases where these occur women have to wait for the implant to wear off—which can further add to their existing burden of symptoms. For women who still have their uterus, the hormone progesterone must also be taken in conjunction with oestrogen in order to prevent the risk of cancer of the uterus. Implants are best reserved for older women with PMS symptoms who are also approaching the menopause.
- ◆ **Hormone injections.** These are now on offer to some women,

but once again they can often precipitate side-effects which have to be lived with until the effect of the injection wears off, usually three months at least.

♦ Other hormone-related products. Danazol and Bromocriptine are powerful agents that are not suitable for long-term use. Danazol, for example, suppresses ovulation and may bring side-effects of hair growth and deepening of the voice.

### The oral contraceptive

This can improve PMS symptoms in some, but in others it makes matters worse or has no effect at all. Perhaps a useful treatment for mild PMS in younger women.

### Diuretics

Water pills have been popular treatments in the past. However, many of the older preparations lead to loss of important minerals that may already be in short supply. Spironolactone, a newer type of diuretic, has been shown to be moderately helpful with water retention, but is not recommended by the manufacturers for long-term use in younger women. The good news, however, is that most of the symptoms of fluid retention respond to dietary adjustments anyway, especially salt restriction, within a few months.

### Antidepressants

These are not regarded as an appropriate treatment for PMS, but some of the newer preparations may be helpful for severely depressed or suicidal women.

### Vitamin B6

Pyridoxine is prescribed by some doctors, but has not been shown to be consistently effective in clinical trials. PMS is a multi-factorial condition that is unlikely to respond to one single nutrient in the long term.

### Efamol (evening primrose oil)

Efamol has been shown to be effective in clinical trials for pre-menstrual breast tenderness. It needs to be taken every day of the cycle at a dose of between 2–4 g per day, for at least four months.

## *What You Can Do*

Here are some simple dietary recommendations.

◆ Never miss a meal. You will need to eat little and often in order to maintain optimum blood sugar levels, and to keep a constant supply of good nutrients flowing through to the brain and the nervous system.

◆ In your premenstrual week, your kilojoule requirements increase by up to 2100 additional kilojoules per day. In order to avoid dips in blood sugar, and temptation to eat chocolate or other processed sweet food, you will need to eat both a mid-morning and a mid-afternoon snack as well as your breakfast, lunch and dinner.

◆ Ensure you have a daily salad, three portions of vegetables— including one green leafy vegetable, which is particularly rich in magnesium and iron—and at least three portions of fruit per day.

◆ Aim to eat three portions of oily fish per week—mackerel, herring, salmon, pilchards and sardines are all good examples. These can be eaten fresh—or tinned for convenience—with a salad at lunchtime.

◆ If you follow a vegetarian diet ensure you eat plenty of vegetarian protein each day—unsalted nuts, seeds, beans, lentils, peas, brown rice, soya bean products and sprouted beans.

◆ Eat some protein with your lunch and again with your dinner— chicken, fish, lean meat, low-fat cheese, eggs or a vegetarian protein.

◆ Avoid caffeine in the form of tea, coffee, cola or chocolate and chocolate drinks. Do not drink more than two decaffeinated drinks per day as they contain other chemicals called methylxanthines that can aggravate other symptoms. Use alternatives like Rooitea, which is a tea lookalike, other herbal teas or coffee substitutes like Ecco, Caro and dandelion coffee.

◆ Sodium salt and salty food should be avoided as salt tends to drag fluid into the cells and can make you feel bloated. You can use a potassium-rich salt substitute in small amounts, or fresh herbs, garlic, ginger, spices and black pepper to flavour your food.

◆ Instead of eating foods that contain a large amount of sugar, like cakes, biscuits, puddings, chocolate and sweets, aim to eat intrinsically sweet foods, like dried or fresh fruit, nuts and seeds, as these are much more nutritious. The PMS diet is not a weight-loss diet, and so it is acceptable to eat wholesome cakes and biscuits. You will find a further selection of menus and recipes in our *Beat PMS Cookbook*.

◆ Keep your dairy consumption down to the equivalent of milk in your cereal, milk in your drinks and one other serving of dairy per day, like yoghurt or cheese.

◆ Concentrate on eating a diet rich in the minerals magnesium, iron, zinc and chromium, and vitamins B, C, E and essential fatty acids. For details about rich sources of these nutrients refer to the Nutritional Content of Foods.

### Constipation, *abnormal wind and bloating*

It is best to avoid products that contain phytic acid such as wheat and bran and, in some extreme cases, oats, barley and rye, for an initial period of at least six weeks. If you suffer with constipation take 2 tablespoons of linseeds with your breakfast cereals each day. You may also need to take some additional supplements of magnesium—up to 800 mg per day. Magnesium needs to be taken to gut tolerance level as eventually it will cause diarrhoea. See Constipation, Abdominal Wind and Bloating, plus refer to the Menu for Irritable Bowel Syndrome.

### Migraine headaches

Women commonly experience cyclical migraine headaches, which are sometimes associated with diet. Root or crystallised ginger taken as the headache begins often helps to relieve symptoms. There are also a number of foods associated with migraine headaches which you can read about under that heading.

### Other causes

Thrush, fatigue, craving for sweet food, acne, eczema, loss of libido and panic attacks often occur premenstrually. Details of how to overcome these problems can be found in the relevant sections. See Candida and Thrush, Fatigue and Chronic Fatigue Syndrome, Food Craving, Acne, Eczema, Libido, Loss of, and Anxiety. See also the menus for PMS, Fatigue, Sugar Craving and Acne.

## Exercise

You will need to do three or four sessions of exercise per week, to the point of breathlessness. Following aerobic exercise, when the heart increases its number of beats per minute, the brain releases chemicals called endorphins, which raise mood and energy levels, and influence the hormones positively.

Cycling, swimming, brisk walking, jogging, skipping, racquet sports, gym work or a workout are all suitable forms of exercise. Choose the sort of exercise you will enjoy, and make yourself an exercise schedule that fits in with your lifestyle. If you cannot easily get out of the house to exercise, try using an exercise video at home.

## Nutritional Supplements

In the short term at least, until the symptoms are well under control, it is likely that you will need to take some nutritional supplements to speed up your recovery. There are a few scientifically based supplements which we recommend at the WNAS which have been through properly conducted clinical trials.

◆ Use a magnesium-rich multi-vitamin and mineral preparation which also contains B vitamins and zinc. Severe sufferers will need to take supplements with breakfast and with lunch, making a total of at least two tablets every day of the cycle.

◆ To help patients suffering with premenstrual cravings for food, and in particular sweet snacks like chocolate, we have found supplements containing the minerals chromium, magnesium and B vitamins particularly helpful, as all of these nutrients have been shown to be necessary for normal blood sugar control. These supplements should be taken on an empty stomach before lunch, and if symptoms are severe they may also be taken either before breakfast or the evening meal, depending on the time of day the cravings are at their worst.

◆ Efamol Evening Primrose Oil has been shown to be extremely effective in helping to alleviate premenstrual breast tenderness and eczema. It is the only form of evening primrose oil that has been subjected to extensive research, and is recommended by the WNAS as part of their programme at a dose of between 6 and 8 x 500 mg capsules per day. The dose should be split between breakfast and lunch, and taken over four months.

| PROBLEM | SUPPLEMENT | DAILY DOSAGE | AVAILABLE FROM |
|---|---|---|---|
| PMS | A,H,C,D PMT | 2 tabs | Chemists, health-food shops |
| Breast problems | Efamol/Efamast evening primrose oil, natural vitamin E | 4–8 500 mg capsules 400 IUs | Chemists, health-food shops |
| Extreme nervous tension, drug withdrawals | High-potency vitamin B complex | 1–2 tabs | Health-food shops |
| Sugar cravings | Bio magnesium | 1–2 tabs | Health-food shops, chemists |
| Eczema | Efamol/evening primrose oil | 4–8 mg tabs | Chemists, health-food shops |
| Dry, rough skin/ dandruff | Cold-pressed linseed oil | 2 tbsp with fruit at night | Health-food shops |
| Period pains/ palpitations/ insomnia | Magnesium tablets | | Health-food shops and chemists |

## Complementary Therapies

Herbal medicine may be useful in helping to normalise hormone levels. Herbs such as black cohosh, damiana, raspberry leaf, vitex agnus castus, wild yam and dong quai are all used to correct hormone levels. Herbal 'tranquillisers' like Hypericum or Nervaids, a combination of soothing herbs, may help to reduce symptoms of anxiety, irritability and nervous tension.

Cranial osteopathy is a particularly good method of getting your body into correct balance. Tension in the neck and back, or trauma following childbirth, can prevent the body from functioning normally. If you have had a neck or back injury or feel this is a weak area, it may be worth having a consultation with a cranial osteopath. Unlike ordinary osteopathy, this form of treatment is extremely gentle and relaxing. To find the address of your nearest practitioner, contact the Australian Osteopathic Association (see Useful Addresses, Appendix V).

Acupuncture and acupressure are two valuable ways of helping to return your body to normal function. These traditional Chinese methods can be used at two levels, self-help with acupressure which involves finger pressure, or acupuncture, with needles, which should be administered by a qualified practitioner. Acupuncture is particularly valuable for stubborn, chronic and severe problems. For details of your nearest qualified practitioner contact the Acupuncture Association of Australia (see Useful Addresses, Appendix V).

Massage is a lovely way of helping to relax your mind and body, and is easily accessible and inexpensive. You could either treat yourself to a massage, or persuade your partner or a friend to volunteer their hands, or you could literally reach many parts yourself. Aromatherapy massage oil makes the massage extra soothing. Try using a combination of ylang-ylang, clary sage and neroli.

A combined programme of diet, exercise and scientifically based nutritional supplement has been shown to be the most effective approach to overcoming symptoms of PMS. Following these recommendations is likely to help you over your PMS and to leave you feeling better than you have felt for some time.

Further information about the WNAS programme for PMS can be found in our books *Beat PMS Through Diet*, and *Beat PMS Cookbook*. Details of these and other books can be found on the Recommended Reading List.

........................................................................

## Eleanor's Story

Eleanor was a thirty-two-year-old wife and mother of two who worked as a nanny in Surrey. Her PMS began after the birth of her second daughter, and the final straw came when she was found screaming and naked in the road in the middle of the night by her husband. She was unable to control her behaviour before her period, and as a result her relationship with her husband and children was severely threatened.

*I felt as if an alien had taken over my body each month, as I struggled to control my raging temper and mood swings. I was a real Jekyll and Hyde. I am usually pretty laid back and sociable, but about ten days before my period I'd turn into a 'hag from hell' and refuse to go out of the house. I was also plagued by headaches and water retention. I'd snap and shout at my husband and the children for no real reason. I began throwing plates, and wrote off a car. I was lucky I didn't kill myself, but things got so bad I did seriously contemplate suicide.*

*My husband read an article about the WNAS and phoned them in desperation. I reluctantly went with him to a consultation at their clinic, during which time a programme was tailor-made for me. I changed my diet, took supplements of Optiv-ite and regular exercise, and within three months my symptoms completely disappeared. At first I was wary as I was sure it was a fluke, but to our utter delight I have remained symptom-free. PMS is gone and I've got my family back.*

*See also*: Depression, Breast Pain, Food Craving, What's Wrong with Present-day Diet and Lifestyle?, Nutrition is the Key to Health, Menu for PMS, Menu for Breast Tenderness. Plus Recommended Reading List (*Beat PMS Through Diet*) and References.

# PSORIASIS

Psoriasis is a common, often chronic, skin complaint where red patches of variable size are covered with fine scales. The patches, which are well demarcated, are found most commonly on the trunk or concentrated over the elbows and knees. Other areas that can be affected are the scalp, which becomes very scaly, shedding large amounts of dandruff, and the nails which may be thickened with scales at their edge or pitted by minute craters. The face is rarely affected. Very often the disease varies from month to month, with spontaneous remissions occurring. Some patients develop an associated arthritis. The affected skin is very active, growing at ten times the rate of normal skin and can contain a very high concentration of chemicals that are produced in situations where there is a lot of inflammation. Just what triggers this change is uncertain.

## Who Gets It?
Psoriasis affects 2 per cent of the white population, and is less common in populations originating near the equator. Some forms of the rash may develop in childhood, especially the form that looks like a series of raindrops.

## *What Causes It?*

◆ It may follow an infection such as a sore throat.
◆ It can run in families, and is commoner in smokers, especially when it affects the palms or soles of the feet.
◆ Deficiencies of folic acid, selenium, possibly zinc and sometimes calcium are known to occur, especially if the skin involvement is widespread and severe.

## *What Your Doctor Can Do*

A number of different medicines seem to help, although certain drugs can worsen psoriasis. Long-term use is usually the order of the day.

◆ Creams based on coal tar, like Dithranol, are smelly but effective. High concentrations burn the skin.
◆ Steroid creams and ointments can be used but are often limited if the psoriasis is widespread.
◆ Calcipotriol (Dovonex) and ketoconazole (Nizoral) cream and ointment are derived from vitamin D and are quite effective at reducing the inflammation and scaling of psoriasis. They cause less irritation and are less smelly than some of the tar preparations.
◆ Phototherapy with ultraviolet light is highly effective. UVA light is used and the patient given a dose of a medicine called apsoralen that sensitises the skin to light. The treatment is thus often called PUVA.
◆ Shampoos usually based on tar preparations are useful for excessive scalp scaling. Sometimes an anti-fungal shampoo (Nizoral) is worth trying, and oral antifungal agents are sometimes effective too.
◆ A powerful vitamin A derived drug, Etretrinate, is occasionally used.
◆ Powerful anti-inflammatory drugs or immune-altering drugs are now used for severe cases.

## *What You Can Do*

◆ Stop smoking. This can worsen psoriasis.
◆ Sunbathe. This is helpful in up to 75 per cent of patients. Some sun-beds may be helpful too (check with your specialist).
◆ Eat a diet rich in essential fatty acids. These fats influence skin

quality and inflammation. A high intake of the Omega-3 essential fatty acids is known to help psoriasis. Follow The High Essential Fatty Acid Diet. If you are overweight then you will need to lose weight as well for this to be effective.

- Take supplements of fish oils. Usually 4–6 high-strength fish oil capsules will suffice. It is the content of EPA (eicosapentaenoic acid) and DHA (docosahexaenoic acid) that you are interested in, not the vitamins A and D.

- Try avoiding wheat, oat, barley and rye foods. A recent report noted that 10 per cent of those with psoriasis may have evidence of sensitivity to these types of cereals. Generally exclusion diets do not seem to work well in psoriasis in the way that they do for eczema, but it might be worth trying to exclude these cereals for six to eight weeks to see if this helps.

- Try taking supplements of multi-vitamins, zinc and selenium. The first two may influence skin quality, and the requirement of all three may well be increased in long-standing widespread psoriasis. Zinc at a dose of 30 mg per day might be particularly useful for psoriasis affecting the palms and soles, and is known to help the arthritis associated with this skin condition.

## Complementary Therapies

Homoeopathy and herbalism are perhaps the two most worth considering. These therapies can be comfortably combined with both conventional and nutritional approaches.

# RAYNAUD'S DISEASE AND POOR CIRCULATION

Sometimes poor circulation is due not to furring up of the arteries but to a reversible spasm of the muscles in their wall. Typically this happens in the hands and feet. These extremities change colour, become cold and tingle. The skin changes follow a sequence of pale then blue then a dusky red. This phenomenon

was first described by a French physician, Raynaud, in the nine-
teenth century.

## Who Gets It?

Typically young women are affected. Both hands are usually
involved and there are a number of triggering factors and sometimes causative diseases. Some researchers have associated this
problem with irritable bowel syndrome and migraine, two conditions where spasm of muscles in the gut wall and the blood vessels
of the head may play a part.

## What Causes It?

Common trigger factors include:

- cold weather
- emotional upset
- trauma
- smoking a cigarette

Sometimes the condition is associated with other illnesses such as
arthritis, skin diseases, pressure on nerves in the neck (following
use of vibrating equipment, chain saws, for instance), in association
with an increased stickiness of the blood which may sometimes
follow an infection.

## What Your Doctor Can Do

- Mainly examine you for some of the rare underlying causes.
- Prescribe a vasodilating drug, but they are not usually very
  effective.

## What You Can Do

- Wear gloves. Obvious but effective.
- Wear a silk scarf around your neck.
- Regular physical exercise may improve cold tolerance.
- Stop smoking.
- Try some nutritional supplements. None are of proven value
  but the following might help:
  - Fish oils and plenty of oily fish in the diet (see The High
    Polyunsaturated Fat Diet).
  - Supplements of magnesium might help. They could in

theory reduce the tendency to spasm of the blood vessels.
◊ Supplements of nicotinic acid, up to 300 mg per day; try it as 100 mg three times a day. This form of vitamin B3 can cause a flush reaction so always take it after food other than on an empty stomach.

*See also*: Standard References.

# STRESS

More than half the adult population claims to be suffering from stress to some degree. It's not only the high-flying executives that are suffering, but exhausted mothers, the unemployed and the homeless as well. And it's not just 1990s hype either. A paper published recently in the *British Medical Journal* confirmed that women who developed breast cancer were far more likely to have experienced bereavement, redundancy, homelessness, violent crime or family crises within the past five years than their healthy counterparts. We also know from a study of Danish bus drivers that those who faced the worst traffic died earlier than their colleagues who drove country routes.

There is scientific evidence linking stress to certain diseases, perhaps not as a cause, but certainly as an underlying factor, although the nature of the link between stress and disease is not fully understood. These stress-related diseases include:

◆ high blood pressure
◆ headaches
◆ facial pain
◆ irritable bowel syndrome
◆ ulcerative colitis
◆ stomach ulcers
◆ infections
◆ rheumatoid arthritis
◆ anorexia nervosa
◆ asthma

◆ period problems, including irregular periods and PMS

There is a fine line between stress and distress. Professor Hans Selye, the founder of modern research into stress, described it as 'the rate of wear and tear on the body'. He distinguished between good and bad stress. Good stress can be reasonably healthy as it stretches us to capacity and keeps us on our toes. Dealing with challenges as they present themselves is good for our morale. However, when we get to the point of overload, the stress becomes bad. The product of modern-day lifestyle is that it leaves many of us feeling overwhelmed and under par. If these conditions continue for anything other than a short period of time, it can take its toll on our health.

## What Are the Symptoms?

The rational ones amongst us do not usually take on our 'case load' all at once; we don't ask to be overwhelmed, it just grows on us gradually. We collect our responsibilities as we go along. Perhaps we have been coasting along quite successfully, then a promotion comes along which demands more from us, and at the same time a close relative gets sick, or our partner gets made redundant, and then we find we are pregnant again and so on. Additionally, when asked to commit to a project some of us have not learned to say 'no'. And so we soldier on as martyrs, believing that we can manage somehow, until one day our body sends out the warning. Whilst this scenario is occurring we are snacking instead of eating properly and not doing much in the way of exercise or relaxation.

The most common symptoms include:

◆ disturbed sleep and early morning waking
◆ insomnia
◆ panic attacks
◆ palpitations
◆ headaches
◆ loss of appetite
◆ compulsive eating
◆ desire to increase consumption of alcohol
◆ excessive smoking
◆ fatigue

◆ irrational thoughts
◆ minor illnesses

The first warning for some of us could be a bout of flu, or the onset of headaches. Alternatively our digestive system or our energy levels could be affected. Were we to re-evaluate our runaway lifestyle at this point, and invest time in getting our body back in to shape, we may well be able to circumvent the health crisis brewing. Invariably, though, we get up from our sick bed, and go into the ring for the next round. Many of us feel that we have to soldier on, no matter what. There does not seem to be an obvious alternative. Women are particularly prone to this form of martyrdom.

And so we continue, until our body says 'no'. We all have both physical and mental limits, and the body can only tolerate so much abuse. It is a vicious circle. Because we feel so awful, usual tasks are more demanding, and looking after ourselves is even less likely at that point. When something goes wrong with the car the warning light goes on, and when the computer doesn't like the conditions it makes a noise or flashes a message, but our poor body fails to communicate its troubles. Most of us wouldn't recognise the body's signal anyway until it was too late.

We may not necessarily have a nervous breakdown, but we can develop a weakness in some area of our body as a result of an immune system dysfunction. Some of us develop migraine headaches, others get recurrent thrush, irritable bowel syndrome, panic attacks, depression, chronic fatigue or a nervous rash. The unlucky minority will simply have a fatal heart attack or develop a serious medical condition. New research reported in the *Lancet* show that people who bottle up their emotions are more likely to die early, and in particular to have heart attacks.

## What Your Doctor Can Do
◆ Eliminate the possibility of any underlying cause to your symptoms by giving you a physical examination, and performing routine tests to check your iron levels, thyroid function, plus checking for underlying infection or early diabetes.
◆ Suggest some counselling to help you sort out the stressful situations you face.

◆ If you are suffering with panic attacks, your doctor may prescribe a low dose of beta-blockers to help you cope with anxiety symptoms.
◆ Alternatively you may be offered tranquillisers, but these should not be taken for longer than a few weeks.

Whilst all this has been going on it is likely that many of us will have become regular visitors to our doctor's surgery, and have begun taking the 'appropriate' medication. So we are now treating the symptoms, and at best suppressing them. You might even get labelled as 'neurotic' if you are really persistent. What we actually should be doing at this point is looking seriously for the root cause of the problem and addressing it. Whilst some doctors are enlightened and may question you about your troubles or refer you for counselling, they are used to dishing out 'a pill for an ill'. They do not usually have the time in their short consultation to really find out what underlies your symptoms. (At the WNAS we take a whole hour for our first consultation in our clinics, and we have to be organised about using the time wisely in order to get the measure of the real problem.)

There is plenty of medical evidence to support the fact that persistent stress (distress) can affect us both physically and mentally. Let us look at the following case history to demonstrate the point.

....................................................................................................

## Bernice's Story

Bernice was a thirty-four-year-old mother of two who, despite her apparently normal life, was at breaking point through stress.

*My husband, a conservative, high-powered, executive, said I should have been able to 'pull myself together', but I was unable to. He wouldn't discuss my upset over the termination I had had after the birth of our last child, or the problems we were experiencing with our sex life, which was non-existent. I was so anxious and tearful, I honestly don't know how I got through each day. Everything seemed too much, I couldn't even bring myself to answer the telephone when it rang. The most frightening thing of all, which I didn't bring myself to tell anyone, was that I kept seeing 'little people' out the corner of my eyes. I knew they weren't there, but they seemed so real. I really thought I was going insane.*

Formerly I was such an organised and rational person. I have a very idealistic brain and usually like things to be just so. I used to entertain a lot and loved doing activities with my two children. I have many friends and lots of close family, but I couldn't cope with seeing them as I felt antisocial. One minute I'd feel violent and aggressive, and then I'd think morbid thoughts about dying. I also had chronic back pain and as well as the sleeping pills I took regularly, most days I took at least eight painkillers, which made me very constipated.

My doctor suggested that I got in touch with the WNAS, and in sheer desperation I did. My diet was overhauled, I was sent off to the cranial osteopath, and took Optivite and Efamol. Once my back was feeling better I started to exercise gently and was able to stop taking all the painkillers and sleeping pills. I found the WNAS programme hard to stick to for the first few weeks, but was determined to give it my best as I honestly felt this was the last resort for me.

It did get easier and within a month I was feeling considerably better. Miraculously the osteopath sorted out my back problem, so that I no longer suffered constant pain. My constipation cleared up and the 'little men' disappeared, thank goodness. After following the programme for three months my symptoms had vanished, and my husband felt that his wife had returned. I was relieved too. I hate to think what might have happened to me and to my family if I had not been pointed in the right direction when I was at such a low ebb.

## What You Can Do

Many of us have the ability to cope with near tragedy or disaster, and it is not until it is over, and the dust has settled, that we feel it is safe to 'fall apart'. With hindsight, the warning signals were all there and we could have reversed the situation had we come to our senses soon enough.

Here are some tips to help you next time!

- Make sure you have some sacred time for yourself: time to think, and time to switch off from your responsibilities.
- Tell your family how you feel, and ask for their support whilst you get yourself sorted out.
- If your stress comes from work, discuss with colleagues how you can make changes, or if you are self-employed you will need to re-evaluate.
- Try to get away, even if it's only for a few days. Sometimes we can see things more clearly from a distance.
- Learn not to take on too much—if you feel fully committed learn to say no.

◆ Prioritise your responsibilities and see if you can off-load or delegate some of the less important tasks.

◆ Eat regular wholesome meals and have a supply of nutritious snacks. Don't fall into the trap of missing meals and eating junk food or chocolate instead. Follow the recommendation for The Very Nutritious Diet.

◆ Take time each week to exercise—you should be doing three or four sessions of exercise per week, even if it's just skipping or a work-out to a video at home.

◆ Make time each day to relax formally—you will need 15 minutes, with no interruptions. Really switching off is an art, you may need some instruction or to read a book on the subject.

◆ Get your partner or a close friend to give you a massage, preferably using some relaxing aromatherapy oils like geranium or lavender.

◆ Watch an entertaining film or make time to read a good book.

◆ Make sure you laugh occasionally. Laughter is so good for us, and yet when we get absorbed with problems in life we forget about our sense of humour.

◆ If you can't see a solution to your current stresses find someone to talk it through with, or get some professional help.

## Complementary Therapies

When the symptoms you are experiencing are related to stressful events in life, the most effective thing to do is handle the stress—but it is not always that simple or instantaneous. As well as following the recommendations suggested here there are several complementary therapies that would be helpful. Massage and any method of relaxation would be good to incorporate into your lifestyle on a regular basis. Acupuncture will help to boost your immune system so that you feel more able to cope, and cranial osteopathy may help to ease the tension that has built up in your body as a result of being stressed.

There are homeopathic remedies to try, or even the Bach Rescue Remedy to help you cope with stressful moments. There are also some very effective herbal tranquillisers like Lanes Quiet Life which can be taken when needed, and do not have any addictive properties.

# THYROID DISEASE

The thyroid is a gland in the neck which produces a hormone that essentially controls the metabolic rate of all cells throughout the body. A fall in the production of the thyroid leads to an underactive thyroid, also termed hypothyroidism. An excessive production produces an increase in metabolic rate and is termed hyperthyroidism.

## What Are the Symptoms?

Symptoms of hyperthyroidism include:

- weight loss
- rapid pulse rate
- palpitations
- fine tremor of the hands
- increased sweating
- intolerance to heat
- increased appetite

Symptoms of underactive thyroid may cause:

- fatigue
- muscular aches and pains
- weight gain
- intolerance to cold
- slow pulse rate
- an elevation in blood pressure
- dry skin
- hair loss and a variety of other changes if the disease is prolonged
- changes in facial appearance, especially puffiness, which may be noticed by friends and relatives

## Who Gets It?

Thyroid disease is common and often runs in families. It can be associated with diabetes, rheumatoid arthritis and pernicious anaemia, and either an under- or over-active thyroid gland can affect over 1 per cent of the adult population. These disturbances occur more easily in women than they do in men. In women of child-bearing age menstrual disturbance, including premenstrual syndrome, may occasionally be due to an under-active thyroid.

## What Causes It?

- Antibodies against the thyroid gland are a common cause of an under-active thyroid gland and they also may lead to over-stimulation of the thyroid. This is termed auto-immune thyroiditis. This can be detected by blood tests which are different to the measurements of the actual level of thyroid hormone.
- An over-active 'nodule' in the thyroid.
- A virus infection which may produce a temporary rise in the production of thyroid hormone. This is often associated with painful swelling of the thyroid gland.
- Radiation treatment for an over-active thyroid gland. The thyroid may become under-active many years later.

## What Your Doctor Can Do

- Tests for thyroid function are very sensitive and will easily detect an over- or under-active thyroid gland.
- Tests for thyroid antibodies will help decide on the cause and best treatment available.
- Treatment for an over-active thyroid involves either:
  ◇ drugs to control the level of thyroid hormone
  ◇ surgical removal of part of the thyroid
  ◇ use of radioactive iodine to partially destroy part of the thyroid gland
- Treatment for an under-active thyroid gland involves giving replacement thyroid hormones usually as thyroxine and occasionally as triiodothyronine.
- Continual blood tests to monitor progress of treatment are vital. Complicated patients may require the services of a thyroid specialist. This is especially true for those with an over-active thyroid.

## What You Can Do

- Be a good patient. This is one situation in medicine where standard medical treatment produces excellent results.
- Do not take kelp or other forms of iodine. These do not boost

or lower thyroid function and may disturb the test that your
doctor wishes to do.

◆ If you are not making satisfactory progress, let your doctor
know. Especially in the treatment of an under-active thyroid,
hypothyroidism, the adjustment of the dosage of thyroid
hormone depends upon not only your thyroid hormone tests,
but how you feel.

### Complementary Therapies
Don't even think about it!

*See Also*: Diabetes, Rheumatoid Arthritis, Anaemia. Plus Standard
References.

# TONSILLITIS

The tonsils are swellings formed by white cells, blood vessels and
supporting tissues, which lie at the back of the mouth on either
side. They are essentially lymph glands of the mouth, and are
there to fight infection. Sometimes they become badly infected
themselves, either by a virus or a bacterium called *Streptococcus*.
These infections can also occur even after the tonsils have been
removed. Infected tonsils are common in childhood and should be
treated as influenza, although a number will require treatment
with antibiotics, most commonly penicillin, if bacterial infection is
suspected. Sometimes the tonsils remain enlarged though they are
not always infected.

Removal by operation is appropriate for enlarged, repeatedly
infected tonsils. If they are not infected, but just large, they can
still cause problems of pressure in the throat, discomfort on swallowing, and snoring! (Snoring is also related to being overweight,
high blood pressure, alcohol consumption or other distortions of
the upper airway.)

## What You Can Do

For enlarged, repeatedly infected tonsils, treat as for recurrent infections. For those who have enlarged non-infected tonsils it may sometimes be worthwhile trying The Simple Exclusion Diet. Sensitivity to dairy products seems to be the most likely situation in such cases, and avoidance for as little as a week may make a noticeable difference.

You can also follow the advice about supplements given in the section on Influenza, Recurrent Coughs, Colds and Sore Throats. To relieve the pain, gargling with aspirin is quite effective.

# ULCERATIVE COLITIS

Ulcerative colitis is a chronic non-infective disease, producing inflammation of the lining of the colon and the rectum. It is a relatively common disorder with about five to ten new cases per 100 000 of the population per year. Adults aged twenty to forty years are especially vulnerable, but children, including infants, may be affected.

## What Are the Symptoms?

Diarrhoea with blood and mucus are typical symptoms. Abdominal pain and weight loss are not as commonplace as they are in Crohn's disease. Often the symptoms start gradually but may be of sudden onset. Sometimes constipation is a feature if the disease is confined to the rectum; this is termed proctitis. In more severe cases there may be inflammation in other organs, causing arthritis, mouth ulcers, liver problems, eye pains and skin rashes.

## What Causes It?

As with Crohn's disease, there appears to be a mixture of genetic and environmental factors. The genetic element seems to be smaller than that for Crohn's disease. Some 10–20 per cent of sufferers have a near relative also with the disease. It is more common in some Jewish communities around the world. The possible environmental factors include:

- Infection. The bacteria in the colon are continually changing, and some relatively normal bacteria, present in the colon of those with colitis, have the potential to produce chemicals that could damage the lining of the colon. Whether they actually cause colitis is not clear.
- Allergy to foods. This is possible in a minority of adults. Cows' milk appears the most likely culprit. Intolerances to wheat and other foods are a possibility too (see below). In infantile colitis, food allergy is in fact the rule.
- An intolerance to some strong vitamins. A side effect of high-dose vitamin E in infants is colitis. We have seen a few patients experience abdominal pain with passage of blood in the stools after taking either vitamin E or a strong multi-vitamin preparation containing it. This is rare though.
- Not smoking cigarettes or being an ex-smoker. This is one of the great oddities in medicine. Several studies show that smokers are protected against ulcerative colitis. Ex-smokers, however, have a particularly high incidence. For them we cannot recommend re-starting cigarettes, but nicotine patches may be a possible therapy. We await further research on this.
- Following use of painkillers. These do not cause colitis but they may account for its aggravation. This applies to paracetamol and anti-arthritic drugs. Occasionally there may be marked sensitivity to aspirin and food containing salicylates. Such patients are made much worse if they take aspirin or are given a drug often used in colitis called sulphasalazine. If this makes the bowel condition worse, then a low salicylate diet is worth a try. This can occasionally lead to a complete resolution. Such a diet is complicated and requires expert management as many fruits, vegetables and spices need to be avoided.

## What Your Doctor Can Do

- Assess the extent of the disease, using a barium enema X-ray or colonoscopy (examination of the large bowel with a flexible telescope).
- Assess the severity of the disease from blood tests, frequency of bowel movements, the presence of blood in the stool and if there is a fever.
- Exclude the presence of any bowel infection, including home-grown as well as tropical infection.

- Prescribe drug treatment with:
  - ◇ Steroid by mouth, or in the form of an enema for those with disease confined to the last part of the bowel. Steroids are useful for controlling a flare up, but have no benefit as a maintenance therapy, so every attempt should be made to withdraw them from the patient once the disease is controlled.
  - ◇ Anti-inflammatory drug based on 5-aminosalicylic acid (sulphasalazine and related compounds). Again this comes as tablets or as an enema and is useful for maintenance therapy.
- Suggest hospital treatment, which may involve blood transfusions and fluids and specialised feeding intravenously.
- Recommend surgical treatment to remove a diseased colon or part of it. Cancer can develop in the colon usually after fifteen years of disease. Regular examinations of the whole of the colon are recommended for many patients with colitis, even if their disease is quiet.

## What You Can Do

- In theory there should be a diet or diets for colitis, but this has not really proved to be the case. There are a number of possibilities to consider, though it is probably best to discuss these with your specialist first.
- A diet free of cows' milk products and lactose is perhaps worth most sufferers trying at some stage. Calcium supplements are necessary if followed long-term.
- Ask your doctor about a low-salicylate diet for those made worse by drug treatment, or if there is a history of aspirin sensitivity (see Asthma, and Hayfever and Allergic Rhinitis).
- A diet avoiding foods that commonly irritate the gut, which include coffee, wholemeal bread, bran and other wholegrain products, corn, beans and other high-fibre foods. It may be useful to avoid these foods during an attack and when in remission. Even when the disease is not active, the bowel habit is often erratic, and this may respond to the avoidance of these or other foods.
- A diet low in sulphur-containing foods could work if there is a lot of foul-smelling wind due to hydrogen sulphide (bad eggs gas). These sort of compounds are found at a high level in those with active disease, and the drug 5-aminosalicylic acid inhibits

their production. It may therefore be prudent to avoid the main sulphur-containing foods which are: sulphite preservatives E220–227, wine and beer, bread, eggs and dried fruit.

◆ Take supplements if there has been significant weight loss, or you need to follow a restricted diet. The following may be needed:

  ◇ iron, if there is anaemia from blood loss
  ◇ multi-vitamin and multi-mineral, if there is weight loss
  ◇ folic acid, if on 5-aminosalicylate
  ◇ calcium, if on a dairy-free diet long term
  ◇ fish oils may help to reduce the inflammation slightly, and may reduce the need for steroids. They are perhaps worth considering if there is an associated arthritis and you cannot take anti-arthritic drugs

## Complementary Therapies

There is a real possibility that some herbal preparations might influence the degree of inflammation in the colon. Expert advice from a qualified herbalist is needed.

*See also*: Standard References.

# URTICARIA

Urticaria—also known as nettle rash—is an itchy skin rash, characterised by short-lived, sometimes severe, swellings called weals. It may occur as a one-off episode, or several episodes may happen over the course of a few weeks. Sometimes it is chronic, lasting for three or more months with the eruption appearing suddenly, then disappearing and changing from day to day. In these instances there is a strong need to try and identify the cause. The rash and irritation are due to the release of histamine and other chemicals into the skin. Allergies often play a part but are by no means the only cause. A severe form, where there are large deep swellings which may affect the lip, tongue or airways is called angioedema, may occasionally be life-threatening.

## What Causes It?

There are many possibilities to consider and often in one-off episodes no clear cause may be identified.

- A food allergy. Egg white, fish, tomatoes and cows' milk are known possibilities.
- A food intolerance reaction. This can happen with strawberries, artificial colours (tartrazine E 102 and Sunset Yellow E 110), the preservative benzoate (commonly found in fizzy drinks), salicylates in food, and shellfish.
- Reaction to a drug. Antibiotics, aspirin (a salicylate) and, rarely, others are all possibilities.
- Contact allergies to housedust and animal fur, saliva and, rarely, semen.
- Genetic factors, as this condition may run in families.
- Exercise can be a trigger, and this may interact with other triggers, especially foods.
- Exposure to cold and occasionally heat.
- Pressure may trigger localised urticaria.
- Infection, especially hidden parasitic infection causing chronic urticaria.
- Candida infection is another known, albeit rare, trigger.
- Insect bite or sting, jellyfish sting and, of course, stinging nettles.
- In association with various diseases.

## What Your Doctor Can Do

Investigations are only necessary for those with chronic urticaria (lasting three months or more), if the reactions are very severe or if there is a family history. Usually the likely trigger is decided from the history and an awareness of the events and circumstances preceding repeated attacks. Allergy tests are not very helpful but may uncover a food allergy or sensitivity to *Candida albicans* (thrush). Treatment, as a rule, is by use of one of several antihistamines. Many of these are now available without prescription. Their use is limited by drowsiness which is the main side-effect and by their inability to control all of the reaction. Many chemicals other than histamine are released in a reaction and thus antihistamines do not always control the reaction. Other drugs with antihistamine-like effects can be used, and adrenaline by injection is needed for the severe life-threatening reactions.

## What You Can Do

◆ Try and find the cause. Make a list of all activities, food and drink consumed, and any medicines or other pills (including vitamins) consumed in the 24 hours before an attack. Collect several of these, and go and discuss them with your doctor.

◆ Exclude common likely triggers such as all drugs, aspirin, foods containing artificial colouring agents, beverages containing benzoates, foods rich in yeast and yeast-derived beverages (all forms of alcohol except those that are filtered, e.g. gin and vodka).

◆ Take some supplements. Vitamin C at a dose of 1 g twice a day can halve the level of histamine in the blood after two weeks. So it may be useful for those with chronic urticaria. It probably won't replace a good antihistamine in the short term.

◆ Magnesium helps to stabilise the allergy cells called mast cells that release histamine and other chemicals. Supplements of this mineral at a dose of 300–400 mg per day combined with The Very Nutritious Diet might reduce the intensity of the rash after two or more months. Zinc may also help in a similar fashion (supplements of 10–20 mg) and vitamin B6, pyridoxine, is needed by the body's own enzymes that break-down and detoxify histamine.

◆ Be patient. It sounds terrible but many resolve spontaneously, disappearing as mysteriously as they came.

## Complementary Therapies

Again homoeopathy is perhaps the most promising. Homoeopathic preparations of bee sting and stinging nettle are available, and are worthy of use for symptomatic relief at least.

## Veronica's Story

For twelve years Veronica, a thirty-seven-year-old teacher, had experienced recurrent itchy red swellings on her face. Urticaria had been diagnosed but no cause had been found, though she herself was suspicious that there were a number of dietary triggers. In fact she felt better when following a high protein, high dairy product diet. Her rash had been so severe that she had used steroids in the past, but had stopped these.

A few simple skin allergy tests did not reveal any obvious potential triggers. It therefore seemed possible that she had a degree of salicylate sensitivity. These compounds are found widely distributed in a number of fruits, vegetables and yeast-derived products. She began a low salicylate diet and took supplements of vitamin C and magnesium for their antihistamine effects.

Over several months her skin reactions diminished, though occasional episodes still occurred for reasons that were not entirely clear. The general conclusion was that she was likely to have a degree of salicylate sensitivity though there is no specific test to confirm this.

# VAGINAL PROBLEMS

In women of child-bearing age the secretions of the vagina vary throughout the cycle. During the first part of the cycle, when the hormone oestrogen is predominant, the vaginal fluid is thin and almost watery. From ovulation onwards, which usually occurs at approximately mid-cycle, when the levels of the pregnancy hormone progesterone increase, the vaginal mucus becomes much more noticeable, and is considerably thicker and opaque. It is sometimes referred to as 'friendly' mucus, as this is the environment that sperm thrive in.

When the vaginal fluid deviates from this pattern, this usually signifies that trouble is brewing. Abnormal vaginal discharge and vaginal discomfort often indicate that infection is present and medical attention is needed. There is a variety of common vaginal complaints which can be overcome, provided adequate measures are taken.

## *Vaginitis*

When the vaginal cells stop secreting fluid, either because of infection or at the time of the menopause when oestrogen levels are falling, the vaginal walls and tissue naturally become dry, and sometimes itchy. Sexual intercourse then becomes painful, as there is no natural fluid being produced, possibly placing a strain on a relationship, and wrecking sexual enjoyment.

## What Your Doctor Can Do

♦ Prescribe some hormone cream to insert into the vagina.
♦ Suggest a course of hormone replacement therapy. (Refer to page 352 before making a decision about taking HRT.)

## What You Can do

♦ Concentrate on eating a diet rich in phytoestrols, naturally occurring oestrogen, as these have been shown to bring about the same changes in the lining of the vagina as HRT.
♦ Follow the recommendations for The Very Nutritious Diet, unless you are approaching or going through the menopause, in which case you need to refer to the recommendations on page 312 and the WNAS plans on pages 487–90.
♦ Use a vaginal lubricant in the short term like Replens or KY Jelly before attempting to make love.
♦ As well as vitamins and minerals, it is advisable to take herbal supplements of ginseng and dong quai which also contain naturally occurring oestrogen.
♦ Do daily pelvic floor exercises.

# Vaginal Infections

Apart from the falling levels of oestrogen at the time of the menopause, causing vaginal dryness, there are three main types of infection that cause vaginitis:

*Candida albicans*, which causes thrush; *Trichomonas vaginalis*, a sexually transmitted infection; *Bacterial vaginosis*, which may co-exist with other vaginal and sexually transmitted infections.

# Trichomonas Vaginalis

This is the name of the organism causing this common infection. It is estimated that there are 180 million new cases per year worldwide. In men infection is often without symptoms; in women, however, common symptoms include:

♦ vaginal discharge, which may be yellowish-green and frothy
♦ an unpleasant odour
♦ swelling and redness of the vaginal walls

◆ inflammation of the cervix may also be seen on internal examination which may cause spotting or bleeding between periods. Some women may carry the infection with relatively few symptoms, or it may be associated with other sexually transmitted diseases

## What Your Doctor Can Do

◆ There is good response to a single oral dose of metronidazole, 2 g. Do not drink alcohol whilst taking this medicine.
◆ Check for other infections.
◆ Screen your partner.

## What You Can Do

◆ Ensure your partner either uses a condom, or has been cleared as a carrier of *Trichomonas vaginalis*.
◆ If your infection is slow to clear, supplements of zinc, 30 mg daily, and a multi-vitamin preparation, may be helpful.

## Mary's Story

Mary had known for years that she had a number of food allergies. Mouth tingling and swelling occurred when she consumed a variety of foods, especially certain fruits and thus she was easily aware of the connection. Curiously one of her sensitivities was to avocado, an unusual but known sensitivity.

Her main complaint, however, was of vaginal irritation, which she had noticed was worse after intercourse. She had been carefully checked for vaginal infection, and this was not the problem. Furthermore, her husband always used a condom and so it seemed unlikely her irritation could be related to his semen.

There is in fact a botanical similarity between rubber and avocado plants, which she was aware of. It was suggested that she might be sensitive to rubber and that she change to using hypo-allergenic condoms which are now widely available. This appeared to improve the problem greatly. Unfortunately her wish to be desensitised to food, especially fruit allergies, could not be fulfilled, and it is likely that these will persist for some time.

# Bacterial Vaginosis

This was also known as *Gardenerella*, and is due to an infection with a variety of co-existing organisms. In this condition there is no inflammation of the vagina, hence irritation is normally absent. There is usually a whitish discharge which may have a distinctive fishy smell, due to the presence of ammonia. The odour may be more noticeable after sexual intercourse, because of the chemical effect of semen. Again, many women may have this condition without knowing as there are few symptoms. Recent research has shown that this condition is associated with an increased risk of:

- having a premature baby
- having low birthweight babies
- infections during pregnancy, after delivery, following a hyster-ectomy and after an abortion

Some women will need to be screened before conceiving, during pregnancy and before planned gynaecological operations.

Male partners may be carriers for similar bacteria, but transmission has not been proved.

## What Your Doctor Can Do

Prescribe antibiotic treatment, with either metronidazole or clindamycin. Both can now be given as vaginal preparations as well as tablets.

Screen both you and your partner for sexually transmissible disease.

## What You Can Do

Some women may be predisposed to this type of infection and may be helped by:

- Eating well. Follow the recommendations for The Very Nutritious Diet.
- Applications of plain live yoghurt into the vagina daily for two or three weeks.
- Avoiding alcohol and cigarettes completely.
- Taking supplements of multi-vitamins and zinc.

## Allergic Vaginitis

Believe it or not allergy is a possible cause of vaginal irritation. This should only be considered after infection has been excluded.

Curiously, one of the first reports of this came from a study of migraine in over ninety children. Not only did the headaches often improve following the exclusion of certain foods but ten of the eleven girls in the study who were observed to have a vaginal discharge also noticed that this complaint resolved. Sensitivity to wheat, dairy products and yeast-rich foods, both baker's and brewer's, seem particularly likely. It may therefore be useful to try an exclusion diet.

Finally, it is possible to be allergic to your man! A report from America (where else) revealed that some men's semen may have high levels of antibodies which react with the woman's vaginal proteins. Improvement will occur if the woman takes an antihistamine or if her partner uses a condom.

One of the women in this study noticed her vaginitis was worse after her husband drank beer, and allergy to brewer's yeast is not impossible. It may be possible to test for this using a modified skin prick test technique.

# Vaginismus

A minority of women experience this unpleasant condition, which involves spasm of the muscles at the entrance to the vagina. This makes intercourse or even the insertion of a tampon difficult, painful or impossible. In severe cases routine gynaecological examination may even require an anaesthetic.

## What Causes It?

◆ Anxiety about intercourse or the possibility of becoming pregnant.
◆ Following episiotomy—an incision made during labour to widen the birth canal.
◆ Psychological trauma following rape.
◆ In association with irritable bowel syndrome.

## What Your Doctor Can Do

◆ Discuss the problem and potential trigger factors with you. Understanding the workings of the sexual organs and how the problem occurs is very important.
◆ Perform a physical examination.
◆ Refer you for some counselling.
◆ Suggest the use of graded dilators which you can gently introduce into the vagina on a daily basis.

## What You Can Do

- ◆ Discuss the problem with your partner to generate more understanding.
- ◆ Prolonged foreplay may help to relax the muscles.
- ◆ Treat any irritable bowel syndrome. Resolving associated constipation is particularly important.
- ◆ Take daily supplements of magnesium, between 300–400 mg per day.
- ◆ Do pelvic floor exercises at regular intervals throughout the day.
- ◆ Make sure you take time out each day, 15–20 minutes at least, to relax formerly.

## Complementary Therapies

Vaginal problems need to be addressed by conventional means initially, and any underlying infection cleared. The strength of complementary therapies is that they are good at helping to boost the immune system, which then makes your resistance to a recurrence that much better.

Massage is particularly relaxing; you could even administer some self-massage to tight muscles with some almond oil, if you suffer with vaginismus. Acupuncture, herbal therapy and homoeopathy may or may not be helpful, but they are certainly worth a try if all else fails.

## Joanne's Story

Joanne, a fifty-four-year-old mother of four, approached the WNAS for help with her menopause problems. She had also experienced vaginal and pubic itching following treatment years before for erosion of the cervix, which still persisted.

*I had an abnormal smear twenty-nine years ago which needed attention. When I went to the hospital for a cauterisation I turned out to be pregnant. I noticed during the pregnancy that I had continuous itching around the pubic area and vagina and assumed that I had picked up some infection in the hospital. My doctor took swabs but could not find any abnormal organism and when the problem continued after the pregnancy it was felt it was hormonal. The doctor suggested it was worse before my period due to a rise in my body temperature.*

*Five years ago I saw a dermatologist who suggested it might be a form of eczema although I have never suffered with eczema before.*

*I read about the work of the WNAS, and I was recommended to seek their advice about my menopausal problems, as I was experiencing hot flushes, night sweats, palpitations and was generally feeling exhausted. I went along to the clinic and had a very thorough consultation. I left with a detailed plan for a modified diet, exercise and a specific nutritional supplement regime. I did not imagine that the vaginal and pubic symptoms would be influenced by the programme I was given, but I am pleased to say that everything has cleared up. I occasionally get a mild version of flushes when I am not practising my relaxation regularly, but I feel a million times better, and I'm delighted to say that after all those years the pubic itching and vaginal discomfort seem to be a thing of the past.*

*See also*: References.

# VARICOSE VEINS

If you read the section on haemorrhoids, which are the equivalent of varicose veins, but in the tail end, you will recall that veins contain valves, which shut off to prevent the backflow of blood. When these valves malfunction, a pool of blood collects, weakening the walls of the vessel, which eventually balloon out and appear swollen. The veins at the back of the legs and thighs are often affected, giving an appearance of a shrivelled bunch of black grapes, and a tendency to this often runs in families.

Varicose veins can also occur in the vulva during pregnancy which is usually due to the increased weight of the uterus, the size of the baby and the fact that blood vessels relax because of the pregnancy hormone relaxin.

Sometimes the blood in the veins may clot, especially if there is a superficial injury or skin infections; it may be associated with the oral contraceptive pill, and with smoking. This leads to further damage to the valves and worsening of the varicose veins.

## What Are the Symptoms?

◆ aching in the legs, which is worse at the end of the day
◆ swelling of the ankles
◆ episodes of thrombosis (blood clotting) with further pain and swelling
◆ eczema of the overlying skin (called varicose eczema)
◆ ulceration of the skin, if the varicose veins are severe and long-standing

## What Your Doctor Can Do

◆ Recommend support stockings which are not very sexy, but they are effective.
◆ Inject fluid to shrink the worst of the varicose veins, which takes several weeks to effect.
◆ Operate to tie off and remove the worst of the veins. Heavy support bandages are worn after the operation and support stockings may be needed subsequently until healing is complete.
◆ Treat any varicose ulcer, which includes leg elevation to reduce any swelling, a non-stick antiseptic dressing, compression bandage, antibiotics if infected and possibly low-dose aspirin.

## What You Can Do

◆ Lose weight if you need to.
◆ Follow a low-salt diet if ankle swelling is a particular problem.
◆ Take supplements of vitamin C, 1 g twice daily, with bioflavonoids, as these may help to strengthen the vessel walls.
◆ If you have a varicose ulcer, take supplements of multi-vitamins and zinc, 30 mg per day, which may aid ulcer healing.
◆ Avoid standing for long periods of time.
◆ Keep your legs elevated whenever possible so that the fluid can drain away from the varicose vein.
◆ Wear the support stockings, don't just keep them in the drawer!

## Complementary Therapies

Acupuncture, homoeopathy, herbal medicine and cranial osteopathy all have something to offer in their own way. Improving the flow of fluid around the body will help to unlock the areas of stagnation. Additionally acupuncture may also be able to help strengthen the walls of the vessels.

*See also*: Standard References.

# PART THREE

## The Nutritional Answers

# THE VERY NUTRITIOUS DIET

Each person's needs differ. Women are particularly likely to be short of certain nutrients at certain times in their lives, which affects not only their metabolic rate and their hormones, but also their mental and physical well-being. Inadequate nutrition and lack of exercise are two known ways of adversely affecting hormone function and energy levels, and of perpetuating common symptoms like mood swings, depression and headaches. The appearance of our skin, the health of our hair and nails, our hormone function and our general sense of well-being are all directly affected by our diet, lifestyle and environment.

There is also plenty of scientific evidence to show that there is a direct link between hormone function and what we eat. Japanese women, whose diets contain a large amount of soya protein (rich in natural oestrogen) and oily fish (rich in essential fatty acids), have far fewer health problems than women living on a Western diet. Women, who have changing needs throughout life, need to be aware of the real dietary rules that can greatly influence their quality of health and longevity.

Two essential parts of looking at diet are whether the intake is adequate in amount, and whether the balance is correct. Nowadays lack of intake is not usually a problem. The Very Nutritious Diet has been designed to provide a healthy diet, with a good balance of all the important nutrients, and the portion sizes should be adjusted according to your appetite and activity level. One major point worth noting about this diet is that it is supposed to be enjoyable, and can be adapted to individual taste. Use the recommendations as a basic guideline. Additionally, look over the Nutritional Content of Food lists, which begin on page 495, for other appealing foods to include in your diet.

## Food Allowances and Cooking Instructions

- ◆ Meat and fish. Always use lean cuts and trim the excess fat.
- ◆ Fried food. Use the stir-fry method with a minimum of oil, and keep fried foods to a minimum.
- ◆ Oils and fats. Use polyunsaturated oils, e.g. sunflower, rape, walnut and sesame. Polyunsaturated spreads like Flora are

preferable to butter. Small amounts of butter can be used on toast or crackers if preferred.

◆ Sugar and sweet foods. Keep sugar-rich foods to a minimum, and always consume after a wholesome meal. Options for cooking include fructose, concentrated apple juice and small amounts of honey.

◆ Bread. Try to incorporate a variety of grains into your diet as well as wheat including rye, oats, corn and rice. Health-food shops often stock a good variety of breads.

◆ Bran. Avoid bran and foods containing bran completely as it impedes the absorption of good nutrients.

◆ Salt and salty foods. Try not to add salt to cooking or at the table especially if fluid retention is a problem as it tends to drag fluid into the cells. We already consume too much salt.

◆ Fruit. Preferably fresh, although tinned in fruit juice is permitted. Aim to eat three portions of fresh fruit per day (one bowl of berries = one portion).

◆ Vegetables. Aim to consume three portions of fresh vegetables daily including one green leafy vegetable, i.e. cabbage, spinach, broccoli, kale, Brussels sprouts, etc. Where possible have raw vegetables in salads and raw vegetable crudités. Cook in the minimum amount of water, or steam if possible.

◆ Tea and coffee. Avoid caffeine and keep decaffeinated to a maximum of four cups per day. Ideally try some of the alternatives.

◆ Milk and yoghurt. Aim to use milk, preferably reduced fat, which is available from supermarkets now. Try to consume live yoghurt (preferably containing acidophilus and bifidus cultures). Aim to consume between 450–600 ml of milk per day.

◆ Cheese. A variety of cheeses are permitted, a portion daily if desired.

◆ Eggs. Preferably free-range may be consumed daily if desired.

## Sample Menu

### Breakfast options

A substantial bowl of cereal, i.e. muesli, oat or wheat based, or Cornflakes with added nuts, seeds and dried fruit plus a portion of chopped fresh fruit, yoghurt and semi-skimmed milk;
or

A bowl of porridge and a large egg boiled, scrambled or as an omelette, with sautéed or grilled mushrooms and tomatoes;
and/or
One slice of toast with polyunsaturated spread and sugar-free jam or marmalade

*Mid-morning snack*
See below.

*Lunch options*
A salad with meat, poultry, fish, egg, cheese, beans or nuts or a salad with jacket potato with filling, i.e. tuna and sweetcorn, baked beans and cheese
or
A bowl of soup, ideally home-made, vegetable based with either peas, beans, lentils fish or meat
or
Sandwich containing lean meat, fish, chicken, egg, cheese, etc.
or
Pasta with tomato and meat or fish sauce with salad

*Mid-afternoon snack*
See below.

*Dinner option*
A portion of lean meat, poultry, fish or vegetarian protein weighing approximately 175–225 g. Three portions of vegetables or salad. Root vegetables, rice and pasta are an optional extra, followed by a fresh fruit dessert

*Snacks and desserts*
- Fresh fruit
- A combination of dried fruit, nuts and seeds
- Yoghurt with fruit and nuts
- Raw vegetables with dips like hummus, taramasalata or guacamole
- Fruit, nut and oat bar/flapjack
- Cheese and biscuits
- Scone with sugar-free spread
- Yoghurt and fruit

◆ Baked apple stuffed with dried fruit

*Beverages*
◆ Moderate amounts of tea and coffee, ideally no more that two or three cups or mugs per day
◆ Limited amounts of decaffeinated drinks, as these contain other chemicals, no more than two or three cups or mugs per day
◆ Unlimited amounts of herbal teas and coffee substitutes—see The Caffeine-free Diet
◆ Unlimited amounts of fresh fruit juice, water (preferably filtered) or a combination of the two
◆ Instead of cola-based drinks or lemonade, regular consumption of the healthy varieties of fruit juice and mineral water. Try several until you find the ones that suit your taste

## Basic Dietary Guidelines
◆ Eat three proper meals a day.
◆ Always start the day with breakfast—it is the most important meal of the day.
◆ Plan your meals ahead, preferably a week in advance, so that when you go shopping you can make sure you purchase the correct ingredients.
◆ Eat wholesome snacks between meals to keep your blood sugar constant particularly in your premenstrual week if you are still menstruating.
◆ Avoid convenience foods and junk food which are high in sugar, salt or fat.
◆ Go shopping at least twice a week to buy fresh fruit and vegetables.
◆ Don't go shopping on an empty stomach as you may end up buying the wrong foods. Take a list with you and try to stick with it.
◆ Arrange to eat with family and friends as often as possible.
◆ Savour your food as you eat, and chew it well.

# THE CAFFEINE-FREE DIET

It is particularly important for people suffering with nervous tension, mood swings, irritability, headaches, breast tenderness or insomnia to avoid caffeine. Many alternatives are listed below but beware the withdrawal symptoms. In the first week of avoiding caffeine people often experience extra symptoms of headaches, anxiety, irritability, mood swings, insomnia and sometimes fatigue. These symptoms will pass within the space of a few days to a week, so do persist.

Follow the instructions for The Very Nutritious Diet but avoid caffeine in the form of tea, coffee, drinking chocolate, cola-based drinks and other products containing chocolate. Read labels carefully, as painkillers often contain caffeine.

Look out for alternative products to tea and coffee and other drinks which are available from the supermarket and the health-food shop.

- Herb teas. There is a wide variety of choices of fruit teas like raspberry and ginseng, lemon verbena, mixed berry teas, etc., and they are sold in single sachets so that you can buy and try without being committed to a whole box of tea bags.
- Rooitea. A very tea-like alternative to tea when made with milk but contains no caffeine, very little tannin and a mild muscle relaxant. There are a number of other teas available in the health-food shop that fit into this category.
- Coffee. There is Nature's Cuppa, Caro, Ecco and dandelion coffee. The latter comes in two varieties: the instant in a jar which is sweet; and the dandelion root which can be ground in a coffee grinder and stored in a jar. This is best used through a coffee filter or strainer either over a cup or through a coffee filter machine. It makes a very strong malted drink.
- Fizzy drinks. There are many sparkling drinks that do not contain caffeine.
- Chocolate. The bad news is there are no real alternatives, although some people find carob acceptable and this can be purchased in the health-food shop. Fresh fruit or dried fruits, nuts and seeds, which are intrinsically sweet, are a much more nutritious alternative.

# The Dairy-free Diet

The dairy-free diet is particularly indicated for people with allergies, eczema and asthma. Irritable bowel symptoms can be aggravated by dairy products as can skin problems, catarrh and arthritis.

Follow the instructions for The Very Nutritious Diet with the following modifications.

◆ Milk. There are numerous varieties of soya milk available, some more palatable than others. Vita Soy and Aussie Soy are good brands to try.
◆ Butter. Use polyunsaturated spreads sparingly.
◆ Oil. Use sunflower, safflower, or canola for cooking and oils like sesame, walnut, and olive oil for dressing salads.
◆ Yoghurt. There are some very acceptable soya yoghurts on the market now.
◆ Ice-cream. Use sorbet or soya ice-cream made from natural ingredients.
◆ Cheese. There is a soya version of cheese which is available from health-food shops. It is reasonably acceptable sliced with crackers. It does not seem to cook at all well, however.

*Note: Although soya is a rich source of calcium those following a dairy-free diet should ensure they have an adequate intake of calcium. It is advisable to refer to the calcium food list on page 500.*

# The High-protein Diet

A high-protein diet is particularly indicated for people who have a high energy output like manual workers or athletes, for those suffering with recurrent infection, or recovering from a period of weight loss.

Follow the directions for The Very Nutritious Diet with the following modifications.

- Have some protein at each meal.
- Include nuts and seeds, or eggs and cheese with your breakfast.
- Increase your protein portion size at your main meal from 175–225 g to 225–350 g.
- Eat plenty of high-protein snacks like cheese and biscuits, cheese and apple, and nuts and seeds.
- Consume between 600 ml and 1.2 litres of milk a day, and include eggs and cheese in your diet on a regular basis.

# THE TUNATARIAN DIET (VEGETARIAN PLUS FISH)

A tunatarian diet is particularly indicated for those who wish to avoid red meat and poultry, and those directed to a diet rich in essential fatty acids who do not wish to consume meat or poultry.

Follow the directions for The Very Nutritious Diet with the following modifications.

- Replace meat or poultry with fish, beans or eggs.
- Consume fish, beans or eggs every day.
- Eat plenty of nuts, particularly walnuts.
- Consume green leafy vegetables regularly.
- Use walnut, canola, sunflower or safflower seed oil in salad dressings.
- Consume at least three portions of oily fish per week, i.e. mackerel, herring, salmon, pilchards or sardines.

# THE HIGH ESSENTIAL FATTY ACID DIET

A diet rich in essential fatty acids is particularly suitable for some patients with cardiovascular disease, patients with peripheral vascular disease, patients with multiple sclerosis, patients with rheumatoid arthritis and patients with psoriasis.

Follow the directions for The Very Nutritious Diet with the following modifications.

- Use polyunsaturated rich soft margarine.
- Consume plenty of green leafy vegetables daily.
- Take marine fish oils, and use walnut, canola, sunflower and corn oils in your salad dressings.
- Consume game meat.
- Consume plenty of oily fish, such as herring, mackerel, salmon, pilchards and sardines.
- Aim to consume some game meat or oily fish daily.

# THE YEAST-FREE DIET

This is particularly suitable for thrush sufferers, those with an itchy bottom, bloated abdomen, cracking at the corners of the mouth, excessive wind, cystitis and often depression.

Two or more episodes of thrush and/or any other two symptoms certainly qualify you for the yeast-free diet.

## Food Allowances and Cooking Instructions

It is surprising how many foods actually contain yeast, and yeast itself is often used in the food preparation process, in which case it is generally marked on the label of the product. However, yeast is a fungus which grows on food, particularly leftover food, even if well covered. It is also fond of foods with an acid base like citrus fruits and vinegar, and of course foods that contain sugar.

Follow the instructions for The Very Nutritious Diet whilst avoiding the yeast-based foods and drinks listed.

Aim to avoid:

- All foods containing sugar or honey, as yeast thrives in sugary or starchy food.
- All bread, buns, biscuits, cakes, etc.
- Most alcoholic drinks. These often depend on yeast to produce the alcohol, especially beer.
- Citrus fruit, juices—only fresh home-squeezed juice is yeast-free.
- Malted cereals, malted drinks.
- Pickles, sauerkraut and chilli peppers.
- Blue cheese (Roquefort etc.).
- Mushrooms and mushroom sauce.
- Hamburgers, sausages and cooked meats made with bread or breadcrumbs.
- Yeast extract (miso and soy sauces, Bovril, Marmite, Vegemite).

# THE VEGETARIAN OR VEGAN DIET

Strictly speaking, a 'vegetarian' should strictly mean someone who eats only vegetable-derived foods, but a strict vegetarian is now more usually referred to as a vegan. Vegetarian is often usually used to describe somebody who simply avoids meat, fish and poultry, but this can be further subdivided.

Those who consume dairy products as well are known as lacto-vegetarian, and those who consume eggs as well as dairy products are known as ovo-lacto-vegetarian.

## Food Allowances and Cooking Instructions
Avoid refined carbohydrates as they are low in essential minerals and vitamins. It is advisable they should only be consumed in very small quantities by vegetarians and vegans. The intake of essential nutrients, particularly iron and zinc, may be borderline in some vegetarians and vegans, and this will only be further hindered by consuming refined carbohydrates.

Ensure an adequate balance of protein in your diet. A major

problem with vegetarian and vegan diets has been borderline or poor-quality protein intake. This is particularly true in those who have not taken care to learn the protein-rich foods or their combinations that vegetarians and vegans should eat. Protein-rich foods include nuts, seeds, peas, beans, lentils, wholegrains, brown rice, sprouted beans and soya bean preparations. Vegetarians and vegans should not rely heavily upon any one source of vegetable protein. In particular, they should not rely heavily upon soya protein, as it alone is not a complete protein.

If you are not a strict vegan, make use of other protein-rich foods. High-quality, well-balanced protein is found in eggs, which are also rich in iron. One or two eggs can be consumed quite easily per day and would be beneficial.

*Good protein combinations*
◆ rice with legumes, sesame or cheese
◆ wheat with legumes or mixed nuts and milk or sesame and soya bean
◆ corn with legumes
◆ mixed nuts with sunflower seeds
◆ sesame seeds with beans or mixed nuts and soya beans or wheat and soya beans

The addition of any first-class protein i.e. milk, or particularly eggs, may substantially enhance the protein value of the vegetable food. Not all members of the legume family are high in protein. Those that are particularly nutritious include mung beans, red kidney beans, haricot beans, butter beans, chickpeas, pinto beans, lentils, peas and split peas.

Sprouted beans may be more appetising. Soaking beans for 24 hours and de-husking them may reduce the problem of wind which occurs in some bean eaters.

## Avoid Foods That Block Mineral Absorption

Many foods contain substances which bind with essential trace minerals and prevent their absorption. Such foods include bran, unleavened wheat—particularly wholewheat as in pastry or when used as a thickening agent—tea, coffee, soft drinks and foods containing phosphate additives. Alcohol also causes increased certain losses of trace minerals. Iron and zinc absorption may be inhibited by the above foods and drinks. Accordingly such foods should be avoided or consumed in small quantities. It should never be necessary for a vegetarian or vegan to eat bran as there is plenty of fibre in other foods. Also tea should not be consumed with a vegetarian meal because of its powerful effect in reducing iron absorption. It is suggested, therefore, that tea consumption should be minimal, two or less cups per day, particularly in female vegetarians.

Ensure an adequate supply of mineral- and vitamin-rich foods. Usually if you are careful to balance the quantities of protein in your diet, and avoid mineral-depleted convenience foods, then your intake of trace minerals would, on the whole, be good. It is strongly recommended that vegetarians and vegans learn which foods are nutritious. The worst possible combination is a poor quality vegetarian diet together with a high intake of sweets, chocolates, and other nutrient-depleted foods.

## Vegetarian and Vegans in Special Situations

There are certain situations when a vegetarian or vegan diet may be distinctly inadvisable, or should only be undertaken if one has a very good knowledge of what a healthy vegetarian diet is. Particularly at risk are:

◆ infants under the age of one year as well as young children
◆ the elderly, pregnant or breast-feeding women
◆ people who are ill or who have nutritional deficiencies

Usually medical advice should be sought, in particular to determine whether any additional supplements may be required by people in such situations. Infants, for example, may frequently become short of iron on a strict vegetarian or vegan diet. Severe vegan diets may in fact lead to rickets in young children because of lack of vitamin D and calcium in the diet.

The nutritional requirements of pregnant and breast-feeding women must be met and a poor-quality vegetarian diet will often not satisfy the additional needs at these times. The specific advice about nutrient intake and the use of supplements in the preconception phase and pregnancy can be found in the relevant chapters. See Preconception and Pregnancy.

The elderly have a declining food intake and so the quality of their dietary intake must be very high in order for them not to develop deficiencies.

While there are certain medical conditions that would benefit from a vegetarian or vegan diet, patients who are ill or who have nutritional deficiencies should seek medical advice before embarking on such a programme.

## Food Allergy/Intolerance and Vegetarians/Vegans

Food allergies are increasingly common and the major foods that appear to cause trouble are wheat, milk, yeast and soya, many of which may be staple foods in a vegetarian or vegan diet. Thus if your health deteriorates after embarking upon a vegetarian or vegan diet, this may be because of inadequacies in the diet or the presence of food allergies or intolerances. On the other hand, certain aspects of vegetarian or vegan diets may be beneficial for people with food allergies or intolerances, in particular the high consumption of salads and vegetables. If you suspect you may have food allergies refer to the section on Allergy, The Simple Exclusion Diet, and The Strict Exclusion Diet.

## Vitamin B12

Many experienced vegetarians and vegans appreciate the importance of ensuring adequate vitamin B12 in the diet. The major source of vitamin B12 is meat. Other reasonably good sources include eggs, brewer's yeast and dairy produce. Only strict vegans may need a vitamin B12 supplement. However, anyone who develops vitamin B12 deficiency, should receive appropriate investigations to precisely determine the course of their deficiency and it should not be presumed to be due to dietary inadequacy.

## Sample Menu

*Breakfast*
Glass of orange juice
Wheat- or oat-based muesli with additional nuts, seeds, dried fruit, chopped fresh fruit
Toast with nut butter or low-sugar spread or marmalade
Mug of either decaffeinated tea or coffee, or herbal tea or coffee substitute

*Lunch*
Salad made with sprouting alfalfa and other mixed salad
Home-made soup or jacket potato with filling

## Vegetarian option
Cheese or eggs may be added, with a glass of milk
Fresh fruit juice, herb tea or decaffeinated coffee

*Dinner*
Protein and vegetable combinations such as:
Nut roast with baked parsnips, carrot and boiled spinach
or
Beanbake with mixed vegetables
or
Stir-fry vegetables and nuts or beans, followed by
Fruit dessert, i.e. baked apple, rhubarb crumble or apple pie

## Vegetarian option
Cauliflower and broccoli cheese with jacket potato
Fresh fruit mousse followed by herb tea, decaffeinated coffee or
fruit juice
Note: Pasta should be accompanied by protein as it is not suffi-
ciently nutritious by itself.

*Snacks*
There are many wholesome vegetarian snacks that can be included
into your diet, encompassing both sweet and savoury options.
Examples are:

- oat, fruit and nut flapjacks
- dried fruit, nuts and seeds
- fresh fruit and soya yoghurt
- raw vegetable crudités and dips
- nut butter on toast or crackers

# THE HIGH-FIBRE DIET

This is particularly useful for patients with benign breast disease, constipation or diverticulosis. Portion sizes according to energy levels and size.

## *Food Allowances and Cooking Instructions*

Despite the wide use of wholemeal cereal and bran, it is now recognised that the phytic acid content of these foods may impede the absorption of good nutrients and can also produce an antibody reaction resulting in worsening symptoms. Fruit and vegetable fibre are preferable as these speed up gut transit time, so avoid excessive consumption of foods containing wholewheat, wholegrain pasta and bran.

Concentrate on vegetables, fruit and salad and grains that contain low phytic acid like corn, rice and buckwheat.

## *Sample Menu*

*Breakfast*
Fruit juice, grapefruit or fresh fruit salad
Oat-based muesli or oat crunchy cereal
or
Home-made muesli with rice, corn, nuts, seeds, dried fruit with added fresh fruit, bio yoghurt and milk
or
Brown rice cake, Ryvita or oatcakes with nut butter or low-sugar spread
Decaffeinated tea or coffee or herbal alternative

*Mid-morning snack*
Raw vegetables with dip
Fresh fruit, dried fruit, nuts and seeds
Oat crunchy bar

*Lunch*
Vegetable soup including plenty of chopped fresh vegetables, peas, lentils and barley
or

Jacket potato with baked beans and cheese filling or tuna and sweetcorn
or
Salad with protein, i.e. meat, fish, chicken or vegetarian protein, cheese, egg, nuts, seeds, beans, lentils
or
Raw vegetable crudités and dips like hummus, taramasalata or guacamole

*Mid-afternoon snack*
Oat flapjack
Fresh fruit or dried fruit, nuts and seeds

*Dinner*
Portion of meat, fish, poultry or vegetarian protein
Baked jacket potato
3 portions of vegetables and/or salad
Fresh fruit or fresh fruit dessert like baked apple, fruit salad
Herb tea or decaffeinated tea or coffee

# THE LOW-SALT DIET

Sodium chloride—table salt—has long been used as a natural flavour-enhancer and preservative. Compared with the diets consumed by primitive man, we consume ten to fifty times as much salt and not all of us have had the ability to adapt to making such a change. It is now appreciated that high intakes of sodium salt may cause or aggravate a variety of different conditions, including:

- high blood pressure
- kidney disease
- heart failure
- liver disease
- fluid retention, especially in women
- patients on high doses of steroids
- certain types of asthma

Benefit may be experienced by many of those troubled by the above conditions if they reduce their sodium intake. Unfortunately, this is not just simply a matter of not adding salt to meals, or not using it in cooking. Some two-thirds of our sodium intake now comes from processed and prepared foods, rather than that which is added to the cooking or at the table.

## How to Reduce Your Salt Intake

1. Do not add salt or sodium bicarbonate when cooking foods. If cooking savoury dishes or vegetables, try adding herbs instead, to help give more flavour.
2. Do not add salt at the table. At first, food may taste a little bland or unexciting, without its usual spray of salt. After four to six weeks, your tastebuds should adjust, and food will regain its original flavour, and you may even develop a dislike for salty foods.
3. Avoid foods rich in sodium salt. As a rule, all fresh vegetables and fresh fruits are low in sodium and high in its healthy mineral counterpart, potassium. Many processed and prepared foods are rich in sodium. Often they will not give the sodium content, but if on the listed ingredients they include the words 'salt', 'sea-salt' seasoning, it should be avoided completely. Also, some additives, especially monosodium glutamate, sodium benzonte or any other sodium compound means the food should be avoided.
4. Avoid all foods in 'brine'—e.g. some tinned foods and tinned vegetables—as brine is simply salted water.

The following foods are high in sodium, and should not be consumed as part of a low-sodium diet.

- ◆ Vegetables. Baked beans, tinned peas, potato crisps, instant potato, salted peanuts, any canned vegetables (unless stated as being salt-free). Fresh vegetables have a low sodium content and can be eaten in abundance.
- ◆ Meats. Almost all preserved meats, including bacon, ham, corned beef, sausages, frankfurters, tinned meat and meat sauces, pork pies, sausagemeat, sausage rolls, pâté, meat or poultry pies, tongue.
- ◆ Fish. Tinned, frozen or cooked shellfish, including cockles,

shrimps, lobster and crab, unless alive and uncooked. Tinned fish, e.g. tuna, anchovies, salmon (unless stated to be salt-free).

♦ Cheese and butter. All types of cheese, salted butter. Foods made with cheese, e.g. pizza.

♦ Bread and grain products. All bread (unless stated to be salt-free). Other wheat products, e.g., naan, rolls, most crackers.

♦ Cakes, puddings and desserts may all contain moderate quantities of sodium, and if salt is an ingredient on the packet, they should be avoided.

♦ Breakfast cereals are low in sodium, unless it is stated as an ingredient on the packet. Allbran, Cornflakes and Rice Bubbles contain substantial amounts of sodium, and should be avoided. Most mueslis and shredded wheat are low in sodium. Nuts and seeds are low in sodium, unless it is added, e.g. salted peanuts.

♦ Condiments. Sauces and pickles should be regarded as being high in sodium, unless it is not listed as an ingredient. Many packet soups and canned soups are also high in sodium, and should all be avoided. Bovril, Marmite, Vegemite and Oxo cubes and similar savoury products are high in sodium.

♦ Baking powder.

♦ Soft drinks are low in sodium, except tomato juice, unless it is stated to be salt-free.

♦ Sugar and sweet foods. Sugars and sugar products, e.g. toffees, sweets, etc. contain small amounts of sodium, but should not be consumed in anything other than small quantities, as they themselves may enhance fluid retention in some people.

♦ Alcoholic beverages are low in sodium, but again should only be consumed in moderation.

## Sample Menu

*Breakfast*
Fruit or fruit juice
Low-salt cereal, e.g. puffed rice, salt-free Cornflakes
or
Home-made muesli using salt-free Cornflakes, puffed rice, dried fruit, sunflower seeds, nuts with chopped fresh fruit, yoghurt and semi-skimmed milk
or
1 egg, unsalted, with low-sodium bread or crackers, unsalted butter

and low- or sugar-free jam or marmalade
Decaffeinated tea or coffee with milk

*Mid-morning snack (if desired)*
Any unsalted snack from the snack list on page 444.

*Lunch*
Fruit juice if desired
Salad with low-sodium or home-made salad dressing with unsalted
meat, poultry or fish
Potato or rice or pasta cooked without salt
Fresh vegetables
Low-sodium bread or crackers
or
Home-made soup (salt-free)

*Mid-afternoon snack (if desired)*
Any unsalted snack from the snack list on page 444.

*Evening meal*
Grapefruit or avocado or home-made unsalted soup
Unsalted meat, fish, chicken or vegetarian protein like nuts, beans
or lentils
3 portions of vegetables or salad if desired
Low-sodium bread, roll or crackers
Herb tea or decaffeinated coffee

# THE GLUTEN-FREE DIET

Foods containing gluten are most commonly the grains wheat, oats,
barley and rye. Whilst those suffering with coeliac disease know
that they must avoid gluten, according to recent research there are
many pre-coeliacs or gluten-sensitive individuals who also would
do well to avoid gluten.

## Food Allowances and Cooking Instructions

Avoiding foods that contain gluten is not necessarily as easy as it sounds, for wheat in particular is used as a thickening agent in the form of modified starch in so many types of foods, ranging from yoghurts to sauces. In order to avoid gluten completely you will need to arm yourself with alternatives, and to read food labels carefully before making your purchases. There are plenty of alternatives, it is just a question of knowing what to look for.

### Bread

There are now many alternatives to ordinary bread, some of which can be purchased and others which you need to bake yourself. Health-food shops usually have some stocks of the alternative grain products. Rice cakes are also very acceptable. It is possible to make something that resembles bread using a combination of rice, corn, potato and gram flour.

### Pasta

Although you will need to avoid the pasta made with wheat, there are many reasonable alternatives you can try. Most of these are available from health-food shops or Asian supermarkets.

Rice noodles are available in a wide variety from supermarkets. There are wide, flat rice noodles that resemble tagliatelli, spaghetti-like noodles, and the very skinny variety that only need soaking in a covered pan in boiling water for a few minutes. You will probably find that these are cheaper than the alternative pastas available from health-food shops.

### Breakfast cereal

Any rice or corn cereals will be fine, even ordinary Rice Bubbles and Cornflakes from the supermarkets. Add some chopped fruit and some crumbled nuts, perhaps a few seeds and a little dried fruit to your cereal to make it a bit more wholesome, or make a museli using nuts, seeds, rice, corn and dried fruit. There are some alternative mueslis available, but they are usually very expensive for only a small packet.

*Home-made cakes*

If you enjoy cooking there are plenty of very acceptable biscuits, cakes, pastries, sponges and pancakes you can make using alternative flours. If you have never used any of the alternative flours before it may take you a little time to find the consistency that you like.

◆ Sponge. Brown rice flour is probably the best for making a sponge. Make it up to the weight given in the recipe by mixing it with a little ground almond and a raising agent (cream of tartar and bicarbonate of soda).

◆ Raising agents. As baking powder contains wheat, you will need to use an alternative. Either use a combination of one part bicarbonate of soda to two parts of cream of tartar, or use wheat-free baking powder.

◆ Savoury pancakes. These can be made with pure buckwheat flour, which is part of the rhubarb family and tends to be quite heavy, or buckwheat mixed with a little white rice flour, which is very light.

◆ Sweet pancakes. These are best made with a combination of brown rice flour, or ground rice and cornflour, purchased from a health-food shop or Asian supermarket. Use half cornflour and half rice flour to replace the normal quantity of flour in the ordinary pancake recipe.

◆ Breadcrumbs or batter. A crisp coating for fish or meat can be made with maize meal, which can be found in health-food shops. Coat the fish or meat with maize meal, then with beaten egg, and once again with maize meal. You can then bake, grill or even fry the food, which should emerge with a crispy coat.

◆ Biscuits. There is a variety of biscuits that you can make using brown rice flour, or ground rice, and ground nuts or coconut. If you make plain biscuits you can flavour them with lemon or ginger. Recipes for almond macaroons and coconut biscuits are very acceptable. and at the same time more nutritious than the average biscuit, as they are full of eggs and nuts. It is a good idea to make some and keep them in the freezer, so that you can take a few out when you really feel you need something sweet to eat.

There are many other flours that you can use in your cooking. Gram flour made from chickpeas, potato flour, soya flour, tapioca flour and millet flour are all good examples.

*Shop-bought cakes and biscuits*
Acceptable cakes and biscuits can now be purchased in health-food shops.

*Snacks*
It's nice to have something to crunch on when you are avoiding wheat. There are lots of corn products available, but do remember to read the labels, as some have added wheat. Try corn chips, crisps and wafers, and look in the Mexican section of the supermarket. Also, poppadoms are fine, and little mini spiced poppadoms are nice to nibble on or dip.

## Sample Menu

*Breakfast*
Puffed rice, Cornflakes, chopped almonds, sunflower seeds, raisins, chopped apricots, with a chopped banana, yoghurt and fat-reduced milk
Rooitea, or decaffeinated tea

*Mid-morning snack*
Gluten-free bread or crackers with nut butter or fruit spread with a glass of orange juice or milk

*Lunch*
Jacket potato with protein filling, i.e. fish, poultry, cheese or beans, with mixed salad
or
Home-made soup and salad
or
Fish, meat, poultry, egg, cheese and salad with gluten-free bread or crackers
Decaffeinated coffee or herbal tea

*Mid-afternoon snack*
Wheat-free cake or biscuits with tea, decaffeinated or herbal tea
or
Raw vegetable crudités with hummus dip and corn wafers

*Dinner*
Grilled or steamed fish with spring onions and ginger, zucchinis, carrots and snow peas
or
Chicken or nut and mixed vegetable stir-fry with rice noodles
Fresh fruit salad, fruit mousse or baked apple stuffed with dried fruit and nuts
Herbal tea or coffee substitute

# THE SIMPLE WEIGHT-LOSS DIET

This is a simple weight-loss diet which aims to achieve three things:

- a reduced intake of kilojoules
- a good intake of essential nutrients including protein, vitamins and minerals, and
- the avoidance or reduction of intake of common foods that are often associated with weight gain and certain health problems.

## Food Allowances and Cooking Instructions
- Meat and fish. Always lean, trim excess fat, remove skin and cook by grilling or baking.
- Fried foods. Ideally none, or use stir-fry method with the minimum of oil.
- Oils and fats. Use low-fat polyunsaturate spread, e.g. Flora Light—2 teaspoons per day—and one of oil, e.g. sunflower or canola, per day.
- Sugar and sweet foods. Ideally none, use artificial sweeteners. 1–2 teaspoons of honey per day may be allowed.
- Bread. Limited to two pieces of bread, white or wholemeal, per day. Use slimmer's bread without bran, if available.
- Bran. Do not eat bran, or foods or breakfast cereals containing it.
- Pasta. One portion of white pasta only and three of white rice per week.

- Salt and salty foods. Avoid, especially if fluid retention is a problem.
- Fruit. Preferably fresh, if canned then drain off the syrup. Eat three pieces of fresh fruit per day. A banana counts as two pieces.
- Vegetables. Eat fresh vegetables daily. Cook in the minimum of water and without salt if possible. Green vegetables are virtually unlimited.
- Tea and coffee. Allow a total of four cups (2½ mugs) per day of either ordinary or decaffeinated. No sugar allowed, use sweeteners.
- Milk and yoghurt. Use skimmed or reduced-fat milk and low fat yoghurt. (Allow a total of 300–450 ml per day).
- Cheese. Low-fat cheese only, e.g. Cheddar or Gouda, 75 g per week only.
- Eggs. Allow four per week. Boiled, poached or scrambled and not fried.

*Breakfast options*
One of the following:
A bowl of Cornflakes or Rice Bubbles, 40 g and milk, with fruit if desired
A bowl of porridge without sugar
A large egg boiled or scrambled, and bread/toast
One rasher of bacon, grilled, and two tomatoes
Sautéed mushrooms 50 g and toast or a small egg
One piece of toast and low-fat spread and low-sugar marmalade

*Lunch options*
One of the following:
A baked potato 175 g, no butter, and baked beans, sweetcorn, tuna/ham/chicken 75 g with onion/capsicum/olives and low-kilojoule mayonnaise or occasionally cheese.
A large salad, either green or made from cold rice with 75 g of chicken breast/lean ham or beef/tinned tuna or mackerel. Use low-kilojoule mayonnaise or oil-free dressing.
A bowl of soup, ideally home-made vegetable based, with either peas/beans/lentils or approximately 75 g lean meat.
A sandwich, one round containing lean meat, fish, chicken, egg, cheese etc., and always a lot of salad, e.g. tomato, lettuce, cucumber.

*Dinner options*
One each of the following:
A protein portion of lean meat, poultry or fish, 120–175 g
Green vegetable or salad portion, 225–350 g
Root vegetable, pasta or rice portion (optional), 120–175 g cooked weight
Or any of the Lunch options

*Desserts and snacks*
You may have one dessert and two snacks per day. Choose from the following:
A piece of fresh fruit or fruit salad
A low-fat yoghurt, with some fresh fruit or a little dried fruit
Two rice cakes spread with low-sugar jam or a little peanut butter
An apple and a few nuts, e.g. almonds, brazil or walnuts
A little cold rice salad with 25 g cold meat and mixed nuts
A bowl of Cornflakes or Rice Bubbles 25 g only, and low fat milk

## Basic Dietary Guidelines
Here are some pointers to eating well and tips to help you keep to a diet, regardless of its type.

◆ Eat regularly—have three meals per day.
◆ Always have breakfast. Missing it may cause you to eat more later.
◆ Plan your meals for the day or week. Make sure that you can have the right foods in the house or you will land up eating the wrong ones.
◆ If you are hungry between meals have a snack, a nutritious low-kilojoule one. Convenient foods are high in fat, sugar and kilojoules.
◆ Make sure that you have a cooked main meal every day and that this contains plenty of vegetables.
◆ Enjoy your food and eat your main meal with family or friends where possible. Don't eat it while watching the television.
◆ Go shopping twice a week to buy fresh fruit and vegetables and never go shopping when you are hungry. Take a list and stick to it.

- ◆ Tell your friends that you are on a diet. Some will want to join you and it will help to stop them leading you astray.
- ◆ If necessary have the occasional cheat. A few small pieces of chocolate after a good meal is not the end of the world or the diet.
- ◆ Finally, make sure that you do have a very good reason for losing weight. It may be to look better, to feel more comfortable or for a medical reason. In case you don't know, being seriously overweight is strongly linked to heart disease, high blood pressure, strokes, diabetes and even some types of cancer.

# THE SIMPLE EXCLUSION DIET

The Simple Exclusion Diet is divided into three stages. In the first four weeks, during Stage I, it is very important to eat only the permitted foods. If you introduce other foods you will lose the beneficial effects of the diet and it will be necessary for you to begin again! In Stage II, also four weeks, you start trying out groups of foods to see whether they push your weight up or produce unwanted symptoms or side-effects. During the final two-week period you will be eating a diet composed of the foods you have selected through trial and error in the preceding four weeks.

## Stage 1 Permitted Foods

### Meat and poultry
For non-vegetarians: all meat, including lamb, beef, pork, chicken, turkey, other poultry and game, and offal, such as liver, kidneys, sweetbreads and hearts, can be eaten if desired. Meat and poultry can be fresh or frozen.

Meat must be lean, with all visible fat trimmed before cooking. Do not eat the skin of chicken or other poultry; it should be removed before or after cooking.

*Fish and shellfish*

For non-vegetarians: all types are included and they may be fresh or frozen. Do not eat the skin of fish as it is high in fat.

Note: all meat, poultry and fish should be cooked by grilling, dry-roasting, steaming, baking, or stir-frying with low-fat ingredients, e.g. tomatoes or vegetables.

*All vegetables*

You can and should eat larger amounts of vegetables, especially green ones or salad foods daily. Your allowance will be detailed in the daily menus.

Root vegetables, e.g. potatoes and parsnips, are limited to 120–175 g per day. Beans and peas, which are protein-rich vegetables, are also included in moderate amounts.

*Vegetarian proteins*

For vegetarians and vegans these are an essential part of the diet. You are allowed all types of nuts, beans, peas, lentils, seeds, corn maize, rice and potatoes. Vegans in particular should have two or three portions of these per day. Some people experience abdominal bloating and wind with beans, and these should be well soaked and cooked, if necessary de-husked.

*Fruits*

All fruits are allowed, except dried fruits, glacé fruits, dates, figs, mangoes, and tinned fruits with sugar. Keep tinned fruits without sugar to a minimum also.

Aim to consume three portions of fruit per day. Fruit can either be eaten whole or as a fruit salad.

*Vegetable oils and vegetable mayonnaise*

A small amount of these is allowed daily. You can have up to 2 teaspoons of a low-fat, polyunsaturate-rich margarine per day. There are no fried foods on the diet (you didn't really expect them, did you?), but there are some stir-fry dishes and here you just wipe the inside of the pan or wok with a piece of kitchen roll dipped in sunflower or corn oil.

### Nuts and seeds

Peanuts, Brazil nuts, almonds, pistachios, cashews, sunflower seeds, and sesame seeds are very nutritious. Nuts and seeds can help to liven up a salad or be used as a nutritious snack, combined with an apple or another fruit.

### Rice and other salads

White or brown rice of any variety—long-grain, short-grain or basmati—is allowed. It will often be used instead of potatoes. Rice cakes (a rice crispbread) can be used in place of bread. Additionally, buckwheat, millet, sago and tapioca can be used from time to time, but these are not usually very popular.

### Breakfast cereals

Only Cornflakes and rice cereals are included in Stage I. They contain a good amount of protein and are fortified with extra vitamin B and iron. Other breakfast cereals are not allowed.

### Eggs

Up to seven eggs per week are allowed, unless you are known to have a very high cholesterol level or allergy to egg. Free-range eggs are highly nutritious and very good value for money.

## Stage I Foods to Be Avoided or Severely Limited

### Wheat, oats, barley, and rye

All foods made with these, apart from the exceptions given below, are to be avoided. This means no ordinary cakes, biscuits, puddings, pasta, pastry, pies, porridge or breakfast cereals (apart from Cornflakes or rice cereals). Bread is severely limited to two slices of white French bread.

### Dairy products

Cream and cheese are forbidden—even low-fat cottage cheese is out. Your milk allowance is very low, only 75 ml per day of skimmed milk, 600 ml per week. You can use dried skimmed milk instead, or low-fat plain yoghurt.

Butter or a polyunsaturated low-fat spread is allowed: 2–3 teaspoonfuls per day. However, if you have premenstrual tension, painful breasts, or an elevated blood cholesterol level, you should have a low-fat polyunsaturated spread instead of butter.

Foods containing milk, cream, cheese, milk solids, non-fat milk solids, lactalbumin, whey and caseinates should be avoided. The only exception to this is polyunsaturated margarine which often contains a very small amount of milk protein, lactalbumin or whey.

Vegetarians, i.e. non-meat or fish eaters can have up to 250 ml cows' milk per day and probably they should have either one egg per day or good portions of beans, peas, lentils and some nuts or seeds on most days. If you are known to have problems with cows' milk you can use soya milk instead—most supermarkets and health-food shops stock it.

### Animal fats and some vegetable fats

Animal fats, some vegetable fats, hard margarines, lard, dripping and suet are out, as are palm oil and coconut oil, and foods containing them. Chemically, these vegetable oils are much more like saturated animal fats than good quality sunflower or corn oil which are high in the healthier polyunsaturates. Hard margarines, which are made from hydrogenated vegetable oils, are also off the menu.

### Sugar, honey, glucose, and fructose (fruit sugar)

Any food made with these should be avoided in the main. This means cakes, biscuits, most ice cream, sweets of all kinds, chocolate, and puddings. This is not as depressing as it sounds. There are plenty of fresh fruit desserts, as you will see on the suggested menus. Leave the large helpings of honey for the bees!

### Alcoholic beverages

You name it—alcohol's out. Sorry! Don't do this diet over Christmas. Even low-kilojoule alcoholic drinks, though they are a great improvement, present too many complications for Stage I. You will, however, get the chance to try out alcohol in the third week of Stage II of the diet.

### Yeast-rich foods

This includes any foods containing yeast extract: Bovril, Marmite, Oxo, Knorr and other stock cubes, vinegar, any pickled food, chutneys, piccalilli, sauces, or condiments containing yeast extract or vinegar.

## Salt

Salt should not be used in cooking or at the table. This is particularly true if you experience fluid retention or high blood pressure. Salty foods such as ham, bacon, and any other salted meats should be eaten sparingly. Crisps, peanuts and many convenience dinners are not on the menu at all. If you really cannot do without salt, then use a very small amount only. Put it on the side of your plate. Try flavouring any salads, vegetables, or cooked main dishes with pepper or herbs instead of salt. You should find that your taste for salt becomes less as you progress through the diet programme.

## Foods with additives

These cannot be avoided completely, but it is best to avoid those with some types of colouring and preservatives which can cause asthma, urticaria (nettle-rash), eczema, and possibly migraine.

Avoid the following additives where possible:

E102 Tartrazine

E104 Quinoline Yellow

E110 Sunset Yellow FCF or Orange Yellow

E122 Carmoisine or Azorubine

E123 Amaranth

E124 Ponceau 4R or Cochineal Red A

E127 Erythrosine BS

E131 Patent Blue V

E132 Indigo Carmine or Indigotine

E142 Green S or Acid Brilliant Green BS or Lissamine Green

E151 Black PN or Brilliant Black PN

E180 Pigment Rubine or Lithol Rubine BK

E220–227 Sulphites—these may worsen asthma in very sensitive individuals.

Other colourings are not likely to cause any adverse reactions.

## Suspect foods

Avoid any foods that you know or suspect do not suit you. For example, many people find some fruits, such as oranges or pineapples, too acidic. Even though they are not particularly high in kilojoules you should avoid them. A not-infrequent problem is an inability to digest beans, peas and some vegetables properly, resulting in excessive wind. Possible vegetables in this group include cabbage, cauliflower, onions and sweetcorn. At this point, trust your own knowledge and experience. After all, it is this that we want to increase, so let's not go against anything you know already. Accordingly you may have to adapt the day's menu to recipes to suit yourself.

## *Modifications*
Vegetarians/vegans should also allow peas, beans, lentils, soya milk, non-fermented soya produce, and increased amounts of nuts, seeds and rice.

## *Symptoms*
You may notice during the beginning of Stage I that you experience some withdrawal symptoms as a direct result of giving up certain foods and drinks that you usually consume. These symptoms may be anything from headaches to fatigue or even depression. This will depend on your existing diet. For example, if you are consuming lots of cups of coffee or tea, cola drinks, or refined sweet foods, you may find the first week of the diet is quite a challenge!

It is probably best to begin the diet when you have a quiet week to spare. A word of advice to women of child-bearing age is to begin the diet just after your period has arrived and not in the week your period is due. The reason for this is to prevent additional symptoms occurring at a time when you might be suffering from PMS.

You will need the time to accustom yourself to your new way of eating and to get plenty of relaxation. This doesn't mean that you should take time off work; quite the opposite, as it is preferable that you remain occupied while on the diet. Just keep social engagements that involve eating to a minimum. Then, if you feel tired or experience any withdrawal symptoms, you can go off to rest without any guilty feelings of having let others down.

After the first week or so of following the diet, with any possible withdrawal symptoms behind you, things should look up. By Week 3, you may notice that a number of minor health problems have begun to improve. By Week 4, you should be feeling quite well, perhaps better than you have felt for some time and, you may notice that you have shed a few kilos without really trying. In fact those underweight will need to work at maintaining their weight by consuming nuts, seeds, oily salad dressing and alternative cakes and biscuits.

## Stage II

You start becoming a 'nutritional detective' during the second four-week period: trying out groups of foods to see whether they push your weight up or produce unwanted symptoms or side-effects. See the Food List for Reintroduction (page 475).

For each week there are different instructions. You will need to follow these very carefully as this is an important stage of the diet. If you follow the instructions precisely, you will end up with a diet that is really tailored to suit your own body.

You may experience some symptoms or side-effects from the foods under test. These should pass off within two or three days. There are a large number of symptoms that could be experienced, but these should only be those that cleared up in Stage I. They include migraine, headaches, eczema, urticaria (nettle-rash), rhinitis, asthma, abdominal bloating and discomfort, constipation, diarrhoea, wind, anxiety, irritability, insomnia, and possibly premenstrual tension. If and when you do have a reaction to individual food groups, you may feel that you have had a setback. On the contrary, any reaction should be regarded as a positive step. It means that you have discovered some foods that don't really suit your body at the moment. Any reaction, should it occur, is unlikely to be worse than you have already experienced, and probably will not last more than three days. If you do experience a reaction, you will need to stop eating the foods that are causing the problem. Keep a diary each day and score any reaction you get on a scale of 0–3, 0 = none, 1 = mild, 2 = moderate and 3 = severe. Keep an ongoing list of foods you react to and another list of suspect foods.

## Stage III

During the final two-week period you will be eating a diet composed of the foods you have selected through trial and error in the preceding four weeks. You should continue to lose weight and to feel more and more healthy as the weeks go by.

You will have gained the knowledge of how to tell when a particular food does not suit your body and how to deal with any bloating or other symptoms that may occur as a result. By that stage, you should feel totally at home with your new diet and confident that you can maintain it as a life-style with ease in the place of your former diet. Every so often you can reintroduce the foods that were on your Suspect List to see whether you can tolerate them, perhaps in small quantities. Sometimes, once the body has had a rest from a previously irritating substance, it can cope with reintroduction without any problems.

# THE STRICT EXCLUSION DIET

This diet is based on considerable work done in the USA and the UK, especially at the hospital for Sick Children, Great Ormond Street, London and at Addenbrooke's Hospital, Cambridge. We recommend it for adults only.

Follow this diet (see page 474) exactly. If a food is not mentioned, it is not allowed. Only those foods in the *Included* list are allowed.

This diet needs to be followed for one to three weeks, and must be undertaken with medical supervision.

## *Your Progress on an Exclusion Diet*

If your symptoms are due to a food reaction, then there should have been some improvement or even complete disappearance of your symptoms whilst following the appropriate diet. It is now important to reintroduce foods, and by so doing, determine which foods, if any, are responsible for your symptoms. In so doing, it is important to bear the following points in mind.

◆ On introducing foods, reactions can occur within minutes, hours or several days of consuming a new food. The speed with which symptoms occur depends to some degree upon the types of symptoms. Nettle rash or facial swelling due to food allergy can occur within minutes or hours. With muscle aches and pains, or even arthritis, it can sometimes take three or four days before the symptoms appear.

| EXCLUDED | INCLUDED |
|---|---|
| Beef, pork, preserved meats, bacon, sausages | Lamb, turkey, rabbit |
| All fish and shellfish, except trout | Trout, fresh or frozen |
| Potatoes, onions, sweetcorn, and many other vegetables. Only those mentioned are allowed | Carrots, parsnips, swedes, spinach, celery, leeks, lettuce and sweet potatoes |
| All fruits, except those listed opposite | Peeled bananas, pears, mangoes, pomegranates, paw-paws |
| Wheat, oats, barley, rye, corn | Rice (white only), rice flakes, rice flour, sago, tapioca, millet, buckwheat and rice cakes |
| Corn oils, soya oil, vegetable oil, nuts, especially peanuts | Sunflower oil, safflower oil and olive oil |
| Cows' milk, butter, most margarines, cows' milk yoghurt, cheese, eggs. All goats', sheep's and soya milk products | |
| Tea, coffee (beans, instant and decaffeinated), fruit squashes, orange juice, grapefruit juice, alcohol, tap water | Herbal teas, e.g. camomile, etc. without milk. Water—filtered or bottled mineral |
| Chocolate, yeast, preservatives. All food additives (see separate list). Herbs, spices, sugar, honey | Sea salt, unless fluid retention, asthma or high blood pressure are present |

◆ If the reaction occurs, stop consuming the food that you have just introduced, and wait for it to settle down before reintroducing a further food. This may take two or three days.

◆ If your symptoms are severe, particularly if it is a migraine, you may try taking a drink of 2 teaspoons bicarbonate of soda dissolved in water. Also breathing into a paper bag may help abort a migraine attack. Such measures can be useful in reducing the severity of a reaction.

◆ If you only consume a small amount of the test food, a positive reaction may be missed. It is important that you consume a normal to large portion, not excessive, of the food in question.

◆ If you are uncertain whether there has been a reaction or not, it is usually advisable to leave the food off, assuming that a positive reaction has occurred. It can be tested later. If, however, you are on a very restricted diet, it may be unwise to do this.

◆ If on a very restricted diet, it is usually advisable to reintroduce relatively safe foods, i.e. further vegetables, meat and fruits. It is often better to leave common high-risk foods, such as wheat and dairy produce, until later in the diet.

Remember that an exclusion diet is done to determine whether or not you have a food sensitivity. Only by reintroducing foods can this be determined. It is very often the case that a considerable amount of weight is lost on such a diet. It is important that this amount is not excessive, and that before starting an exclusion diet, you do not have any physical signs or symptoms attributable to nutritional deficiencies. If so, your doctor will advise you to take appropriate supplements for several weeks before commencing an exclusion diet.

In the long run, reactions to various foods might be diminished by avoiding excessive consumption of salt, sugar and alcohol, even if you are not sensitive to these. Factors such as cigarette smoking, that interfere with normal digestive processes, could also be a contributory factor. Long-term avoidance of those foods to which one reacts may sometimes result in a reduction of the sensitivity to various foods. It is not uncommon that, with appropriate management, those who were previously sensitive to a food, can after several months of appropriate dietary management, tolerate small quantities of the foods to which they reacted. This is not, however, always the case.

## Food List for Reintroduction

This list of foods is for people who have been on one of the exclusion diets, and are now ready to test out some foods. By now you should have experienced a significant improvement, and unfortunately, may well experience a return of your old symptoms on testing some of these foods. It is important that you proceed in a strictly ordered fashion, otherwise the picture may become confused.

◆ Add the following foods or food groups at intervals of five days.
◆ Eat a normal to large portion of these on each day of the trial.

♦ The foods should be fresh, if possible, and not contain any additives.

*Vegetables*

Carrots, parsnips, celeriac, fennel, parsley
Brussel sprouts, cabbage, broccoli, cauliflower, kale, mustard, turnip, watercress
Cucumber, zucchinis, melon, marrow, pumpkin
Potato
Tomato, capsicum, chilli, eggplant, paprika
Sweet potato
Onion, leeks, spring onions, garlic, asparagus, chives
Spinach
Peas, beans (dry and green), lentils
Nuts, walnuts, Brazil nuts, hazelnuts
Peanuts (plain, no additives), roasted or unroasted
Soy beans, soy sauce

*Fruits*

Apples, pears with skins (and juices)
Oranges, lemons, grapefruit, lime, mandarin, tangerine, satsuma, etc. (and juices)
Peach, apricot, nectarine, prune, cherries
Raspberry, loganberry, strawberry, blackberry
Bananas
Bilberry, blueberry, cranberry
Blackcurrant, redcurrant, gooseberry
Pineapple
Dried fruits

*Meats, chicken and fish*

Test plain meats, not meat products, such as pies, sausages, salami, etc.
Beef, plain, e.g. steak, roast joint, hot or cold
Pork, not bacon, ham and gammon or pâtés
Fish
Shellfish
Chicken and eggs

*Grains*
Wheat as wholemeal pasta and pastry, not wholemeal bread
Oats
Rye, e.g. Ryvita
Wholemeal bread
Corn maize

*Dairy*
Cows' milk, cream, yoghurt, butter
Cows' cheese
Goats' milk
Goats' cheese
Soya milk

*Other*
Tap water
Oxo, Marmite, Bovril, stock cubes
Alcohol, vinegar
Mushrooms
Tea
Coffee
Chocolate
Sugar

It may well help to keep a written record of any reactions you experience after testing various foods.

❖

# Menu for PMS

## *Mild to Moderate*

*Breakfast*
Oat-based muesli with fresh chopped fruit and semi-skimmed milk
Rooitea

*Mid-morning snack*
Fresh banana and raisins

*Lunch*
Glass of orange juice
Jacket potato with cheese and sweetcorn with a mixed salad

*Mid-afternoon snack*
Toast with low-sugar spread or nut butter

*Dinner*
Grilled trout with cauliflower, carrots and mixed root vegetables
Fresh fruit salad

# Menu for PMS

## *Severe*

*Breakfast*
Muesli made with Cornflakes, puffed rice, chopped almonds, dried apricots, sunflower seeds and raisins with chopped fresh fruit, yoghurt and semi-skimmed milk.
Rooitea

*Mid-morning snack*
Almonds, raisins and apple slices

*Lunch*
Glass of orange juice
Jacket potato with tuna and sweetcorn with a mixed salad

*Mid-afternoon snack*
Wheat-free cake or biscuit or fresh fruit and herbal tea

*Dinner*
Stir-fry chicken and vegetables with chilli and ginger
Berry mousse and fruit tea

*Variations*

## Premenstrual Cravings for Sweet Food
- ◆ Concentrate on eating foods rich in the minerals chromium and magnesium and B vitamins (see pages 495–8, 502).
- ◆ Your kilojoule requirements in your premenstrual week increase by up to 2100 kilojoules per day so you will need to eat little and often.
- ◆ In your premenstrual week have a wholesome mid-morning and mid-afternoon snack (see snack list on page 444).

## Premenstrual Breast Tenderness
- ◆ Cut down on animal fat and increase your consumption of fruit and vegetable fibre.
- ◆ Eat a low-salt diet.
- ◆ Cut out caffeine in the form of tea, coffee, chocolate and cola-based drinks.
- ◆ Keep alcohol consumption to a minimum.
- ◆ Cut down or better still cut out cigarettes.
- ◆ Restrict your intake of dairy products.
- ◆ Take daily supplements of Efamol Evening Primrose Oil (6–8 × 500 IU capsules per day).

## Premenstrual Constipation
- ◆ Avoid all foods containing wheat and modified starch.
- ◆ Eat plenty of fruit and vegetables.

- Take regular exercise.
- Massage your tummy and lower back with sweet almond oil with a few drops of lavender or geranium essential oil.
- Take 2 tablespoons of organic linseeds every day with your cereal.
- Spend 15–20 minutes relaxing each day.

### Period Pains

- Concentrate on foods rich in magnesium and B vitamins (see pages 495–8, 502).
- Take regular exercise.
- Massage the tummy and lower back with sweet almond oil with a few drops of lavender or geranium essential oil.
- Take extra supplements of magnesium (preferably amino acid chelate).
- Apply a heat pad to help relax the muscles.

# Menu for Fatigue

Diet and nutrition play a very important part in causing—and alleviating—fatigue. Many people need extra iron, magnesium and vitamin B in their diet, especially women of child-bearing age. Eating a more nutritious, high-protein diet should give you more vitality.

Drinking too much tea, coffee and alcohol, and eating too much sugar or sweet and processed foods, can also contribute to fatigue. So eat good food, with three regular meals per day and nutritious energy-sustaining snacks.

*Breakfast*
Oat crunch cereal
Scrambled egg on toast
Decaffeinated coffee

*Mid-morning snack*
Plain yoghurt with grated apple and sunflower seeds
Mixed berry tea

*Lunch*
Jacket potato with grated cheese or tuna filling
Mixed salad
Dandelion coffee

*Mid-afternoon snack*
Wholemeal toast and peanut butter
Herb tea or Rooitea

*Dinner*
Chicken curry with rice, mixed vegetables and poppadoms
Apple pie
Jasmine tea

# Menu for Migraine

A variety of factors can trigger a migraine attack, including stress, diet, hormonal changes, missing meals, drinking too much tea or coffee—or cutting back on them too suddenly—high blood pressure and, in rare cases, neurological problems. Key foods are known to cause attacks. Try avoiding:

Cheese
Chocolate
Tea
Coffee
Alcohol
Yeast extract
Pickled foods
Soya sauce
Liver
Oranges
Artificial colourings
Monosodium glutamate

After a few weeks, add these items back to your diet one by one. If you experience a headache discontinue that particular substance, wait a few days until you feel well again before introducing the next type of food or drink. Keep careful records to avoid confusion.

*Breakfast*
Boiled egg and two slices of Ryvita
Rooitea

*Mid-morning snack*
Apple and walnuts
Dandelion coffee

*Lunch*
Stir-fry prawns and vegetables with ginger
Fruit tea

*Mid-afternoon snack*
Almond macaroon
Rooitea

*Dinner*
Lean ham with a portion of hummus and mixed salad
Rhubarb and ginger mousse
Apple and cinnamon tea

# Menu for Acne

Acne sufferers should have a low-fat and low-sugar diet, and concentrate on eating foods that are high in B vitamins and the minerals zinc and selenium.
Rich sources of zinc are:

Liver
Wholegrains
Nuts
Beans
Lentils
Pilchards
Spinach
Milk
Cheese
Oysters
Cockles

Selenium-rich foods are:
Herring
Cod
Scallops
Shrimps
Brazil nuts
Wheatgerm
Milk
Brown rice
Eggs
Steak
Lamb
Turnips
Garlic
Orange juice

Many of these foods are also rich sources of B vitamins.
For further details see Nutritional Contents of Food list.

*Breakfast*
Fresh grapefruit and orange salad with sunflower seeds
Toast and dried fruit conserve
Dandelion coffee

*Mid-morning snack*
Brazil nuts and raisins
Rooitea

*Lunch*
Mackerel in spicy tomato sauce
Mixed salad with mung beans
Ecco or Dandelion coffee

*Snack*
Dried apricots and figs
Cranberry and apple tea or herbal tea

*Dinner*
Lamb steak with jacket potato, spring greens and cauliflower
Carrot cake
Decaffeinated coffee

# MENU FOR IRRITABLE BOWEL SYNDROME

A growing number of people are reported to have irritable bowel syndrome, and suffer with abdominal pain, constipation or diarrhoea, and sometimes indigestion. The causes are thought to be related to stress, lack of fibre and, for some, food intolerance.

Eat lots of fibre in the form of fruit and vegetables, and not in the form of wholewheat and bran which can aggravate the symptoms.

It is important to isolate the foods that irritate your condition. Many books on diet and allergies suggest using exclusion diets to relieve symptoms.

*Breakfast*
Rice Bubbles with chopped banana and soya milk
Rooitea

*Snack*
Apple and pecan nuts
Cranberry and apple tea or herbal tea

*Lunch*
Sardines in tomato sauce with jacket potato and green salad
Dandelion coffee

*Mid-afternoon snack*
Two rice cakes with low-sugar jam
Rooitea

*Dinner*
Grilled lamb chop with French beans, carrots and peas
Baked apple
Mixed berry tea or fruit or herbal tea

# MENU FOR BREAST TENDERNESS

For every one woman with breast cancer there are ten other
women who suffer with benign lumps (non-cancerous) or breast
tenderness. Any breast problem should be checked out with your
doctor. Once you have established that nothing sinister is going
on then you would be advised to change your diet.

◆ Eat leaner cuts of meat, avoid processed meats like pies and
sausages which have a high-fat content, and leave the chicken
or fish skin on your plate.
◆ All meat and fish should be grilled and your dairy intake should
be limited, replacing full-cream milk with skimmed or semi-
skimmed. Eat low-fat cheese, polyunsaturated spreads instead
of butter, and avoid cream altogether.
◆ Eat plenty of fibre in the form of fruit, vegetables and salads
and steer away from alcohol, sugar, tea, coffee and tobacco.
◆ Evening primrose oil can be helpful—but you need to take
6–8 × 500 ml capsules per day.

*Breakfast*
Cornflakes with chopped apple, crumbled pecan nuts and
skimmed milk
Rooitea

*Mid-morning snack*
Two carrots and two sticks of celery with a hummus dip
Dandelion coffee

*Lunch*
Selection of mixed vegetables and brown rice stir-fry, with 2 table-
spoons of mixed nuts or beans
Herbal or fruit tea

*Mid-afternoon snack*
Rye crackers and mashed banana
Rooitea

*Dinner*
Poached salmon with zucchinis, boiled potatoes and green salad
Fresh fruit salad
Mixed berry tea

# MENU FOR SUGAR CRAVING

In order to overcome sugar cravings, you need to eat three nutritious meals per day, and two or three wholesome snacks in
between meals. You will not need to worry about your weight as
many nutritional foods like fruit are intrinsically sweet and much
lower in kilojoules than all those bisucuits and chocolate you have
been eating.

B vitamins, and the minerals magnesium and chromium, are all
important for maintaining normal blood sugar levels. Eat plenty
of:

Wholegrains
Green leafy vegetables
Salad
Chicken
Liver
Potatoes

Green capsicums
Chilli
Bananas
Unsalted nuts
Black pepper

*Breakfast*
Poached eggs on toast with grilled tomatoes
Decaffeinated coffee

*Mid-morning snack*
Small bag of nuts and raisins

*Lunch*
Tuna fish with coleslaw salad and potato salad
Dandelion coffee

*Mid-afternoon snack*
Rye crackers with peanut butter
Decaffeinated tea

*Dinner*
Stir-fry chicken with mixed vegetables
Dried fruit compote
Mango and peach tea

# Sample WNAS Programme: Normal Menopause (late forties/early fifties)

If you are not particularly planning to take HRT, and have no real family history of osteoporosis you should concentrate on:

◆ dietary changes and including phytoestrols, foods rich in oestrogen

- a supplement programme
- relaxation
- weight-bearing exercise

## Sample Menu

### Breakfast
Cornflakes with chopped fresh fruit, pecan nuts, sunflower seeds, linseeds and semi-skimmed milk
Rooitea

### Mid-morning snack
Yoghurt, apple and raisins

### Lunch
Sardines with a celery, fennel and pine-nut salad and jacket potato
Stewed rhubarb and a glass of milk

### Mid-afternoon snack
Carrot cake or rice cakes with sugar-free spread

### Dinner
Stir-fry vegetables with almonds and prawns
Lemon mousse or yoghurt and fresh fruit
Raspberry and ginseng tea or fruit tea
Note: This menu provides approximately 1600 mg of calcium.

## Supplement Programme
- Multi-vitamins and minerals to correct nutrient balance.
- Natural vitamin E and ginseng to help control the hot flushes and night sweats.
- Efacal to increase calcium absorption and reduce the chances of osteoporosis, especially if not taking HRT.

## Relaxation
15–20 minutes per day to help control the hot flushes.

## Exercise
At least three 30-minute sessions of low-impact aerobic and weight-bearing exercise per week, to help keep the heart healthy and prevent osteoporosis.

# SAMPLE WNAS PROGRAMME: EARLY MENOPAUSE (NATURAL, CHEMICAL OR SURGICAL)

If you have a family history of osteoporosis or a history of fractures we suggest:

◆ a bone density scan
◆ a blood test to determine if a 'fast-loser'
◆ you consider taking HRT if severe symptoms or low bone mineral density
◆ you follow the WNAS recommendations

You should also concentrate on:

◆ dietary changes and including phytoestrols, foods containing naturally occurring oestrogen
◆ consuming extra calcium
◆ five sessions of exercise per week

## Sample Menu

*Breakfast*
Orange juice
Oat-based muesli with linseeds, chopped fresh fruit, yoghurt and reduced fat milk
Rye toast and sugar-free spread

*Mid-morning snack*
Dried apricots, ginseng slices and melon

*Lunch*
Cheese omelette and a salad of sprouted soya beans, alfalfa, fennel and celery
Fresh banana with a glass of milk

*Mid-afternoon snack*
Almond macaroon or almonds and raisins

*Dinner*
Grilled salmon with broccoli, zucchinis, carrots and new potatoes
Crème caramel and fresh berries with a glass of milk
Note: This menu provides approximately 1700 mg of calcium.

*Supplement Programme*
- Multi-vitamins and minerals to correct nutrient balance
- Natural vitamin E and ginseng to help control the hot flushes and night sweats
- Efacal to increase calcium absorption and reduce the chances of osteoporosis, especially if not taking HRT

*Relaxation*
15–20 minutes per day to help control the hot flushes.

*Exercise*
At least three 30-minute sessions of low-impact aerobic and weight-bearing exercise per week, to help keep the heart healthy and prevent osteoporosis.

# SAMPLE WNAS PROGRAMME: PREVENT OSTEOPOROSIS (HEAVY EXERCISER/ATHLETE)

If you are menstruating regularly, we suggest you follow the plan below. If you have no periods or irregular ovulation, we suggest:

- a bone density scan
- if established osteoporosis exists, you consider taking one of the bisphosphates
- you follow the WNAS recommendations

You should also concentrate on:

◆ consuming extra kilojoules to meet your energy output
◆ consuming a diet rich in calcium
◆ reducing your exercise to five sessions per week if it is a hobby
◆ taking regular supplements of multi-vitamins and minerals and Efacal to increase the uptake of calcium and help to prevent osteoporosis

## Sample Menu

*Breakfast*
Muesli, with fresh fruit and yoghurt
Cheese omelette and toast

*Mid-morning snack*
Rye crackers and nut butter spread

*Lunch*
Jacket potato with cheese and bean filling
Salad of sprouted soya beans, fennel, celery and walnuts
Glass of milk

*Mid-afternoon snack*
Yoghurt, almonds and fresh fruit, or cheese and biscuits with grapes

*Dinner*
Raw vegetable crudités with hummus or taramasalata
Grilled fish with broccoli, carrots, zucchinis and new potatoes
Berry mousse or fresh fruit salad with yoghurt
Note: This menu provides approximately 2300 mg of calcium.

## Sample High-calcium Menu

*Breakfast*
Cornflakes with chopped fresh fruit, a tablespoon of linseeds, and semi-skimmed milk
Toast with almond butter spread

A mug of either decaffeinated tea or coffee, or herbal tea or coffee substitute

*Lunch*
Baked beans on toast
Low-fat yoghurt with chopped almonds and grapes
Glass of milk

*Dinner*
Sardines, with baked potato, and fennel and mixed pepper salad
Cheddar cheese and biscuits with fresh grapes
Herb tea or decaffeinated coffee

This menu will provide over 1800 mg of calcium, as well as a good quantity of naturally occurring oestrogen. Bear in mind that up to two-thirds of dietary calcium fails to be absorbed by the body, so it may be that you will benefit from approximately 600 mg.

# POSTSCRIPT: GETTING THE BALANCE RIGHT

Both orthodox and complementary medicine have a great deal to offer us. However, as there is so much published medical literature, it would be almost impossible for any one doctor or practitioner to become familiar with it all. Searching for medical papers in an attempt to get educated is probably a time-consuming luxury which some busy practitioners forego. We know from our surveys on doctors that by their own admission some 90 per cent have little or no nutritional training, so it is hardly surprising that important research rarely gets translated for the lay public.

From the years we have spent combing medical journals in postgraduate libraries, reading books and treating patients, we have come to realise that, for many conditions, not only does medical science have a lot to offer, but there is a great deal that a well-informed person can do to help themselves. Lack of knowledge, and confusion arising from conflicting unscientific writing, can deny the 'sufferer' the key to renewed health.

In this book we have tried to present you with scientifically based information that will enable you to make an informed choice about your treatment. There is no substitute for knowledge and knowing the options that are available to you.

By now you will have gathered that your health prospects lie, to a large degree, in your own hands, and that your diet, lifestyle and environment play an important role in your well-being. Getting the balance right is the secret for good health. You can work hard, but you must allow for having fun too. Taking regular exercise and relaxation and making time for your friends is every bit as important as meeting a deadline. Our priorities must be balanced and we need to be mindful that life is not a rehearsal, it is the real thing!

There is a wealth of tried and tested self-help measures contained within this book for your use. Often these will be sufficient to help you over your problem. However, if you feel overwhelmed at the thought of helping yourself, don't be afraid to consult your doctor, or a complementary practitioner. There is a list of addresses in Appendix V designed to help you locate a qualified practitioner. Just ensure that you make an appointment with someone who has recognised qualifications and plenty of experience.

We hope that the information contained in this book will provide you with the key to a long and healthy life.

# APPENDIX I

## *Nutritional Content of Foods*

Unless stated otherwise, foods listed are raw
Source: McCance and Widdowson, *The Composition of Foods*, HMSO

### *Vitamin A—Retinol*
*(Micrograms per 100 g)*
Skimmed milk 1
Semi-skimmed milk 21
Grilled herring 49
Whole milk 52
Porridge made with milk 56
Cheddar cheese 325
Margarine 800
Butter 815
Lamb's liver 15 000

### *Vitamin B1—Thiamin*
*(Milligrams per 100 g)*
Peaches 0.02
Cottage cheese 0.02
Cox's apple 0.03
Full-fat milk 0.04
Skimmed milk 0.04
Semi-skimmed milk 0.04
Cheddar cheese 0.04
Bananas 0.04
White grapes 0.04
French beans 0.04
Low-fat yoghurt 0.05
Cantaloupe/Rockmelon 0.05
Tomato 0.06
Green capsicums, raw 0.07
Boiled egg 0.08
Roast chicken 0.08
Grilled cod 0.08
Haddock, steamed 0.08
Roast turkey 0.09
Mackerel, cooked 0.09
Savoy cabbage, boiled 0.10
Oranges 0.10
Brussels sprouts 0.10
Potatoes, new, boiled 0.11
Soya beans, boiled 0.12
Red capsicums, raw 0.12
Steamed salmon 0.20
Corn 0.20
White spaghetti, boiled 0.21
Almonds 0.24
White self-raising flour 0.30
Plaice, steamed 0.30
Bacon, cooked 0.35
Walnuts 0.40
Wholemeal flour 0.47
Lamb's kidney 0.49
Brazil nuts 1.00
Cornflakes 1.00
Rice Bubbles 1.00
Wheatgerm 2.01

### *Vitamin B2—Riboflavin*
*(Milligrams per 100 g)*
Cabbage, boiled 0.01

Potatoes, boiled 0.01
Brown rice, boiled 0.02
Pear 0.03
Wholemeal spaghetti, boiled 0.03
White self-raising flour 0.03
Orange 0.04
Spinach, boiled in salted water 0.05
Baked beans 0.06
Banana 0.06
White bread 0.06
Green capsicums, raw 0.08
Lentils, boiled 0.08
Hovis 0.09
Soya beans, boiled 0.09
Wholemeal bread 0.09
Wholemeal flour 0.09
Peanuts 0.10
Baked salmon 0.11
Red capsicums, raw 0.15
Full-fat milk 0.17
Avocado 0.18
Grilled herring 0.18
Semi-skimmed milk 0.18
Roast chicken 0.19
Roast turkey 0.21
Cottage cheese 0.26
Soya flour 0.31
Boiled prawns 0.34
Boiled egg 0.35
Topside of beef, cooked 0.35
Leg of lamb, cooked 0.38
Cheddar cheese 0.40
Muesli 0.70
Almonds 0.75
Cornflakes 1.50
Rice Bubbles 1.50

## Vitamin B3—Niacin
*(Milligrams per 100 g)*

Boiled egg 0.07
Cheddar cheese 0.07
Full-fat milk 0.08
Skimmed milk 0.09
Semi-skimmed milk 0.09
Cottage cheese 0.13
Cox's apple 0.20
Cabbage, boiled 0.30
Orange 0.40
Baked beans 0.50
Potatoes, boiled 0.50
Soya beans, boiled 0.50
Lentils, boiled 0.60
Banana 0.70
Tomato 1.00
Avocado 1.10
Green capsicums, raw 1.10
Brown rice 1.30
Wholemeal spaghetti, boiled 1.30
White self-raising flour 1.50
Grilled cod 1.70
White bread 1.70
Soya flour 2.00
Red capsicums, raw 2.20
Almonds 3.10
Grilled herring 4.00
Wholemeal bread 4.10
Hovis 4.20
Wholemeal flour 5.70
Muesli 6.50
Topside of beef, cooked 6.50
Leg of lamb, cooked 6.60
Baked salmon 7.00
Roast chicken 8.20
Roast turkey 8.50
Boiled prawns 9.50
Peanuts 13.80

Cornflakes 16.00
Rice Bubbles 16.00

## Vitamin B6—Pyridoxine
*(Milligrams per 100 g)*
Carrots 0.05
Full-fat milk 0.06
Skimmed milk 0.06
Semi-skimmed milk 0.06
Satsuma 0.07
White bread 0.07
White rice 0.07
Cabbage, boiled 0.08
Cottage cheese 0.08
Cox's apple 0.08
Wholemeal pasta 0.08
Frozen peas 0.09
Spinach, boiled 0.09
Cheddar cheese 0.10
Orange 0.10
Broccoli 0.11
Hovis 0.11
Baked beans 0.12
Boiled egg 0.12
Red kidney beans, cooked 0.12
Wholemeal bread 0.12
Tomatoes 0.14
Almonds 0.15
Cauliflower 0.15
Brussels sprouts 0.19
Sweetcorn, boiled 0.21
Leg of lamb, cooked 0.22
Grapefruit juice 0.23
Roast chicken 0.26
Lentils, boiled 0.28
Banana 0.29
Brazil nuts 0.31
Potatoes, boiled 0.32
Roast turkey 0.33

Grilled herring 0.33
Topside of beef, cooked 0.33
Avocado 0.36
Grilled cod 0.38
Baked salmon 0.57
Soya flour 0.57
Hazelnuts 0.59
Peanuts 0.59
Walnuts 0.67
Muesli 1.60
Cornflakes 1.80
Rice Bubbles 1.80
Special K 2.20

## Vitamin B12
*(Micrograms per 10 g)*
Tempeh 0.10
Miso 0.20
Quorn 0.30
Full-fat milk 0.40
Skimmed milk 0.40
Semi-skimmed milk 0.40
Marmite 0.50
Cottage cheese 0.70
Choux buns 1.00
Eggs, boiled 1.00
Eggs, poached 1.00
Halibut, steamed 1.00
Lobster, boiled 1.00
Sponge cake 1.00
Turkey, white meat 1.00
Waffles 1.00
Cheddar cheese 1.20
Eggs, scrambled 1.20
Squid 1.30
Eggs, fried 1.60
Shrimps, boiled 1.80
Parmesan cheese 1.90
Beef, lean 2.00

Cod, baked 2.00
Cornflakes 2.00
Pork, cooked 2.00
Raw beef mince 2.00
Rice Bubbles 2.00
Steak, lean, grilled 2.00
Edam cheese 2.10
Eggs, whole, battery 2.40
Milk, dried, whole 2.40
Milk, dried, skimmed 2.60
Eggs, whole, free-range 2.70
Kambu seaweed 2.80
Squid, frozen 2.90
Taramasalata 2.90
Duck, cooked 3.00
Turkey, dark meat 3.00
Grapenuts 5.00
Tuna in oil 5.00
Herring, cooked 6.00
Herring roe, fried 6.00
Steamed salmon 6.00
Bovril 8.30
Mackerel, fried 10.00
Rabbit, stewed 1.00
Cod's roe, fried 1.00
Pilchards canned in tomato
    juice 12.00
Oysters, raw 15.00
Nori seaweed 27.50
Sardines in oil 28.00
Lamb's kidney,
    fried 79.00

## *Folate/Folic Acid*
*(Micrograms per 100 g)*
Cox's apple 4.00
Leg of lamb, cooked 4.00
Full-fat milk 6.00
Skimmed milk 6.00

Porridge with semi-skimmed
    milk 7.00
Turnip, baked 8.00
Sweet potato, boiled 8.00
Cucumber 9.00
Grilled herring 10.00
Roast chicken 10.00
Avocado 11.00
Grilled cod 12.00
Banana 14.00
Roast turkey 15.00
Carrots 17.00
Sweet potato 17.00
Tomatoes 17.00
Topside of beef, cooked 17.00
Swede, boiled 18.00
Strawberries 20.00
Brazil nuts 21.00
Red capsicums, raw 21.00
Green capsicums, raw 23.00
Rye bread 24.00
Dates, fresh 25.00
New potatoes, boiled 25.00
Grapefruit 26.00
Oatcakes 26.00
Cottage cheese 27.00
Baked salmon 29.0
Cabbage, boiled 29.00
Onions, boiled 29.00
White bread 29.00
Orange 31.00
Baked beans 33.00
Cheddar cheese 33.00
Clementines 33.00
Raspberries 33.00
Satsuma 33.00
Blackberries 34.00
Rye crispbread 35.00
Potato, baked in skin 36.00
Radish 38.00

Boiled egg 39.00
Hovis 39.00
Wholemeal bread 39.00
Red kidney beans,
    boiled 42.00
Potato, baked 44.00
Frozen peas 47.00
Almonds 48.00
Parsnips, boiled 48.00
Cauliflower 51.00
Green beans, boiled 57.00
Broccoli 64.00
Walnuts 66.00
Artichoke 68.00
Hazelnuts 72.00
Spinach, boiled 90.00
Brussels sprouts 110.00
Peanuts 110.00
Muesli 140.00
Sweetcorn, boiled 150.00
Asparagus 155.00
Chickpeas 180.00
Lamb's liver, fried 240.00
Cornflakes 250.00
Rice Bubbles 250.00
Calf's liver, fried 320.00

## Vitamin C

*(Milligrams per 100 g)*
Full-fat milk 1.00
Skimmed milk 1.00
Semi-skimmed milk 1.00
Red kidney beans 1.00
Carrots 2.00
Cucumber 2.00
Muesli with dried fruit 2.00
Apricots, raw 6.00
Avocado 6.00
Pear 6.00

Potato, boiled 6.00
Spinach, boiled 8.00
Cox's apple 9.00
Turnip 10.00
Banana 11.00
Frozen peas 12.00
Lamb's liver, fried 12.00
Pineapple 12.00
Dried skimmed milk 13.00
Gooseberries 14.00
Raw dates 14.00
Melon 17.00
Tomatoes 17.00
Cabbage, boiled 20.00
Canteloupe/Rockmelon 26.00
Cauliflower 27.00
Satsuma 27.00
Peach 31.00
Raspberries 32.00
Bran flakes 35.00
Grapefruit 36.00
Mangoes 37.00
Nectarine 37.00
Kumquats 39.00
Broccoli 44.00
Lychees 45.00
Unsweetened apple juice 49.00
Orange 54.00
Kiwi fruit 59.00
Brussels sprouts 60.00
Strawberries 77.00
Blackcurrants 115.00

## Vitamin D

*(Micrograms per 100 g)*
Skimmed milk 0.01
Whole milk 0.03
Fromage frais 0.05
Cheddar cheese 0.26

Cornflakes 2.80
Rice Bubbles 2.80
Kellogg's Start™ 4.20
Margarine 8.00

## Vitamin E
*(Milligrams per 100 g)*
Semi-skimmed milk 0.03
Boiled potatoes 0.06
Cucumber 0.07
Cottage cheese 0.08
Full-fat milk 0.09
Cabbage, boiled 0.10
Leg of lamb, cooked 0.10
Cauliflower 0.11
Roast chicken 0.11
Frozen peas 0.18
Red kidney beans, cooked 0.20
Wholemeal bread 0.20
Orange 0.24
Topside of beef, cooked 0.26
Banana 0.27
Brown rice, boiled 0.30
Grilled herring 0.30
Lamb's liver, fried 0.32
Baked beans 0.36
Cornflakes 0.40
Pear 0.50
Cheddar cheese 0.53
Carrots 0.56
Lettuce 0.57
Cox's apple 0.59
Grilled cod 0.59
Rice Bubbles 0.60
Plums 0.61
Unsweetened orange juice 0.68
Leeks 0.78
Sweetcorn, boiled 0.88
Brussels sprouts 0.90

Broccoli 1.10
Boiled egg 1.11
Tomato 1.22
Watercress 1.46
Parsley 1.70
Spinach, boiled 1.71
Olives 1.99
Butter 2.00
Onions, dried raw 2.69
Mushrooms, fried in corn
 oil 2.84
Avocado 3.20
Muesli 3.20
Walnuts 3.85
Peanut butter 4.99
Olive oil 5.10
Sweet potato, baked 5.96
Brazil nuts 7.18
Peanuts 10.09
Pine nuts 13.65
Canola oil 18.40
Almonds 23.96
Hazelnuts 24.98
Sunflower oil 48.70

## Calcium
*(Milligrams per 100 g)*
Cox's apple 4.00
Brown rice, boiled 4.00
Potatoes, boiled 5.00
Banana 6.00
Topside of beef,
 cooked 6.00
White pasta, boiled 7.00
Tomato 7.00
White spaghetti, boiled 7.00
Leg of lamb, cooked 8.00
Red capsicums, raw 8.00
Roast chicken 9.00

Roast turkey 9.00
Avocado 11.00
Pear 11.00
Butter 15.00
Cornflakes 15.00
White rice, boiled 18.00
Grilled cod 22.00
Lentils, boiled 22.00
Baked salmon 29.00
Green capsicums, raw 30.00
Young carrots 30.00
Grilled herring 33.00
Wholemeal flour 38.00
Turnips, baked 45.00
Orange 47.00
Baked beans 48.00
Wholemeal bread 54.00
Boiled egg 57.00
Peanuts 60.00
Cottage cheese 73.00
Soya beans, boiled 83.00
White bread 100.00
Full-fat milk 115.00
Hovis 120.00
Muesli 120.00
Skimmed milk 120.00
Semi-skimmed milk 120.00
Prawns, boiled 150.00
Spinach, boiled 150.00
Brazil nuts 170.00
Yoghurt, low-fat,
    plain 190.00
Soya flour 210.00
Almonds 240.00
White self-raising
    flour 450.00
Sardines 550.00
Sprats, fried 710.00
Cheddar cheese 720.00
Whitebait, fried 860.00

## Iron

*(Milligrams per 100 g)*

Semi-skimmed milk 0.05
Skimmed milk 0.06
Full-fat milk 0.06
Cottage cheese 0.10
Orange 0.10
Cox's apple 0.20
Pear 0.20
White rice 0.20
Banana 0.30
Cabbage, boiled 0.30
Cheddar cheese 0.30
Avocado 0.40
Grilled cod 0.40
Potatoes, boiled 0.40
Young carrots, boiled 0.40
Brown rice, boiled 0.50
Tomato 0.50
White pasta, boiled 0.50
Baked salmon 0.80
Roast chicken 0.80
Roast turkey 0.90
Grilled herring 1.00
Red capsicums, raw 1.00
Boiled prawns 1.10
Green capsicums, raw 1.20
Baked beans 1.40
Wholemeal spaghetti,
    boiled 1.40
White bread 1.60
Spinach, boiled 1.70
Boiled egg 1.90
White self-raising flour 2.00
Brazil nuts 2.50
Peanuts 2.50
Leg of lamb, cooked 2.70
Wholemeal bread 2.70
Topside of beef, cooked 2.80
Almonds 3.00

Soya beans, boiled 3.00
Lentils, boiled 3.50
Hovis 3.70
Wholemeal flour 3.90
Muesli 5.60
Cornflakes 6.70
Rice Bubbles 6.70
Soya flour 6.90

## Magnesium
*(Milligrams per 100 g)*
Butter 2.00
Cox's apple 6.00
Turnip, baked 6.00
Young carrots 6.00
Tomato 7.00
Cottage cheese 9.00
Orange 10.00
Full-fat milk 11.00
White rice, boiled 11.00
Semi-skimmed milk 11.00
Skimmed milk 12.00
Boiled egg 12.00
Cornflakes 14.00
Potatoes, boiled 14.00
Red capsicums, raw 14.00
White pasta 15.00
Wholemeal spaghetti,
    boiled 15.00
White self-raising flour 20.00
Green capsicums, raw 24.00
Roast chicken 24.00
Topside of beef,
    cooked 24.00
White bread 24.00
Avocado 25.00
Cheddar cheese 25.00
Grilled cod 26.00
Roast turkey 27.00

Leg of lamb, cooked 28.00
Baked salmon 29.00
Baked beans 31.00
Spinach, boiled 31.00
Grilled herring 32.00
Banana 34.00
Lentils, boiled 34.00
Boiled prawns 42.00
Wholemeal spaghetti,
    boiled 42.00
Brown rice, boiled 43.00
Hovis 56.00
Soya beans, boiled 63.00
Wholemeal bread 76.00
Muesli 85.00
Wholemeal flour 120.00
Peanuts 210.00
Soya flour 240.00
Almonds 270.00
Brazil nuts 410.00

## Selenium
*(Micrograms per 100 g)*
Full-fat milk 1.00
Semi-skimmed milk 1.00
Skimmed milk 1.00
Baked beans 2.00
Cornflakes 2.00
Orange 2.00
Peanuts 3.00
Almonds 4.00
Cottage cheese 4.00
White rice 4.00
White self-raising flour 4.00
Soya beans, boiled 5.00
Boiled egg 11.00
Cheddar cheese 12.00
White bread 28.00
Wholemeal bread 35.00

Lentils, boiled 40.00
Wholemeal flour 53.00

## Zinc
*(Milligrams per 100 g)*
Butter 0.10
Pear 0.10
Orange 0.10
Red capsicums, raw 0.10
Banana 0.20
Young carrots 0.20
Cornflakes 0.30
Potatoes, boiled 0.30
Avocado 0.40
Full-fat milk 0.40
Skimmed milk 0.40
Green capsicums, raw 0.40
Semi-skimmed milk 0.40
Baked beans 0.50
Grilled cod 0.50
Grilled herring 0.50
White pasta 0.50
Tomatoes 0.50
Cottage cheese 0.60
Spinach, boiled 0.60
White bread 0.60
White self-raising flour 0.60
Brown rice 0.70
White rice 0.70
Soya beans, boiled 0.90
Wholemeal spaghetti,
    boiled 1.10
Boiled egg 1.30
Lentils, boiled 1.40
Roast chicken 1.50
Boiled prawns 1.60
Wholemeal bread 1.80
Hovis 2.10

Cheddar cheese 2.30
Roast turkey 2.40
Muesli 2.50
Wholemeal flour 2.90
Almonds 3.20
Peanuts 3.50
Brazil nuts 4.20
Leg of lamb, cooked 5.30
Topside of beef, cooked 5.50

## Essential Fatty Acids
Exact amounts of these fats
are hard to quantify. Good
sources for the two families of
essential fatty acids are given.

## Omega-6 Series Essential Fatty Acids
Sunflower oil
Canola oil
Corn oil
Almonds
Walnuts
Brazil nuts
Sunflower seeds
Soya products including tofu

## Omega-3 Series Essential Fatty Acids
Mackerel
Herring, fresh cooked or
    smoked/pickled
Salmon
Walnuts and walnut oil
Canola oil
Soya products and soy bean oil

# Appendix II

## References

### Standard References

*Oxford Textbook of Medicine*, 3rd edition, ed. D.J. Weatherall, Ledingham, J.G.G., D.A. Warrell, Oxford Medical Publications, 1996.

*Nutritional Influences on Illness*, M.R. Werbach MD, Thorsons, 1989.

*Nutritional Influences on Mental Illness*, M.R. Werbach, MD, Third Line Press, Inc. (California), 1991.

*Human Nutrition and Dietetics*, R. Passmore & M.A. Eastwood, 8th edition, Churchill Livingstone, 1986.

*Nutritional Medicine*, Dr Stephen Davies & Dr Alan Stewart, Pan Books, 1987.

*Hysterectomy—New options and advances*, L. Dennerstein, C. Wood & A. Westmore, 2nd edition, Oxford University Press, 1995.

### Abdominal Wind and Bloating

Maxton, D.G., Martin, D.F., Whorwell, P.J., Godfrey, M., 'Abdominal distension in female patients with irritable bowel syndrome; exploration of possible mechanisms', *Gut*, 1991; 32: 62–4.

Cummings, J.H., 'Fermentation in the human large intestine: evidence and implications for health', the *Lancet*, 1983; 1: 1206–9.

Hunter, J.O., 'Food allergy—or enterometabolic disorder?', *The Lancet*, 1991; 2: 495–6.

Calloway, S.P. , Fonagy, P., 'Aerophagia and irritable bowel syndrome', *The Lancet*, 1985; 2: 1368.

Levitt, M.D., Lasser, R.N., Schwartz, J.S., Bond, J.H., 'Studies of a flatulent patient', *The New England Journal of Medicine*, 1976; 295: 260–2.

Editorial, 'The colon, the rumen, and d-lactic acidosis', the *Lancet*, 1990; 336: 599–600.

Trotman, I.F., Price, C.C., 'Bloated irritable bowel syndrome defined by dynamic 99m Tc Bran Scan', the *Lancet*, 1986; 2: 364–6.

Christi, S.U., Gibson, G.R., Cummings, J.H., 'Role of dietary sulphate in the regulation of methanogenesis in the human large intestine', *Gut*, 1992; 33: 1234–8.


## Acne
Standard References

## Acne Rosacea
Standard References

## Ageing
Standard References

## Agoraphobia (see Anxiety)
Standard References
Burns, L.E., Thorpe, G.L., 'Fears and clinical phobias: epidemiological aspects and the national survey of agoraphobics', *Journal of International Medical Research*, Vol. 5(1), 1977.

## Alcoholism
Standard References

## Allergy and Intolerance
Standard References
'Food Intolerance and Food Aversion', Royal College of Physicians and the British Nutrition Foundation, 1984.

## Anaemia
Standard References
Lucas, C.A., Logan, E.C.N., Logan, R.A., 'Audit of the investigation and outcome of iron deficiency anaemia in one health district', *Journal of the Royal College of Physicians of London*, 1996; 33–5.

## Anxiety
Standard References
Durham, R.C., Allan, T., 'Psychological treatment of generalised anxiety disorder: a review of the clinical significance of results in outcome studies since 1980', *British Journal of Psychology*, 1993; 163: 19–26.

## Arthritis and Musculo-skeletal Problems
Standard References

## Asthma, Allergic Rhinitis and Viral Chest Infections

Kaliner, M., Lemanske, R., 'Rhinitis and asthma', *Journal of the American Medical Association*, 1992; 286: 2807–29.

Platts-Mills, T.A.E., Rakes, G.P., Heymann, P.W., 'Role of viral infections in exacerbations of asthma: allergy must also be a factor', *British Medical Journal*, 1995; 311: 629–30.

Peacock, S., Murray, V., Turton, C., 'Respiratory distress and royal jelly', *British Medical Journal*, 1995; 311: 1472.

Royal College of General Practitioners, *Guidelines for the care of patients with asthma*, RCGP Publication, 1993

Britton, J. *et al*, 'Dietary magnesium, lung function, wheezing and airway hyper-reactivity in a random adult population sample', the *Lancet*, 1994; 344: 357–62.

Fantidis, P. *et al*, 'Intracellular (polymorphonuclear) magnesium content in patients with bronchial asthma between attacks', *Journal of the Royal Society of Medicine*, 1995; 88: 441–5.

Wagner, E. *et al*, 'Prostaglandins, leukotrienes and essential fatty acids'. 1990; 39: 59–62.

## Back Pain
Standard References

## Breast Pain

Boyle, C.A. *et al*, 'Caffeine consumption and fibrocystic breast disease: a case control epidemiologic study', *JNCI*, 1984; 72: 1015–19.

London, R.S. *et al*, 'The effect of alpha-tocopherol on premenstrual sympomatology: a double-blind study 2. Endocrine correlates', *Journal of American College of Nutrition*, 1884; 3: 351–6.

Boyd, E.M.F. *et al*, 'The effect of a low-fat, high complex-carbohydrate diet on symptoms of cyclical mastopathy', the *Lancet* 1988; 2: 128–32.

Mansel, R.E. 'Breast Pain, "ABC of Breast Diseases"', *British Medical Journal*, 1994; 309: 866–8.

Gateley, C.A. *et al*, 'Drug treatments for mastalgia: 17 years' experience in the Cardiff mastalgia clinic', *Journal of the Royal Society of Medicine*, 1992; 85: 12–15.

Hughes, L.E. *et al*, *Benign Disorders and Diseases of the Breast*, Baillière Tindal, 1989.

## Cancer

Williams, M.C., and Dickerson, J.W.D., 'Nutrition in cancer—some biochemical mechanisms', *Nutrition Research Reviews*, 1990; 3: 75–100.

## Candida and Thrush

Standard References

## Carpal Tunnel Syndrome

Standard References

## Cerebrovascular Disease

De Keyser, J., De Kippel, N., Merkx, H., Vervaek, M., Herroelen, L., 'Serum concentrations of vitamins A and E and early outcome after ischaemic stroke', the *Lancet*, 1992; 339: 1562–5.

## Coeliac Disease

Standard References

## Constipation

Editorial, 'Constipation in young women', the *Lancet*, 1986; 1: 778–9.

Turnbull, G.K., Lennard-Jones, J.E., Bartram, C.I., 'Failure of rectal expulsion as a cause of constipation: why fibre and laxatives sometimes fail', the *Lancet*, 1986; 1767–9.

Preston, D.M., Lennard-Jones, J.E., 'Severe chronic constipation of young women: "idiopathic slow transit constipation"', *Gut*, 1986; 27: 41–8.

Cann, P.A., Read, N.W., Holdsworth, C.D., 'What is the benefit of wheat bran in patients with irritable bowel syndrome?', *Gut*, 1984; 25: 168–73.

Alun Jones, V., McLaughlan, P., Shorthouse, M., Workman, E., Hunter, J.O., 'Food intolerance: a major factor in the pathogenesis of irritable bowel syndrome', the *Lancet*, 1982; 2: 1115–17.

Also letter, 'Food intolerance and irritable bowel syndrome', the *Lancet*, 1983; 2: 633–4.

Taylor, R., 'Management of constipation', *British Medical Journal*, 1990; 300: 1065–7.

Hojgaard, L., Arffman, S., Jorgensen, M., Kragg, E., 'Tea consumption a cause of constipation', *British Medical Journal*, 1981; 282: 864.

## Crohn's Disease
Standard References

Lennard Jones, L.E., 'Nutrition and Crohn's disease', *Annals of the Royal College of Surgeons of England*, 1990; 72: 152–4.

## Chronic Fatigue Syndrome (see Fatigue)

Stewart, A., *Tired All The Time*, Vermilion, 1993.

Jenkins, R., Mowbray, W. (eds), *Post-viral Fatigue Syndrome*, John Wiley & Sons, 1990.

Behan, P., Goldberg, G., Mowbray, J.F., 'Post-viral fatigue syndrome', *British Medical Bulletin*, 47, No. 4, 1991.

Morrison, J.D., 'Fatigue as a present complaint in family practice', *Journal of Family Practitioners*, 1980; 10: 795–801.

Gold, M.S., Pottash, A.L.C., Extein, I., 'Hypothyroidism in depression', *Journal of the American Medical Association*, 1981; 245: 1919–22.

Marrie, T.J., Ross, L., Mantague, T.J., Doan, B., 'Post-viral fatigue syndrome', *Clinical Ecology*, 1978; 5: 5–10.

Manu, P., Lane T.J., Matthews, D.A., 'The frequency of chronic fatigue syndrome in patients with persistent fatigue', *Annals of International Medicine*, 1988; 109: 554–6.

Kroenke, K., Wood, D.R., Mangelsdorff, B., Meier, N.J. Powell, J.D., 'Chronic fatigue in primary care', *JAMA*, 1988; 260: 929–34.

Valdini, A., Steinhardt, S., Feldman, E., 'The usefulness of a standard battery of laboratory tests in investigating chronic fatigue in adults', *Family Practitioner*, 1989; 6: 286–91.

Lloyd, A.R., Hickie, I., Broughton, C.R., Spencer, O., Wakefield, D., 'Prevalence of chronic fatigue syndrome in an Australian population', *Medical Journal of Australia*, 1990; 153: 522–8.

Wood, G.C., Bentall, R.P., Gopfert, N., Edwards, R.H.T., 'The comparative psychiatric assessment of patients with chronic fatigue syndrome and muscle disease', *Psychological Medicine*, 1991; 21: 619–28.

Sharpe, M., Horton, K., Seagrott, B., Pasvol, G., 'Follow up patients presenting with fatigue to an infectious disease clinic', *British Medical Journal*, 1992; 305: 147–52.

## Cystitis
Standard References
Kilmartin, A., *Understanding Cystitis*, Arrow Books, 1989.

## Dementia
Standard References

## Depression and Mood Swings
Standard References

## Dermatitis
Hunter, J.A.A., Herd, R.M., 'Recent advances in atopic dermatitis', *Quarterly Journal of Medicine*, 1994; 87: 323–7.

## Diabetes Mellitus
McNair, *et al*, 'Hypomagnesemia: a risk factor in diabetic retinopathy', *Diabetes*, 1978; 27: 1075–7.

Moles, K.W., McMullen, J.K., 'Insulin resistance and hypomagnesaemia', case report, *British Medical Journal*, 1982; 285: 262.

Coelingh Bennink, H.J.T., Schreurs, W.H.P., 'Improvement of oral glucose tolerance in gestational diabetes by pyridoxine', *British Medical Journal*, 1975; 3: 13–15.

## Diarrhoea
'Food allergy and intolerance', report by the Royal College of Physicians, 1984.

Cooper, B.T., Holmes, G.K.T., Ferguson, R.A., Thompson, R.N.A., Cooke, W.T., 'Gluten-sensitive diarrhoea without evidence of coeliac disease', *Gastroenterology*, 1980; 79: 801–6.

Arnason, J.A., Gudjonsson, H., Freysodottir, J., Jonsdottir, I., Valdimarsson, H., 'Do adults with high gliadin antibody concentrations have subclinical gluten intolerance?', *Gut*, 1992; 33: 194–7.

Editorial, 'Milk fat, diarrhoea and the ileal brake', the *Lancet*, 1986; 2: 658.

Editorial, 'Hastening Gut Transit', the *Lancet*, 1990; 2: 974.

Merliss, R.R., Hofman, A., 'Steatorrhoea following the use of anti-biotics', *The New England Journal of Medicine*, 1951; 245: 328–30.

Bennett, J.R., Progress report: 'Smoking and the gastrointestinal tract', *Gut*, 1972; 13: 658–65.

## Eating Disorders

Lacey, J.H., 'Bulimia nervosa, binge eating and psychogenic vomiting: a controlled treatment study and long-term outcome', *British Medical Journal*, 1993; 286: 1609–13.

## Eczema

Sloper, K.S., Wadsworth, J., Brostoff, J., 'Children with atopic eczema. 1: Clinical response to food elimination and subsequent double-blind food challenge', *Quarterly Journal of Medicine*, 1991; 80: 677–93.

Morse, P.F. *et al*, 'Meta-analysis of placebo-controlled studies of the efficacy of Epogam in the treatment of atopic eczema; Relationship between essential fatty acid changes and clinical response', *British Journal of Dermatology*, 1989; 121: 75–90.

Turner, M.A., Devlin J., David T.J., 'Holidays and atopic eczema', *Archives of Disease in Childhood*, 1991; 66: 212–21.

## Endometriosis (see Pelvic Pain)

Standard References

Dennerstein, L. *et al*, *Hysterectomy, New Options and Advances*, Oxford University Press, 1995.

*Women's Problems in General Practice*, edited by Ann McPherson, Oxford University Press, 1995.

## Eye Problems

Sedden, J.M. *et al*, 'Dietary carotenoids, vitamin A, vitamin C and E, and advanced age-related macular degeneration', *Journal of the American Medical Association*, 1994; 272: 1413–20.

Hankinson, S.E. *et al*, 'Nutrient intake in cataract extraction in women: a prospective study', *British Medical Journal*, 1992; 305: 335–9.

## Fatigue

Jenkins, R., Mowbray, W. (eds), *Post-Viral Fatigue Syndrome*, John Wiley & Sons, 1990.

Behan, P., Goldberg, G., Mowbray, J.F., 'Post-viral fatigue syndrome', *British Medical Bulletin*, 47, No. 4, 1991.

Manu, P., Lane, T.J., Matthews, D.A., 'The frequency of chronic fatigue syndrome in patients with persistent fatigue', *Annals of International Medicine*, 1988; 109: 554.

Stewart, A., *Tired All The Time*, Vermilion, 1996.

## Fibroids (see Pelvic Pain)

Standard References

Dennerstein, L., Wood, C., Westmore, A., *Hysterectomy—New options and advances*, 2nd edition, Oxford University Press, 1995.

## Fibromyalgia (see Arthritis)

Standard References

Romano, T.J., Stiller, J.W., 'Magnesium deficiency in fibromyalgia', presented at the 7th World Congress of Rheumatology, Paris, Dec. 1993.

## Fluid Retention

Standard References

## Food Craving

Standard References

Stewart, M., *Beat Sugar Craving*, Vermilion, 1992.

## Gallstones

Standard References

## Genital Herpes

Standard References

Oates, J.K., 'Genital herpes', *British Journal of Hospital Medicine*, Jan. 1983; 13–22.

Griffith, R.S., Norrins, R.L., Kagan, C., 'A multi-centred study of lysine therapy in herpes simplex infection', *Dermatologica*, 1978; 156: 257–67.

## Gout (see Arthritis)

Standard References

Stein, H.B., Hassan, A., Fox I., 'Ascorbic acid-induced uricosuria', *Annals of Internal Medicine*, 1976; 84: 385–8.

## Haemorrhoids
Standard References

## Hair Loss
Standard References

## Halitosis
Standard References
Kerr, D.A., Major M. Ash, Jnr, *Oral Pathology*, Lea & Febiger, sixth edition, Philadelphia, 1992.

## Hay Fever (see Asthma)
Standard References

## Headaches
Standard References
Verne, S. *et al*, 'Medical intelligence, current concepts—headache', *The New England Journal of Medicine*, 1980; Vol. 302: 8: 446–50.

## Heart Failure
Standard References

## High Blood Pressure
Standard References

## Hysterectomy
Standard References
Dennerstein, L., Wood, C., Westmore, A., *Hysterectomy—new options and advances*, Oxford University Press, 1995.
Dennerstein, L. *et al*, 'Psychosocial and mental health aspects of women's health', Monograph 1, World Health Organisation, Geneva, 1993.
Bone, K., 'Vitex agnus castus: Scientific studies and clinical applications', Mediherb Newsletter, 1994; 42: 1.
Hirsch, N., 'Technologies for the treatment of menorrhagia and uterine myomas', Australian Institute of Health and Welfare HealthCare Technology Series, Canberra, 1993; 10: 1.
Fraser, I., 'Prostaglandins, prostglandin inhibitors and menstrual disorders. Part 11: Menorrhagia and premenstrual syndrome', *Healthright*, 1988; 8: 31–5.

Morse, C. *et al*, 'A comparison of hormone therapy, coping skills training, and relaxation for the relief of premenstrual syndrome', *Journal of Behavioural Medicine*, 1991; Vol. 14; 5: 469–89.

Helms, J., 'Acupuncture for the management of primary dysmenorrhea'. *Obstetrics and Gynaecology*, Vol. 69; 1: 51–5.

Anon, 'Complementary medicine: A popular adjunct', *Montage* (Monash University, Melbourne), 1994; Vol. 4; 5: 15.

Beecher, H.K., 'The powerful placebo', *Journal of the American Medical Association*, 1995; Vol. 159; 17: 1602–6.

Carlson, K. *et al*, 'The Maine Women's Health Study. 11: Outcomes of nonsurgical managment of leiomyomas, abnormal bleeding, and chronic pelvic pain', *Obstetrics and Gynaecology*. 1994; Vol. 83: 566–72.

Carlson, K. *et al*, 'The Maine Women's Health Study. 1: Outcomes of hysterectomy', *Obstetrics and Gynaecology*. 1994; Vol. 83: 556–65

## Indigestion
Standard References

## Infertility
Healey, D.L., Trounston, A.O., Andersen, A.N., 'Female infertility: causes and treatment', the *Lancet*, 1994; 343: 1539–44.

Editorial, 'Declining fertility: egg or uterus?', the *Lancet*, 1991; 338: 285–6.

Rowe, P.J., Comhaire, F.H., Hargreave, T.B., Mellows, H.J., *World Health Organisation Manual for the Standard Investigation and Diagnosis of the Infertile Couple*, Cambridge University Press, 1993.

Calloway, D.H., 'Nutrition and reproductive function and men', nutrition abstracts and reviews in *Clinical Nutrition*, Series A, 1983; 53(5): 361–80.

Skakkebaek, N.E., Giwercman, A., de Krester, D., 'Pathogenesis and management of male infertility', the *Lancet*, 1994; 343: 1473–9.

Hargreave, T.B., 'Non-specific treatment to improve infertility', in *Male Fertility*, ed. Hargreave, T.B., Springer-Verlag, 1983, 227–45.

## Influenza, Recurrent Coughs, Colds and Sore Throats
Standard References

## Insomnia

Standard References

Coyle, K., Watts, F.N., *The factorial structure of sleep dissatisfaction*, Behave Res Ther, 1991; 29: 315–20.

Ford, D.E., Kamerow, D.B., 'Epidemiological study of sleep disturbances and psychiatric disturbances', *JAMA*, 1989; 262: 1479–84.

*The Medical Management of Insomnia in General Practice*, edited by Malcolm Lader, Royal Society of Medicine, London, 1992.

## Irritable Bowel Syndrome

Connell, A.M., Hilton, C., Irvine, G. et al, 'Variation of bowel habit in two population samples', *British Medical Journal*, 1965; 2: 1095–9

Drossman, D.A., Sandler, R.S., McKee, D.C., Lovitz, A.J., 'Bowel patterns among subjects not seeking health care', *Gastroenterology*, 1982; 83: 529–34.

Heaton, K.W., O'Donnell, L.J.D., Braddon, F.E.M., Mountford, R.A., Hughes, A.O., Cripps, P.J., *Gastroenterology* 1992; 102: 1962–7.

Danivat, D., Tankeyoon, M., Sritratanaban, A., 'Prevalence of irritable bowel syndrome in a non-Western population', *British Medical Journal*, 1988; 296: 17105.

Jones, R., Lydeard, S., 'Irritable bowel syndrome in the general population', *British Medical Journal*, 1992; 304: 87–90.

Isgar, B., Harman, M., Kaye, M.D., Whorwell, P.J., 'Symptoms of irritable bowel syndrome in ulcerative colitis in remission', *Gut*, 1983; 24: 190–2.

Whitehead, W.E. *et al*, 'Effects of stressful life events on bowel symptoms: subjects with irritable bowel syndrome compared with subjects without bowel dysfunction'. *Gut*, 1992; 33: 825–30.

Thompson, W.G., 'Irritable bowel syndrome: pathogenesis and managment', the *Lancet*, 1993; 341: 1569–72.

## Ischaemic Heart Disease

Haq., I.U., Jackson, P.R., Yeo, W.W., Ramsay, L.E., 'Sheffield risk and treatment table for cholesterol lowering for primary prevention of coronary heart disease'. the *Lancet*, 1995; 346: 1467–71.

Stampfer, M.J., Rimm, E.B., 'Epidemiological evidence for vitamin E in the prevention of cardiovascular disease', *American Journal of Nutrition*, 1995; 62(suppl)1365S–9S.

## Kidney Stones
Standard References
Buck, AC., Smellie, WS., Jenkins, A., Meddings, R., James, A., Horrobin, D., 'The treatment of ideopathic recurrent urolithiasis with fish oil and evening primrose oil—a double blind study'. 1996, in press.

## Libido, Loss of
Standard References

## Liver Disease
Standard References

## Mastitis
Standard References

## Menopause
Wilbush, J., 'Climacteric disorders—Historical perspectives', in *The Menopause*, eds Studd, J.W.W., Whitehead, M.I., Blackwell Scientific Publications, 1988; 1–14.

Haas, S., Schiff, I., 'Symptoms of Oestrogen Deficiency', in *The Menopause*, as above, 15–23.

Wilson, R.C.D., *Understanding HRT and the Menopause*, Consumers' Association, 1992.

Jacobs, H.S., Loeffler F.E., 'Postmenopausal hormone replacement therapy', *British Medical Journal*, 1992; 305: 1403–8.

Hunt, K., Vessey, M., McPherson, K., 'Mortality in a cohort of long-term users of hormone replacement therapy: an updated analysis', *British Journal of Obstetrics and Gynaecology*, 1990; 97: 1080–6.

Martin, K.A., Freeman, M.W., 'Postmenopausal hormone-replacement therapy', *The New England Journal of Medicine*, 1993; 328: 1115–17.

Davies, S., Stewart, A., *Nutritional Medicine*, Pan Books, 1987.

McLaren, H.C., 'Vitamin E and the menopause', *British Medical Journal*, 1949; Dec 17: 1378–81.

Punnonen, R., Lukola, A., 'Oestrogen-like effect of ginseng', *British Medical Journal*, 1980; 281: 110.

Wilcox, G., Wahlqvist, M.L., Burger, H.G., Medley, G., 'Oestrogenic effects of plant foods in postmenopausal women', *British Medical Journal*, 1990; 301; 905.

Notelovitz, M., 'The non-hormonal management of the menopause', *in The Modern Management of the Menopause*, eds Berg, G., Hammer, M., Parthenon Publishing, 1994.

Cowan, M.M., Gregory, L.W., 'Responses of pre- and postmenopausal females to aerobic conditioning', *Medical Science, Sports and Exercise*, 1985; 17: 138–43.

Greist, J.H. *et al*, 'Running as treatment for depression', *Comprehensive Psychiatry*, 1979; 20: 41–523.

## Migraine Headaches

Hannington, E., Jones, R.J. *et al*, 'Migraine: a platelet disorder', the *Lancet*, ii, 1981, 720–3.

Egger, J., Carter, C.M. *et al*, 'Is migraine a food allergy? A double-blind controlled trial of oligoantigenic diet treatment', the *Lancet*, ii, 1983, 865–9.

Monro, J., Carini, C., Brostoff, J., 'Migraine is a food-allergic disease', the *Lancet* ii, 1984, 719–21.

Grant, E., 'Food allergies in migraine', the *Lancet*, I, 1979, 966–9.

Lance, J.W., 'Treatment of migraine', the *Lancet*, 1992; 339: 1207–9.

Murphy, J.J., Heptinstall, S., Mitchell, J.R.A., 'Randomised double-blind placebo-controlled trial of feverfew in migraine prevention', the *Lancet*, 1988; 189.

Lockett, D-MC, Campbell, J.F., 'The effects of aerobic exercise on migraine', *Headache*, 1992; 32: 50–4.

Kaiser, H.J., Meienberg, O., 'Deterioration or onset of migraine under oestrogen replacement therapy in the menopause', *Journal of Neurology*, 1993; 240: 195–7.

Iversen, H.K., Nielsen, T.H., Olesen, J., Tfelt-Hansen, P., 'Arterial responses during migraine headaches', the *Lancet*, 1990; 336: 837–9.

Epstein, M.T., Hockaday, J.M., Hockaday, T.D.R., 'Migraine and reproductive hormones throughout the menstrual cycle', the *Lancet*, 1975; 543–8.

Buring, J.E., Peto, R., Hennekens, C.H., 'Low-dose aspirin for migraine prophylaxis', *JAMA*, 1990: 264: 1711–13.

Kew, J., McKeran, R., 'Prophylactic treatment of migraine', *Maternal and Child Health*, 1991: 46–51.

Egger, J., 'Psychoneurological aspects of food allergy', *European Journal of Clinical Nutrition*, 1991: 45 (Suppl. 1), 35–45.

## Miscarriage

Regan, L., 'Recurrent miscarriage', *British Medical Journal*, 1991; 302: 543–4.

Tulppala, N. *et al*, 'Thromboxane dominance and prosta-cyclin deficiency in habitual abortion', the *Lancet*, 1991; 337: 879–81.

Hay, T.E., Lamont, R.P., Taylor-Robinson, D. *et al*, 'Abnormal bacterial colonization of the genital tract and subsequent pre-term delivery and late miscarriage', *British Medical Journal*, 1994; 308: 295–8.

Chard, T., 'Frequency of implantation and early pregnancy loss in natural cycles', *Ballière's Clin Obstet Gynaecol*, 1991; 5: 179–89.

Warburton, D., Fraser, F.C., 'Spontaneous abortion risks in man: data from reproductive histories collected in a medical genetics unit', *Hum Genet*, 1964; 16: 1–25.

Knudsen, U.B., Hansen, V., Juul, S., Secher, N.J., 'Prognosis of a new pregnancy and spontaneous abortions', *European Journal of Gynaecological Reproductive Biology*, 1991; 29: 31–6.

Kline, J., Shrout, P., Stein, Z.A., 'Drinking during pregnancy and spontaneous abortion', the *Lancet*, 1990; 11: 176–88.

Katesmark, M., 'Early pregnancy loss', *Maternal & Child Health*, 1996; 21: 4: 84–90.

## Mouth Disorders

Editorial, 'Aphthous ulceration', *Journal of the Royal Society of Medicine*, 1994; 77: 1–3.

Lamey, P.J., Hammond, A., Allam, B.F., McIntosh, W.B., 'Vitamin status of patients with burning mouth syndrome and the response to replacement therapy', *British Dental Journal*, 1986; 160: 81.

Strean, L.P., Bell, F.T., Gilfillan, E.W., Emerson, G.A., Howe, E.E., 'The importance of pyridoxine in the suppression of dental caries in school children and hamsters', *New York State Dental Journal*, 1958; 24: 133.

Ferguson, M.M., 'Disorders of the mouth in clinical practice', *Medicine in Practice*, 1982; Vol. 1: No. 9: 243–7.

## Multiple Sclerosis
Standard References

## Nail Problems
Standard References

## Obesity
Standard References
Stewart, M., Stewart A., *The Vitality Diet*, Optima, 1992.
Garrow, J. S., *Treat Obesity Seriously, A Clinical Manual*. Churchill Livingstone, 1981.

## Osteoarthritis
Standard References

## Osteoporosis
*The Menopause*, edited by John W. Studd & Malcolm I. Whitehead, Blackwell Scientific Publications, 1988.
*The Modern Management of the Menopause*, edited by G. Berg and M. Hammer, Parthenon Publishing, 1994.
Kanis, J.A. *et al*, 'Evidence of efficacy of drugs affecting bone metabolism in preventing hip fracture', *British Medical Journal*, 1992; 305: 1124–8.
Peel, N., Eastell, R., 'Osteoporosis', *British Medical Journal*, 1995; 310; 989–92.
Ettinger, B., Grady D., 'The waning effect of postmenopausal women', *British Medical Journal*, 1990; 301: 905.
Liberman, U.A., MD PhD *et al*, 'Effect of oral alendronate on bone mineral density and the incidence of fractures in post menopausal osteoporosis', *The New England Journal of Medicine*, 1995; 333: 1437–43.
Wilcox, G. *et al*, 'Osteogenic effects of plant foods in postmenopausal women', *British Medical Journal*, 1990; 301: 905.
Van Papendorp, D.H., Coetzer, H., Kruger, M.C., 'Biochemical profile of osteoporotic patients on essential fatty acid supplementation', *Nutrition Research*, Vol. 15: No. 3., 325–34.
Blumsohn, A. *et al*, 'The effect of calcium supplementation on the

circadian rhythm of bone resorption', *Journal of Clinical Endocrinology and Metabolism*, Vol. 79: 730–5.

Dixon, A.St.J., 'The non-hormonal treatment of osteoporosis', *British Medical Journal*, 1983; 286: 999–1000.

Buck, A.C., Smellie, W.S., Jenkins, A., Meddings, R., James, A., Horrobin, D., Department of Urology, Glasgow Royal Infirmary, Glasgow, 'The treatment of idiopathic recurrent urolithiasis with fish oil and evening primrose oil—a double blind study'. in press.

Notelovitz, M., 'The non-hormonal management of the menopause', in *The Modern Management of the Menopause*, edited by G.Berg and M. Hammer, Parthenon Publishing, 1994.

Martin, D., Notelovitz, M., 'Effects of aerobic training on bone mineral density of postmenopausal women', *Journal of Bone and Mineral Research*, 1993; 8: 931–6.

## Ovarian Cysts (see Pelvic Pain)
Standard References

## Painful Ovulation
Standard References

## Palpitations
Standard References

## Pancreatic Disease
Standard References

## Pelvic Inflammatory Disease (see Pelvic Pain)
Standard References

## Peptic Ulcers
Standard References

## Period Problems
Standard References

## Peripheral Vascular Disease
Standard References

## Polycystic Ovaries (see Pelvic Pain)

Standard References

McCluskey, S.E., Lacey, J.H., Pearce, J.M., 'Binge-eating and polycystic ovaries', the *Lancet*, 1992: 340; 723.

Kiddy, D.S., Hamilton-Fairley, D., Bush, A., Short, F., Anyaoku, V., Reed, M.J., Franks, S., 'Improvements in endocrine and ovarian function during dietary treatment of obese women with polycystic ovary syndrome', *Clinical Endrocrinology*, 1992: 36; 105–11.

Macaulay, J.H., Bond, K., Steet, P.J., 'Epidural analgesia in labor and fetal hyperthermia', *Obstetrics and Gynaecology*, 1992; 80: 665–9.

Polson, D.W., Adams, J., Wadsworth, J., Franks, S., 'Polycystic ovaries—a common finding in normal women', the *Lancet*, 1988: 870.

## Postnatal Depression

Standard References

Riley, D.M., Watt, D.C., 'Hypercalcemia in the etiology of puerperal psychosis', *Society of Biological Psychiatry*, 1985; 20: 479–88.

Dostalova, L., 'Vitamin status during puerperium and lactation', *Annals of Nutrition and Metabolism*, 1984; 28 (6) 385–408 [En 27 ref], Dep. Vitamin and Nutrition Research, F. Hoffmann-La Roche & Co. Ltd, CH-4002, Basle, Switzerland.

Watson, J.P., Elliott, S.A., Rugg, A.J., Brough, D.I., 'Psychiatric disorder in pregnancy and the first postnatal year', *British Journal of Psychiatry*, 1984; 144: 453–62.

## Preconception

Barker, D.J.P., *Mothers, Babies, and Disease in Later Life*, British Medical Journal, Publishing Group, 1994.

Wynn, M., Wynn, A., 'New thoughts on maternal nutrition', The Caroline Walker Lecture 1993, Caroline Walker Trust.

Lucas, A., 'Programming by Early Nutrition in Man', in Bock, G.R., Whelan, J., eds, *The Childhood Environment and Adult Disease*, John Wiley & Sons, 1991; 38–55.

Widdowson, E.M., McCance, R.A., 'A review: new thoughts on growth', *Pediatric Research*, 1975; 9: 154–6.

Barker, D.J.P. *et al*, 'Weight in infancy and death from ischaemic heart disease', the *Lancet*, 1989; ii: 577–80.

Osmond, C., Barker, D.J.P. *et al*, 'Early growth and death from cardiovascular disease in women', *British Medical Journal*, 1993; 307: 1519–24.

Barker, D.J.P. *et al*, 'Foetal nutrition and cardiovascular disease in adult life', the *Lancet*, 1993; 341: 938–41.

Law, C.M. *et al*, 'Initiation of hypertension in utero and its amplification throughout life', *British Medical Journal*, 1993; 306: 24–7.

Barker, D.J.P. *et al*, 'The relation of foetal length, ponderal index and head circumference to blood pressure and the risk of hypertension in adult life', *Paediatric and Perinatal Epidemiology*, 1992; 6: 35–44.

Godfrey, K.M. *et al*, 'Relation of fingerprints and shape of the palm to foetal growth and adult blood pressure', *British Medical Journal*, 1993; 307: 405–9.

McCance, D.R. *et al*, 'Birthweight and non-insulin dependent diabetes: "thrifty geotype", "thrifty phenotype", or "surviving small baby genotype"', *British Medical Journal*, 1994; 308: 942–5.

## Pregnancy

Barker, D.J.P., *Mothers, Babies and Disease in Later Life*, British Medical Journal, Publishing Group, 1994.

*Vitamin A and pregnancy*, Chief Medical Officer, Department of Health letters to all doctors, October 1990 and November 1993.

'Routine iron supplements in pregnancy are unnecessary', *British National Formulary*, April 1994.

Czeizel, A.E., 'Periconceptional multivitamin supplementation in prevention of congenital abnormalities', *Maternal and Child Health*, December 1994; 381–4.

Kirke, P.N., Molloy, A.M., Daly, L.E. *et al*, 'Maternal plasma folate and vitamin B12 are independent risk factors for neural tube defects', *Quarterly Journal of Medicine*, 1993; 86: 703–8.

Laroque, B. *et al*, 'Effects on birth weight of alcohol and caffeine consumption during pregnancy', *American Journal of Epidemiology*, 1993; 137; (9): 941–50.

Spohr, H.L. *et al*, 'Prenatal alcohol exposure and long-term development consequences', the *Lancet*, 1993; 341: 907–10.

Dolan-Mullen, P. *et al*, 'A meta-analysis of randomized trials of prenatal smoking cessation interventions', *American Journal of Obstetrics and Gynaecology*, 1994; 1328–34.

Czeizel, A.E. *et al*, 'Smoking during pregnancy and congenital limb deficiency', *British Medical Journal*, 1994; 308: 1473–6.

Editorial, 'Maternal smoking affects blood pressure in offspring', *Archives of Diseases in Childhood*, 1995; 72: 120–4.

Wei, Dr M., 'Foetal loss and caffeine intake', letter to editor, *Journal of the American Medical Association*, 6 July 1994; 272, No. 1.

Claoo, J.F., 'The effects of maternal exercise on early pregnancy outcome', *American Journal of Obstetrics and Gynaecology*, 1989; 161: 1453–7.

*Dietary Reference Values of Food Energy and Nutrients for the United Kingdom*, Department of Health Report of the Panel on Dietary Reference Values of the Committee on Medical Aspects of Food Policy, HMSO, 1991.

McCance, R.A., Widdowson, E.H., *The Composition of Foods*, HMSO, 1976, supplements 1985, 1988, 1989, 1990, 1991 and 1992.

## Premenstrual Syndrome

Green, R., Dalton, K., 'The premenstrual syndrome', *British Medical Journal*, 1953; 1007–14.

Morton, J.H., Additon, H., Addison, R.G., Hunt, L., Sullivan, J.J., 'A clinical study of premenstrual tension', *American Journal of Obstetrics and Gynecology*, 1953; 55: 1182–91.

Hargrove, J.T., Abraham, G.E., 'The incidence of premenstrual tension in a gynaecologic clinic', *The Journal of Reproductive Medicine*, 1982; 27: 721–4.

Sherwood, R.A., Rocks, B.F., Stewart, A., Saxton, R.S., 'Magnesium in the pre-menstrual syndrome', *Annals of Clinical Biochemistry*, 1986; 23: 667–70.

Yudkin, J., *Pure, White and Deadly*, Viking Press, 1986.

Ashton, C.H., 'Caffeine and health', *The British Medical Journal*, 1987; 295: 1293–4.

Chakmakjian, Z.H., Higgins, C.E., Abraham, G.E., 'The effect of a nutritional supplement, Optivite, for women with pre-menstrual tension syndromes: 2. The effect of symptomatology, using a double-blind cross-over design', *The Journal of Applied Nutrition*, 1986; 37: 1–11.

Mansel, R.E., Pye, J.K., Hughes, L.E., 'Effects of essential fatty acids on cyclical mastalgia and non-cyclical breast disorders', in Horrobin, D.F. (ed), 'Omega-6 Essential Fatty Acids', Wiley-Liss, 1990; 557–66.

Stewart, M., 'Beat PMS Through Diet', Vermilion, 3rd edition, 1994.

## Psoriasis

Menter, A., Barker, J.N.W.N., 'Psoriasis in practice', the *Lancet*, 1991; 338: 231–4.

Maurice, P.D.L., Allen, B.R., Barkley, A.S.J., Cockbill, S.R., Stammers, J., Bather, P.C., 'The effects of dietary supplementation with fish oil in patients with psoriasis', *British Journal of Dermatology*, 1987; 117: 599–606.

Michaelsson, G., Gerden, B., Ottosson, M. *et al*, 'Patients with psoriasis often have increased serum levels of IgA antibodies to gliadin', *British Journal of Dermatology*, 1993; 129: 667–73.

Rowland Payne, C.M.E., 'Psoriatic science', *British Medical Journal*, 1987; 295: 1158–9.

## Raynaud's Disease and Poor Circulation
Standard References

## Rheumatoid Arthritis (see Arthritis)
Standard References

O'Farrelly, C. *et al*, 'Association between villous atrophy in rheumatoid arthritis and rheumatoid factor and gliadin-specific IgG', the *Lancet*, 1988; 2: 819–23.

van der Tempel, H. *et al*, 'The effects of fish oil supplementation in rheumatoid arthritis', *Annals of the Rheumatic Diseases*, 1990; 224: 208–11.

## Stress

Swedlund, J., Sjoden, L., Ottosson, J.O., Doteval, G., 'Controlled study of psychological treatment for the irritable bowel syndrome', the *Lancet*, 1983; 2: 589–91.

Guthrie, E., Creed, F., Dawson, D., Tomensen, B., 'A controlled trial of psychological treatment for the irritable bowel syndrome', *Gastroenterology*, 1991; 100: 450–7.

Whorwell, P.J., Prior, A., Colgan, S.M., 'Hynotherapy in severe irritable bowel syndrome: further experience', *Gut*, 1987; 28: 423–5.

Harvey, R.F., Hinton, R.A., Gunary, R.M., Barry, R.E., 'Individual and group hynotherapy in the treatment of refractory irritable bowel syndrome', the *Lancet*, 1989; 1: 424–5.

## Thyroid Disease
Standard References

## Tonsillitis
Standard References

## Ulcerative Colitis
Standard References

## Urticaria
Standard References

## Vaginal Problems
Standard References

Witkins, S.S., Jeremias, J., Ledger, W.J., 'Recurrent vaginitis as a result of sexual transmission of IgE antibodies', *American Journal of Obstetrics and Gynecology*, 1988; 159: 32–6.

## Varicose Veins
Standard References

# APPENDIX III

## Recommended Reading List

Note: UK, USA and A denotes the following books are currently available in Great Britain, United States and Australia.

### General Health

1. *Pure, White and Deadly* by Professor John Yudkin (a book about sugar), published by Viking. UK A
2. *Coming Off Tranquillizers* by Dr Susan Trickett, published by Thorsons. UK USA A (Lothian Publishing Co.)
3. *The Migraine Revolution—The New Drug-free Solution* by Dr John Mansfield, published by Thorsons. UK USA A (Lothian Publishing Co.)
4. *Understanding Cystitis* by Angela Kilmartin, published by Arrow Books. UK A
5. *The Book of Massage*, published by Ebury Press. UK
6. *Do-it-Yourself Shiatsu* by W. Ohashi, published by Unwin. UK
7. *Candida Albicans: Could Yeast Be Your Problem?* by Leon Chaitow, published by Thorsons. UK USA A (Lothian Publishing Co.)
8. *Candida Albicans* by Gill Jacobs, published by Optima. UK USA A
9. *Nutritional Medicine* by Dr Stephen Davies and Dr Alan Stewart, published by Pan Books. UK A
10. *Bone Boosters—Natural Ways to Beat Osteoporosis* by Diana Moran and Helen Franks, published by Boxtree. UK
11. *The Migraine Handbook* by Jenny Lewis, published by Vermilion. UK A
12. *The Food Scandal* by Caroline Walker and Geoffrey Cannon, published by Century. UK A
13. *Conquering Cystitis* by Dr Patrick Kingsley, published by Ebury Press. UK
14. *Food Allergy and Intolerance* by Jonathan Bristoff and Linda Gamlin, published by Bloomsbury. UK A
15. *Escape from Tranquillisers and Sleeping Pills* by Larry Neild, published by Ebury Press.

16. *Alternative Health Care for Women* by Patsy Westcott, published by Thorsons.
17. *The Well Woman's Self-Help Book* by Nikki Bradford, published by Sidgwick and Jackson.
18. *Food Irradiation*: The Facts by Tony Webb and Dr Tim Lang, published by Thorsons.
19. *Candida—Diet Against It* by Luc de Schepper, published by Foulsham.
20. *Coming Off Tranquillisers* by Dr Shirley Trickett, published by Thorsons. UK USA A (Lothian Publishing Co).
21. *Pain-free Periods* by Stella Weller, published by Thorsons. UK
22. *Osteoporosis* by Kathleen Mayes, published by Thorsons. UK
23. *Natural Hormone Health* by Arabella Melville, published by Thorsons. UK USA A
24. *Fibromyalgia and Muscle Pain* by Leon Chaitow, published by Thorsons.
25. *Alexander Technique* by Chris Stevens, published by Random House.
26. *The Breast Book* by Miriam Stoppard, published by Dorling Kindersley.
27. *Homoeopathy for the First Aider* by Dr Dorothy Shepherd, published by The C.W. Daniel Co. Ltd. UK USA
28. *The Holistic Approach to Cancer* by Ian C.B. Pearce, published by The C.W. Daniel Co. Ltd. UK USA
29. *Evening Primrose Oil* by Judy Graham, published by Thorsons.

## Diet

1. *The Vitality Diet* by Maryon Stewart and Dr Alan Stewart, published by Optima (WNAS Mail Order Service).
2. *The New Why You Don't Need Meat* by Peter Cox, published by Bloomsbury. UK A
3. *Beat Sugar Craving* by Maryon Stewart, published by Vermilion. UK A
4. *The Allergy Diet* by Elizabeth Workman SRD, Dr John Hunter and Dr Virginia Alun Jones, published by Martin Dunitz. UK USA
5. *The Food Intolerance Diet* by Elizabeth Workman SRD, Dr John Hunter and Dr Virginia Alun Jones, published by Martin Dunitz. UK USA

6. *The Salt-Free Diet Book* by Dr Graham McGregor, published by Martin Dunitz. UK USA
7. *Food Allergy and Intolerance* by Jonathan Brostoff and Linda Gamlin, published by Bloomsbury. UK A
8. *The Real Food Shop and Restaurant Guide* by Clive Johnstone, published by Ebury Press.
9. *Organic Consumer Guide/Food You Can Trust*, edited by David Mabey and Alan and Jackie Gear, published by Thorsons.
10. *The New Raw Energy* by Leslie and Susannah Kenton, published by Vermilion. UK A (Doubleday Publishing Co.)
11. *Foresight Index Number Decoder (Pocket Additive Dictionary)* available from Foresight (address in Useful Addresses List). UK

## Stress

1. *Self-Help for your Nerves* by Dr Clair Weekes, published by Angus and Robertson. UK USA (Hawthorn Publishing Co.)
2. *Stress and Relaxation Self-Help Techniques for Everyone* by Jane Madden, published by Optima. UK USA A
3. *Lyn Marshall's Instant Stress Cure* by Lyn Marshall, published by Vermilion. UK A
4. *The Book of Massage* by Lucy Lidell, published by Ebury Press. UK
5. *Do-It-Yourself Shiatsu* by W. Ohashi, published by Unwin. UK
6. *Stress Wise* by Dr Terry Looker and Dr Olga Gregson, published by Headway. UK
7. *Tranquillisation: The Non-Addictive Way* by Phyllis Speight, published by The C.W. Daniel Co. Ltd. UK USA

## Recipe Books

1. *Good Food Gluten Free* by Hilda Cherry Hills, published by Keats. USA
2. *Gluten-Free Cookery* by Rita Greer, published by Thorsons.
3. *The Wheat and Gluten Free Cookbook* by Joan Noble, published by Vermilion. UK A
4. *The Candida Albicans Yeast-Free Cook Book* by Pat Connolly and Associates of the Price Pottenger Nutrition Foundation, published by Keats. UK USA

5. *The Cranks Recipe Book* by David Canter, Hay Canter and Daphne Swann, published by Orion. UK

6. *Raw Energy Recipes* by Leslie and Susannah Kenton, published by Century.

7. *The Reluctant Vegetarian Cook* by Simon Hope, published by Heinemann. UK

8. *Gourmet Vegetarian Cooking* by Rose Elliot, published by Fontana. UK A

9. *Healthy Cooking*, from Tesco Stores. UK

10. *The Gluten-free and Wheat-free Bumper Bake Book* by Rita Greer, published by Bunterbird Ltd. UK

11. *The Single Vegan* by Leah Leneman, published by Thorsons.

12. *Whole Earth Cookbook* by Hilary Meth, published by Vermilion. UK

## General

1. *Getting Sober and Loving It* by Joan and Derek Taylor, published by Vermilion. UK A

2. *The National Childbirth Book of Breast Feeding* by Mary Smale, published by Vermilion. UK USA A

3. *Tired All the Time* by Dr Alan Stewart, published by Optima. UK USA A

4. *Memory Power* by Ursula Markham, published by Vermilion. UK A

5. *Alternative Health Aromatherapy* by Gill Martin, published by Optima. UK USA A

6. *Alternative Health Acupuncture* by Dr Michael Nightingale, published by Optima. UK USA A

7. *Alternative Health Osteopathy* by Stephen Sandler, published by Optima. UK USA A

8. *Aromatherapy for Women and Children* by Jane Dye, published by The C.W. Daniel Co. Ltd. UK USA

9. *A Guide to Herbal Remedies* by Mark Evans, published by The C.W. Daniel Co. Ltd. UK USA

10. *Hysterectomy—New Options and Advances*, by Lorraine Dennerstein, Carl Wood and Ann Westmore, 2nd edition published by Oxford University Press, Melbourne.

11. *Cystitis—Understanding Cystitis*, by Angela Kilmartin, published by Arrow Books.

## Drugs

1. *What Do You Know About Drugs?* by Sanders & Myers, published by Gloucester Press.
2. *Forbidden Drugs—Understanding Drugs and How People Take Them* by Robson, published by Oxford University Press.

## Smoking

1. *How to Stop Smoking and Stay Stopped for Good* by Gillian Riley, published by Vermilion. UK A
2. *Easy Way to Stop Smoking* by Allen Carr, published by Penguin.

## IBS

1. *Beat IBS Through Diet* by Maryon Stewart and Dr Alan Stewart, published by Vermilion. UK A

## Exercise

1. *Diana Moran's 3 in 1 Workout* video by Diana Moran.
2. *The Ys Way to Physical Fitness* by Clayton R. Myers and Lawrence A. Golding.
3. *YMCA Guide to Exercise to Music* by Rodney Cullum and Lesley Mowbray.

## PMS

1. *Beat PMS Through Diet* by Maryon Stewart, published by Vermilion. UK A
2. *Beat PMS Cookbook* by Maryon Stewart and Sarah Tooley, published by Vermilion. UK A

## Menopause

1. *Beat the Menopause Without HRT* by Maryon Stewart, published by Headline. UK A

## Pregnancy and Baby Books

1. *Preparing for Birth with Yoga* by Janet Balaskas, published by Element.
2. *The Complete Book of Relaxation Techniques* by Jenny Sutcliffe, published by Headline. UK
3. *The Complete Book of Massage* by Clare Maxwell-Hudson, published by Dorling Kindersley. UK

4. *A Child is Born* by Lennart Nilsson, published by Doubleday. UK USA A

5. *Planning For a Healthy Baby* by Belinda Barnes and Suzanne Gail Bradley (Foresight), published by Vermilion. UK

6. *Green Babies* by Penny Stanway, published by Century. UK USA

7. *The National Childbirth Trust Book of Pregnancy, Birth and Parenthood* by Shirley Kitzinger, published by Oxford University Press. UK USA

8. *The National Childbirth Trust Book of Breast-feeding* by Mary Swale, published by Vermilion. UK USA

9. *Your Choices for Pregnancy and Childbirth* by Helen Lewison, published by Ebury. UK USA

10. *Breast is Best* by Drs Penny and Andrew Stanway, published by Pan Books.

11. *Breastfeeding Your Baby* by Sheila Kitzinger, published by Dorling Kindersley.

12. *Natural Fertility Awareness* by John and Lucie Davidson, published by Daniel. UK USA

## *Yoga*

1. *The Book of Yoga*, Sivananda Yoga Centre, published by Ebury Press. UK A

2. *Instant Stress Cure* by Lyn Marshall, published by Vermilion.

# APPENDIX IV

# *Further Information About the WNAS*

If you would like some personal help from the WNAS or would like details about our clinics or telephone and postal courses of treatment, please write to the WNAS enclosing $5, and stating your problem clearly, so that the appropriate questionnaire and information can be sent.

Write to WNAS, P.O. Box 268, Lewes, East Sussex, BN7 2QN, or telephone UK 1273 487366.

# APPENDIX V

## Useful Addresses

The following list of useful addresses for Australia and New Zealand was correct at the time this book was sent to the printer. Contact details for key organisations are set out in alphabetical order by topic then by state for Australia and city for New Zealand. We have not been able to include all contact addresses. Many of the organisations listed will refer you to contacts closer to your home if you wish. In addition, various women's advisory services (see under W) will give you information on additional resoources and provide up-to-date contact details.

◆ Telephone numbers will still be changing in Australia during 1997. The 'What Telephone Numbers Change to and When' page in your Telstra White Pages has the details.
◆ 1800 numbers are free calls from outside the metropolitan area

## Australia

### ACUPUNCTURE

Aust       *Acupuncture Association of Australia*
5 Albion Street
Harris Park
SYDNEY NSW 2150
Tel 02 9633 9187

### AGEING

ACT       *Council on the Ageing (COTA)*
Hughes Community Centre
Wisdom Street
HUGHES 2605
Tel 06 282 3777

NSW       *Council on the Ageing (COTA)*
6th Floor
93 York Street
SYDNEY 2000
Tel 02 9299 4100

NT              *Council on the Ageing (COTA)*
18 Bauhinia Street
NIGHTCLIFF 0810
Tel 08 8948 1511

Qld            *Council on the Ageing (COTA)*
Unit 1–3
82 Buckland Road
NUNDAH 4012
Tel 07 3256 6766

SA             *Council on the Ageing (COTA)*
45 Flinders Street
ADELAIDE 5000
Tel 08 8232 0422

Tas            *Council on the Ageing (COTA)*
The Gateway
2 St Johns Avenue
NEWTOWN 7008
Tel 03 6228 1897

Vic            *Council on the Ageing (COTA)*
Mezzanine Floor
Block Court
290 Collins Street
MELBOURNE 3000
Tel 03 9654 4443

WA           *Council on the Ageing (COTA)*
PO Box 7794
Cloisters Square
PERTH 6850
Tel 09 321 2133

## *ALCOHOL and other DRUGS*
*Alcohol and Drug Information Service*
ACT           Tel 06 205 4545

| | |
|---|---|
| NSW | Tel 02 9331 2111<br>*Freecall:* 1800 422599 |
| NT | Tel 08 8981 8030<br>*Freecall:* 1800 629683 |
| Qld | Tel 07 3236 2414<br>*Freecall:* 1800 177833 |
| SA | Tel 08 8274 3387<br>*Freecall:* 1800 131340 |
| Tas | Tel 03 6228 2880<br>*Freecall:* 1800 811994 |
| Vic | Tel 03 9416 1818<br>*Freecall:* 1800 136385 |
| WA | Tel 09 421 1900<br>*Freecall:* 1800 198024 |

## ALLERGIES

| | |
|---|---|
| ACT | Allergies and Intolerant Reactions Association<br>Tel 06 290 1984 |
| NSW | Allergy Prevention Clinic<br>Tel 02 9419 7731 |
| Qld | Queensland Allergy and Hyperactivity<br>Association<br>Tel 07 3848 2321 |
| SA | Allergy and Chemical Sensitivity Association<br>Tel 08 8214 1548 |
| Tas | Allergy Recognition and Management<br>Tel 03 6278 1054 |

Vic          Allergy and Environmental Sensitivity Support
and Research Association
Tel 03 9888 1382

WA         Allergy Association Australia
Tel 09 246 1595

# ARTHRITIS AND RHEUMATISM

ACT         *Arthritis Foundation of ACT*
GPO Box 1642
CANBERRA CITY 2601
Tel 06 257 4842

NSW        *Arthritis Foundation of New South Wales*
PO Box 370
DARLINGHURST 2010
Tel 02 9281 1611

NT          *Arthritis Foundation*
PO Box 37582
WINNELLIE 0821
Tel 08 8983 2071

Qld          *Arthritis Foundation of Queensland*
PO Box 807
SPRING HILL 4004
Tel 07 3831 4255

SA          *Arthritis Foundation of South Australia*
99 Anzac Highway
ASHFORD 5035
Tel 08 8297 2488

Tas         *Arthritis Foundation of Tasmania*
30/84 Hampden Road
BATTERY POINT 7004
Tel 03 6234 6489

Vic                     *Arthritis Foundation of Victoria*
PO Box 130
CAULFIELD SOUTH 3162
Tel 03 9530 0255

WA                   *Arthritis Foundation of Western Australia*
PO Box 34
WEMBLEY 6014
Tel 09 388 2199

# ASTHMA

ACT
and
NSW

*The Asthma Foundation of New South Wales*
82–86 Pacific Highway
ST LEONARDS 2065
Tel 02 9906 3233

NT                    *Asthma Foundation of Northern Territory*
PO Box 40456
CASUARINA 0811
Tel 08 8922 8827

Qld                  *The Asthma Foundation of Queensland*
51 Ballow Street
FORTITUDE VALLEY 4006
Tel 07 3252 7677

SA                   *The Asthma Foundation of South Australia*
329 Payneham Road
ROYSTON PARK 5070
Tel 08 8362 6272

Tas                  *Asthma Foundation of Tasmania*
82 Hampden Road
BATTERY POINT 7004
Tel 03 6223 7725

Vic     *The Asthma Foundation of Victoria*
       101 Princess Street
       KEW 3101
       Tel 03 9853 5666

WA     *Asthma Foundation of Western Australia*
       2/61 Heytesbury Road
       SUBIACO 6008
       Tel 09 382 1666

## BREAST-FEEDING

*Nursing Mothers' Association of Australia*
*Breast-feeding Helpline*

ACT     Tel 06 258 8928

NSW     Tel 02 9639 8686

NT      Tel 08 8988 4616

Qld      Tel 07 3844 8977

SA      Tel 08 8339 6783

Tas      Tel 03 6223 2609

Vic      Tel 03 9878 3304

WA     Tel 09 309 5393

## BREAST SCREENING

Aust     *Breastscreen*
       Tel 132050 (all states)

# CANCER

ACT

> *ACT Cancer Society*
> 15 Theodore Street
> CURTIN 2605
> Tel 06 285 3070

NSW

> *NSW Cancer Council*
> 153 Dowling Street
> WOOLLOOMOOLOO 2011
> Tel 02 9334 1933
> 1800 42 2760

NT

> *Northern Territory Anti-Cancer Foundation*
> Shop 2, Casuarina Plaza
> CASUARINA 0811
> Tel 08 8927 4888

Qld

> *Queensland Cancer Fund*
> 553 Gregory Terrace
> FORTITUDE VALLEY 4006
> Tel 07 3258 2200

SA

> *Anti-Cancer Foundation of the Universities*
> *of South Australia*
> 202 Greenhill Road
> EASTWOOD 5063
> Tel 08 8291 4111

Tas

> *Cancer Council of Tasmania*
> 13 Liverpool Street
> HOBART 7000
> Tel 03 6233 2030

Vic

> *Anti-Cancer Council of Victoria*
> 1 Rathdowne Street
> CARLTON SOUTH 3053
> Tel 03 9279 1111

WA
Cancer Foundation of Western Australia
334 Rokeby Road
SUBIACO 6008
Tel 09 381 4515

## COELIAC
Aust
Coeliac Society of NSW Inc.
1/306 Victoria Avenue
CHATSWOOD NSW 2067
Tel 02 9411 4100

## COUNSELLING—Personal, Relationships, Family
Aust
Relationships Australia (ACT)
15 Napier Close
DEAKIN 2600
Tel 06 285 4466

ACT
Relationships Australia Canberra and Region
15 Napier Close
DEAKIN 2600
Tel 06 281 3600

NSW
Family Life
16 Jersey Road
STRATHFIELD 2135
Tel 02 9745 1288

Relationships Australia (NSW)
5 Sera Street
LANE COVE 2066
Tel 02 9418 8800
Freecall: 1800 801 578

NT
Relationships Australia (NT)
Winlow House
75 Woods Street
DARWIN 0800
Tel 08 8981 6676

Qld          *Relationships Australia (Qld)*
159 St Paul's Terrace
SPRING HILL 4004
Tel 07 3839 9144

SA          *Family Life*
26 Harrow Avenue
MAGILL 5072
Tel 08 8365 4550

*Relationships Australia (SA)*
55 Hutt Street
ADELAIDE 5000
Tel 08 8223 4566

Tas          *Relationships Australia (Tas)*
306 Murray Street
HOBART 7000
Tel 03 6231 3141

Vic          *Family Life*
Rear 314 Camberwell Road
CAMBERWELL 3124
Tel 03 9813 2377

*Relationships Australia (Vic)*
1 Princess Street
KEW 3101
Tel 03 9205 9570

WA          *Relationships Australia (WA)*
755 Albany Highway
EAST VICTORIA PARK 6101
Tel 09 470 5109

# DIABETES
*Diabetes Australia*

| | |
|---|---|
| NSW | 26 Arundel Street |
| | GLEBE 2037 |
| | Tel 02 9552 9900 |
| |     02 9660 3200 |

NT

2 Tiwi Place
TIWI 0810
Tel 08 8927 8488

Qld

Cnr Merivale and Ernest Streets
SOUTH BRISBANE 4101
Tel 07 3846 4600

SA

159 Burbridge Road
HILTON 5033
Tel 08 8234 1977

Tas

79 Davey Street
HOBART 7000
Tel 03 6234 5223

Vic

100 Collins Street
MELBOURNE 3000
Tel 03 9654 8777

WA

48 Wickham Street
EAST PERTH 6000
Tel 09 325 7699

# EATING DISORDERS

ACT

*Anorexia and Bulimia Support Group*
Tel 06 286 3941

NSW

*Eating Disorders Clinic*
Royal Prince Alfred Hospital
CAMPERDOWN
Tel 02 9515 8165

*Eating Disorders Outpatient Assessment*
Westmead Hospital
WESTMEAD
Tel 02 9845 5555

Qld        *Anorexia and Bulimia Support Group*
Tel 07 3358 4988

SA        *Anorexia and Bulimia Nervosa Association*
Tel 08 8212 7991

Tas        *Hobart Women's Health*
Tel 03 6231 3212

Vic        *Anorexia and Bulimia Nervosa Foundation*
Tel 03 9885 0318

WA        *Bulimia and Anorexia Nervosa Group*
Tel 09 474 2598

## ENDOMETRIOSIS
Vic        *Endometriosis Association*
Tel 03 9870 0536 (all states)

## FAMILY PLANNING
ACT        *Family Planning ACT*
Health Promotion Centre
Childers Street
CANBERRA 2601
Tel 06 247 3077

NSW        *Family Planning New South Wales*
328–336 Liverpool Road
ASHFIELD 2131
Tel 02 9716 6099

*Natural Family Planning Services*
2nd Floor, Polding House
276 Pitt Street
SYDNEY 2000
Tel 02 9390 5157
*Freecall:* 1800 114 010

*Natural Fertility Management*
The Jocelyn Centre
1/46 Grosvenor Street
WOOLLAHRA 2025
Tel 02 9369 2047
Fax 02 9369 5179

NT    *Family Planning Northern Territory*
Shop 11, Rapid Creek Shopping Centre
Trower Road
RAPID CREEK 0810
Tel 08 8948 0144

Qld   *Family Planning Queensland*
100 Alfred Street
FORTITUDE VALLEY 4006
Tel 07 3252 5151

*Brisbane Natural Family Planning Centre*
Morgan Street
FORTITUDE VALLEY 4006
Tel 07 3252 4371

SA    *Family Planning South Australia*
17 Phillips Street
KENSINGTON 5068
Tel 08 8431 5177

*Natural Family Planning Centre*
33 Wakefield Street
ADELAIDE 5000
Tel 08 8210 8200

Tas            *Family Planning Tasmania*
73 Federal Street
NORTH HOBART 7002
Tel 03 6234 7200

*Natural Family Planning Centre*
PO Box 369
MOONAH 7009
Tel 03 6278 1660

Vic            *Family Planning Victoria*
270 Church Street
RICHMOND 3121
Tel 03 9929 3500

*Natural Family Planning Centre*
371 Church Street
RICHMOND 3121
Tel 03 9481 1722

WA           *Family Planning Western Australia*
70 Roe Street
NORTHBRIDGE 6003
Tel 09 227 6177

*Natural Family Planning Centre*
27 Victoria Square
PERTH 6000
Tel 09 221 3866

# *GRIEF/LOSS*

Aust          *National Association for Loss and Grief (NALAG)*
PO Box 79
TURRAMURRA 2074
Tel 02 9988 3376
(For national referral)

# HEART DISEASE
*National Heart Foundation*

Aust
PO Box 2
WODEN 2606
Tel 06 282 2144

ACT
Denison Street
DEAKIN 2600
Tel 06 282 5744

NSW
343–349 Riley Street
SURRY HILLS 2010
Tel 02 9219 2444

NT
44 Mitchell Street
DARWIN 8000
Tel 08 8981 1966

Qld
557 Gregory Terrace
FORTITUDE VALLEY 4006
Tel 07 3854 1696

SA
155–159 Hutt Street
ADELAIDE 5000
Tel 08 8223 3144

Tas
86 Hampden Road
BATTERY POINT 7000
Tel 03 6224 2722

Vic
411 King Street
WEST MELBOURNE 3003
Tel 03 9329 8511

WA
334 Rokeby Road
SUBIACO 6008
Tel 09 388 3343

# HERBALISM

Aust              *National Herbalists Association of Australia*
PO Box 61
BROADWAY 2007
Tel 02 9211 6437

# HOMEOPATHY

Aust              *Australian Association of Homeopaths*
Tel 02 9975 6322

NSW          *Sydney College of Homeopathic Medicine*
Tel 02 9564 6731

Qld              *Australian College of Natural Medicine*
Tel 07 32571883

SA               *South Australian College of Classical Homeopathy*
Tel 08 8365 0811

Vic              *Victorian College of Classical Homeopathy*
Tel 03 9877 7399

# INFERTILITY

Aust              *Access National Infertility Network*
PO Box 959
PARRAMATTA 2124
Tel 02 9670 2380
       or 9670 2608 (all states)

*Natural Fertility Management*
The Jocelyn Centre
1/46 Grosvenor Street
WOOLLAHRA 2025
Tel 02 9369 2047

# MENTAL ILLNESS

Aust              *Grow National Office*
209A Edgeware Road
MARRICKVILLE 2204
Tel 02 9516 3733

ACT

Grow ACT
Grow House
9 Anembo Street
NARRABUNDAH 2604
Tel 06 295 7791

NSW

Grow New South Wales
PO Box 64
PETERSHAM 2049
Tel 02 9569 5566

NT

Grow Northern Territory
PO Box 38801
WINNELLIE 0821
Tel 08 8945 4096

Qld

Grow Queensland
PO Box 178
HOLLAND PARK 4121
Tel 07 3394 4344

SA

Grow South Australia
80 South Terrace
ADELAIDE 5000
Tel 08 8231 6566

Tas

Grow Tasmania
82–84 Hampden Road
BATTERY POINT 7004
Tel 03 6223 6284

Vic

Grow Victoria
29 Erasmus Street
SURREY HILLS 3127
Tel 03 9890 9846

WA

Grow Western Australia
3rd Floor, 146 Beaufort Street
PERTH 6000
Tel 09 328 3344

# MYALGIC ENCEPHALOMYELITIS
## *(Chronic Fatigue Syndrome)*

ACT          *ME/CFS Society*
PO Box 717
MAWSON 2607
Tel 06 290 1984

NSW        *ME/CFS Society of New South Wales*
Royal South Sydney Community Complex
Joynton Avenue
ZETLAND 2017
Tel 02 9382 8284

NT          *Darwin ME/CFS Society*
PO Box 1062
PALMERSTON 0831
Tel 08 8932 3503

Qld          *Queensland ME Syndrome Society*
PO Box 938
FORTITUDE VALLEY 4006
Tel 07 3832 9744

SA          *ME/CFS Society of South Australia*
GPO Box 938
ADELAIDE 5001
Tel 08 8373 2110

Tas         *Tasmanian Support Group*
Tel 03 6330 1937

Vic         *ME/CFS Society of Victoria*
23 Livingstone Close
BURWOOD 3125
Tel 03 9888 8798

WA         *Western Institute of Self Help (W.I.S.H.)*
80 Railway Parade
COTTESLOE 6911
Tel 09 383 3188

# NATURAL THERAPIES

Aust                    *The Australian Traditional Medicine Society*
                        PO Box 442
                        RYDE 2112
                        Tel 02 9809 6800 (all states)

ACT                     *ACT College of Natural Therapies*
                        Tel 06 254 0722

NSW                     *Nature Care College*
                        Tel 02 9906 1566

Qld                     *Australian College of Natural Medicine*
                        Tel 07 3257 1883

SA                      *Australian College of Natural Healing*
                        Tel 08 8371 3266

# NUTRITION

*Australian Nutrition Foundation*

ACT                     PO Box 11
                        WODEN 2606
                        Tel 06 244 2211

NSW                     1–3 Derwent Street
                        GLEBE 2037
                        Tel 02 9552 3081

Qld                     PO Box 509
                        ASHGROVE 4060
                        Tel 07 3366 7375

SA                      8th Floor, Samuel Way Building
                        Adelaide Children's Hospital
                        King William Street
                        NORTH ADELAIDE 5006
                        Tel 08 8204 7162

Tas    PO Box 280
      SANDY BAY 7006
      Tel 03 6235 7707

Vic    c/- Caulfield General Medical Centre
      260 Kooyong Road
      CAULFIELD 3162
      Tel 03 9528 2453

WA    Food Centre
      140 Royal Street
      EAST PERTH 6001
      Tel 09 235 6447

## OSTEOPATHY

Aust    Australian Osteopathic Association
      4 Collins Street
      MELBOURNE Vic 3000

## PRECONCEPTION CARE

Aust    *The Foresight Association*
      124 Louisa Road
      BIRCHGROVE 2041
      Fax 02 9818 3734

## PREGNANCY/CHILDBIRTH

NSW    *Childbirth Education Association*
      PO Box 413
      HURSTVILLE 2220
      Tel 02 9580 0399

NT    *Childbirth Education Association*
      Casuarina Plaza
      Trower Road
      CASUARINA 0810
      Tel 08 8927 2575

| Qld | *Childbirth Education Association* |
|-----|-----------------------------------|
|     | PO Box 208                        |
|     | CHERMSIDE 4032                    |
|     | Tel 07 3359 9724                  |

| Tas | *Childbirth Education Association Australia* |
|-----|---------------------------------------------|
|     | PO Box 764                                  |
|     | DEVONPORT 7310                              |
|     | Tel 03 6428 6911                            |

## SEXUAL HEALTH
See FAMILY PLANNING CENTRES for each State under heading 'Family Planning'

## SINGLE PARENTS
*Parents Without Partners*

| ACT | PO Box 465       |
|-----|------------------|
|     | DICKSON 2601     |
|     | Tel 06 248 6333  |

| NSW | PO Box 388           |
|-----|----------------------|
|     | WENTWORTHVILLE 2145  |
|     | Tel 02 9896 1888     |

| Qld | 19 Clarence Street   |
|-----|----------------------|
|     | SOUTH BRISBANE 4101  |
|     | Tel 07 3275 3290     |

| SA | 186 Hampstead Road |
|----|--------------------|
|    | CLAREVIEW 5085     |
|    | Tel 08 8359 1552   |

| Tas | 20 Coraki Street   |
|-----|--------------------|
|     | THIGEELL 7011      |
|     | Tel 03 6249 5215   |

| Vic | PO Box 21          |
|-----|--------------------|
|     | CANTERBURY 3126    |
|     | Tel 03 9836 3211   |

WA                    Oasis House
                      27 Hampden Road
                      NEDLANDS 6009
                      Tel 09 389 8350

## SMOKING
Aust                  *QUIT LINE*
                      CEIDA, Rozelle Hospital
                      ROZELLE
                      Tel 13 1848 (National line)

## SUSTAINABLE AGRICULTURE
Aust                  National Association for Sustainable Agriculture
                      Australia
                      Tel 08 370 8455

## WOMEN'S NATURAL HEALTH
Aust                  *Women's Health Advisory Network*
                      155 Eagle Creek Road
                      WEROMBI 2570
                      Tel 046 531 445
                         or 046 531 199

## WOMEN'S INFORMATION SERVICES
ACT                   *Women's Information Referral Centre (WIRC)*
                      GPO Box 158
                      CANBERRA CITY 2601
                      Tel 06 205 1076
                         or 06 205 107 675

NSW                   *Women's Information and Referral Service (WIRS)*
                      Level 11, 100 William Street
                      WOOLLOOMOOLOO 2011
                      Tel 02 9332 1005
                      *Freecall:* 1800 817 227

NT                                *Women's Infonet*
PO Box 40596
CASUARINA 0811
Tel 08 8989 2717
*Freecall:* 1800 813 631

Qld                               *Women's Infolink*
PO Box 316, Albert Street
BRISBANE 4002
Tel 07 3224 2211
*Freecall:* 1800 177 577

SA                                *Women's Information Switchboard (WIS)*
122 Kintore Avenue
ADELAIDE 5000
Tel 08 8223 1244
*Freecall:* 1800 188 158

Tas                               *Office of the Status of Women (Information Service)*
PO Box 1854
HOBART 7001
Tel 03 6233 2208
*Freecall:* 1800 001 377

Vic                               *Women's Information and Referral Exchange (WIRE)*
First Floor, Ross House
247 Flinders Street
MELBOURNE 3000
Tel 03 9654 6844
*Freecall:* 1800 136 570

WA                               *Women's Information Service (WIS)*
1st Floor, Westralia Street
141 St Georges Terrace
PERTH 6000
Tel 09 264 1900
*Freecall:* 1800 199 174

## YOGA

Aust            *Australian Association of Yoga in Daily Life*
Tel 02 9518 7788 (all states)

# New Zealand

## AGEING
*Age Concern*

Auckland        Tel 09 623 0184

Christchurch     Tel 03 366 0903

Wellington      Tel 04 382 9477

## ALCOHOL and other DRUGS

Auckland       *Alcoholics Anonymous*
Tel 09 366 6688

               *Narcotics Anonymous*
Tel 09 303 1449

Christchurch    *Alcohol and Drug Services*
Tel 03 308 1270

Wellington     *Alcoholics Anonymous*
Tel 04 385 0811

               *Narcotics Anonymous*
Tel 04 496 3365

## ASTHMA

Auckland       *Asthma Society*
581 Mt Eden Road
MT EDEN
Tel 09 630 2293

Christchurch      *Asthma Society*
Cranmer Centre
cnr Armagh and Montreal Streets
CHRISTCHURCH
Tel 03 366 5235

Wellington      *Asthma Foundation of New Zealand*
123 Molesworth Street
WELLINGTON
Tel 04 499 4592

## BREAST-FEEDING/CHILDCARE

New Zealand      *Plunket Society*
Plunket Line (24 hours):
Tel 0800 101 067

## CANCER

Auckland      *Cancer Information Service*
Tel 09 524 2628

Christchurch      *Cancer Society*
Tel 03 379 5835

Wellington      *Cancer Society*
Tel 04 389 8421 (general information)
Tel 04 389 5086 (counselling)

## COUNSELLING

Auckland      *Lifeline* (24 hours)
Tel 09 522 2999

Christchurch      *Lifeline* (24 hours)
Tel 03 366 6743 or
0800 35 3353 (rural areas)

## DIABETES

Auckland      *Diabetes Auckland Inc*
62–64 Valley Road
MT EDEN
Tel 09 623 2508

Christchurch     *Diabetes Society Christchurch*
Deloitte House
32 Oxford Terrace
CHRISTCHURCH
Tel 03 379 5121

Wellington     *Diabetes Wellington Inc*
Betty Campbell Centre
Wakefield Street
WELLINGTON
Tel 04 384 5349

## FAMILY PLANNING
*Family Planning Association (FPA)*
Auckland     Tel 09 377 5049

Christchurch     Tel 03 379 0514

Wellington     Tel 04 499 1992

## HEART DISEASE
Auckland     *Heart Foundation of New Zealand*
17 Great South Road
GREENLANE
Tel 09 524 6005

Christchurch     *Heart Foundation*
255 Madras Street
CHRISTCHURCH
Tel 03 366 2112

Wellington     *Heart Foundation*
10 Gilmer Terrace
WELLINGTON
Tel 04 473 9018

## HOMEOPATHY

New Zealand    *Homeopathic Society (NZ)*
PO Box 67095
MT EDEN
Tel 09 630 5458

## NATURAL THERAPIES

New Zealand    The Association of Natural Therapies
PO Box 1055
PALMERSTON NORTH

Efamol New Zealand Ltd
(nutritional advice and supplements)
Tel 09 415 8477

## NUTRITION

New Zealand    New Zealand Nutrition Foundation
PO Box 33/1409
Takapuna
AUCKLAND
Tel 09 9486 2036

## PREGNANCY/CHILDBIRTH

*Pregnancy Help*
Auckland    Tel 09 373 2599

Christchurch    Tel 03 366 3355

Wellington    Tel 04 384 7979

## SEXUAL HEALTH

*Sexual Health Service*
Auckland    Tel 09 307 2885

Christchurch    Tel 03 364 0485

Wellington    Tel 04 385 5996

# SMOKING

| New Zealand | *ASH—Action on Smoking & Health* |
|---|---|
| | PO Box 99126 |
| | Newmarket |
| | AUCKLAND |
| | Tel 09 520 4866 |

# WOMEN'S INFORMATION SERVICES
*Ministry of Health*

| Auckland | Level 2, 31–35 Hargreaves Street |
|---|---|
| | PONSONBY |
| | Tel 09 309 3035 |

| Christchurch | Ground and First Floors, |
|---|---|
| | National Radiation Laboratory |
| | 108 Victoria Street |
| | CHRISTCHURCH |
| | Tel 03 366 7394 |

| Wellington | 1st Floor, Rossmore House |
|---|---|
| | 123 Molesworth Street |
| | WELLINGTON |
| | Tel 04 496 2000 |

# INDEX

Page numbers in **boldface** refer to reference works